Arthritis

An Alternative Medicine Definitive Guide

by EUGENE R. ZAMPIERON, N.D., A.H.G.,

and ELLEN KAMHI, PH.D., R.N., H.N.C.,

with BURTON GOLDBERG

ALTERNATIVEMEDICINE.COM BOOKS
TIBURON, CALIFORNIA

AlternativeMedicine.com, Inc.
1640 Tiburon Blvd., Suite 2
Tiburon, CA 94920
www.alternativemedicine.com

Editor: John W. Anderson
Associate Editor: China Williams
Research Editor: Gloria St. John
Art Director: Anne Walzer
Production Manager: Gail Gongoll
Layout/Production: Janine White

Cover Photo © 1997, Telegraph Colour Library/FPG International LLC
Illustrations (pp. 31, 33, 38) © 1997 by Jackie Aher

Manufactured in Canada.

10 9 8 7 6 5 4 3

Library of Congress Cataloging-in-Publication Data

Zampieron, Eugene R.
    Arthritis: an alternative medicine definitive guide / by Eugene R.
Zampieron and Ellen Kamhi, with Burton Goldberg
            p.   cm.
    Includes bibliographical references and index.
    ISBN 1-887299-15-7 (pbk.)
    1. Arthritis—Alternative treatment.   I. Title.   II. Kamhi, Ellen
III. Goldberg, Burton 1926-

RC933.Z35   1999
616.7'2206 21--dc21   99-044153

                    CIP

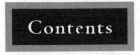

Contents

The Stagnated Lymphatic System
Therapies for Improving Lymphatic Drainage
Supporting the Portals: Kidneys, Skin, and Lungs

About the Authors

Eugene R. Zampieron, N.D., A.H.G., is a licensed naturopathic physician, professional herbalist, and medical botanist specializing in the non-toxic treatment of autoimmune and rheumatological disorders, especially arthritis and fibromyalgia. He received his B.S. in biological and marine sciences from the State University of New York, Stony Brook, and his doctoral degree in naturopathic medicine from Bastyr University of Natural Health Sciences in Seattle, Washington. He is a professional member of the American Herbalists Guild.

Dr. Zampieron also acts as a natural products consultant, syndicated multimedia host, magazine columnist, and professional speaker who lectures to audiences internationally. Along with Ellen Kamhi, Ph.D., R.N., Dr. Zampieron has written *The Natural Medicine Chest* (M. Evans, 1999). The duo also produces syndicated radio programs and appears on television to discuss aspects of natural medicine. He is co-executive with Dr. Kamhi of EcoTours for Cures, which leads educational and botanical eco-excursions into the rainforests around the globe.

Dr. Zampieron serves as an adjunct assistant professor of clinical medicine at the University of Bridgeport College of Naturopathic Medicine, where he is currently teaching doctoral courses in botanical medicine and pharmacognosy. He practices and resides in Connecticut, living on a woodland preserve with his wife and two small children.

A respected authority on natural healing, **Ellen Kamhi, Ph.D., R.N., H.N.C.**, holds a doctorate in public health and degrees in nursing and education. She is certified in reflexology, Bach flower remedies, herbology, darkfield microscopy, and indigenous medicines. She is a member of the Panel of Traditional Medicine at Columbia-Presbyterian Medical Center, in New York City, and The Health Care Consortium at the State University of New York, Stony Brook. She and Dr. Zampieron jointly host health shows on radio in New York and Connecticut as well as America's Health Network on cable television. They also lead groups through New York City's Chinatown district to learn about traditional Chinese medicine, organize outdoor excursions to identify healing wild plants, and teach seminars on edible and therapeutic plants.

Acknowledgements

In the accomplishment of a project such as this one, we have been shaped, inspired, influenced, motivated, supported, and schooled by many great people, who we now acknowledge and thank.

Eugene R. Zampieron, N.D., A.H.G.

I wish to thank the creator, for all healing ultimately comes from the infinite.

To my wife and soulmate, Kathleen, and children, Caitlin and Kevin.

To Ellen Kamhi, for her unending perseverance, patience, and organization amidst many obstacles to bring our vision of this book manifest to reality. May natural alternatives heal the world!

My teachers, friends, and colleagues of natural health who have schooled me in treating the many dimensions of pain and arthritis, including: Ken Bakken, D.O., Joe Pizzorno, N.D., Bill Mitchell, N.D., Douglas Lewis, N.D., Rod Borrie, Ph.D., Kim Vanderlinden, N.D., D.T.C.M., Peter Zilahy, D.C., Ameni Harris, Tom Hudak, L.M.T., Norm Suhu, C.A., Jamba, and Ann Seipt, N.D. To the many hundreds of patients with arthritis and pain whom I coached to wellness and who provided personal and clinical data for this book—thank you for being my patients and teachers, and for your courage and commitment to wellness.

To the staff of AlternativeMedicine.com Books who have shaped this work, and to Burton Goldberg for the incredible opportunity.

Ellen Kamhi, Ph.D., R.N., H.N.C.

To my parents, Julius and Sondra, and my children, Brenda, Titus, and Ali, thank you!

To my friends Dr. Michael and Lois Posner, who were occasionally successful at pulling me away from my work marathons. To Ron Haugen, for his technical and philosophical support; to my teachers, especially Serafino Corsello, M.D., whose intensity, fortitude, and depth of knowledge is always an inspiration; to my partner and soul brother, Eugene Zampieron, without whom this work would not have been possible, and his wife, Kathleen Pye, for her endless patience...and to God almighty.

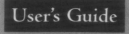

User's Guide

One of the features of this book is that it is interactive, thanks to the following icons:

This means you can turn to the listed pages elsewhere in this book for more information.

Many times the text mentions a medical term that requires explanation. We don't want to interrupt the text, so instead we put the explanation in the margins under this icon.

This tells you where to contact a physician, group, or publication mentioned in the text. This is an editorial service to our readers. All items are based on recommendations from the clinical practice of physicians in this book. The publisher has no financial interest in any clinic, physician, or product discussed in this book.

This sign tells you there may be some risks, uncertainties, side effects, or special contraindications regarding a procedure or substance.

Here we refer you to our best-selling book, *Alternative Medicine: The Definitive Guide*, for more information on a particular topic.

This icon will alert you to an article published in our bimonthly magazine, *Alternative Medicine*, that is relevant to the topic under discussion.

Here we refer you to our book *Alternative Medicine Definitive Guide to Cancer* for more information on a particular topic.

Here we refer you to our book *Alternative Medicine Guide to Chronic Fatigue, Fibromyalgia, and Environmental Illness* for more information on a particular topic.

Here we refer you to our book *The Enzyme Cure* for more information on enzymes and how they can be used to relieve health problems.

Here we refer you to our book *The Supplement Shopper* for more information on nutritional supplements for various health conditions.

You Don't Have to Suffer with Arthritis

AN ILLNESS LIKE ARTHRITIS is not something you have to live with—alternative medicine has practical solutions for identifying and treating the underlying causes and can bring lasting relief to arthritis sufferers. Many people have learned this the hard way, living with discomfort, pain, and inflammation for years before discovering that there is another option. Alternative medicine recognizes that arthritis does not have one cause, but multiple factors that together overload your body systems. Looking at illness and health in this way makes for more effective treatment than the single-cause focus of conventional medicine. In this book, you will learn that once you identify the hidden factors that are combining to produce your arthritis, you can treat each one and permanently eliminate joint pain and inflammation. Patient success stories throughout the book provide practical details on how others were able to reverse their arthritis.

Today, an estimated 43 million Americans have some form of arthritis—rheumatoid arthritis, osteoarthritis, gout, ankylosing spondylitis, psoriatic arthritis, or infectious arthritis. That's one in every six people, making it one of the most prevalent chronic health problems. For many arthritis sufferers, the disease limits their everyday activities and movements—walking or even buttoning a shirt can be a painful experience. And it's estimated that arthritis costs $65 billion per year in health-care costs and lost work time. Conventional medicine offers nonsteroidal, anti-inflammatory drugs (NSAIDs), corticosteroids, and other drug treatments that may temporarily relieve arthritis symptoms, but also introduce side effects that may actually accelerate the destruction of cartilage in the joints.

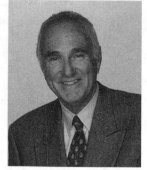

Alternative medicine physicians, on the other hand, focus on finding the root causes, rather than merely trying to alleviate symptoms. In this book, Eugene R. Zampieron, N.D., A.H.G., and Ellen Kamhi,

Ph.D., R.N., H.N.C., show you how to prevent and reverse arthritis using safe, noninvasive, and proven alternative therapies. Alternative medicine looks at the whole person, considering the individual's symptoms, health history, diet, and underlying imbalances. You can then use a combination of alternative treatments to heal these underlying causes leading to arthritis, bringing lasting relief, not a simple masking of symptoms. This is the basic principle of alternative medicine and the reason why it succeeds where conventional medicine often fails in the treatment of chronic disease.

Drs. Zampieron and Kamhi have years of experience treating arthritis and will show you how to keep your joints healthy and, if you already have arthritis, how you can reverse it. You'll learn more about these self-help options:

You don't have to live with pain and inflammation, or with a continuing cycle of drugs and their side effects. By treating what is actually causing the condition, not only can arthritis be reversed but your overall health will be improved.

■ The Arthritis Diet—how to avoid foods that aggravate arthritis and increase foods that nourish joints and support healing (includes arthritis-friendly recipes).

■ Safe and effective pain-stoppers—herbs and nutrients, vitamins and minerals, cartilage-building supplements, and homeopathic remedies.

■ Exercises and physical therapies to improve joint flexibility and relieve pain and stiffness.

■ The role of stress in arthritis and effective mind/body therapies to cope with stress.

This book is here to tell you that you don't have to live with pain and inflammation, or with a continuing cycle of drugs and their side effects. By treating what is actually causing the condition, not only can arthritis be reversed but your overall health will be improved. God bless.

—Burton Goldberg

Visit our website at
www.alternativemedicine.com

Arthritis Can Be Reversed

THE TERM *arthritis* is often used loosely as if it encompassed one entity, although over 100 types of arthritis have been identified. It is not one disease but an aggregate of illnesses whose common features include joint pain, stiffness, and inflammation. For millions of Americans, arthritis limits everyday movements such as walking, standing, or even holding a pencil. Arthritic conditions can progress to complete destruction of the protective covering around joints, brittle bones, loss of mobility, and joint deformities.

Osteoarthritis (OA) is by far the most prevalent form of arthritis, affecting an estimated 20.7 million Americans. Under the age of 45, more men than women are diagnosed with OA, often due to accidents and injuries. The disease becomes three times more prevalent in women than in men after the age of 45.[1] Since aging is a factor in this disease, as many more Baby Boomers turn 50, the number of people afflicted with OA is expected to increase dramatically. According to the National Arthritis Data Workshop, arthritis and other disorders of the musculoskeletal system comprise the most frequently reported cause of impairment affecting the adult population of the United States.[2]

The second most prevalent form of arthritis is rheumatoid arthritis (RA), an inflammatory disease in which the body's immune system attacks its own healthy tissues. RA affects 3%-4% of the population of the United States, striking people of all ages, even children, and women three times as often as men. The likelihood of developing RA increases in women over the age of 30. People with a particular genetic marker (HLA-DR4) tend to have a higher incidence of the illness.

Other forms of arthritis include gout, which occurs in three out of 1,000 adults, or about two million Americans (the majority of whom are men)[3] and less common forms such as ankylosing spondylitis, psoriatic arthritis, and infectious arthritis.

The common conventional medical approach to arthritis relies on anti-inflammatory and pain-killing drugs. While these drugs provide temporary symptom relief, they also have serious side effects of their own. Alternative medicine, on the other hand, offers a wide range of treatment options for eliminating the often hidden causes of arthritis. As with any disorder, especially chronic ones such as arthritis, more than a single cause is usually involved, as the following patient case history graphically demonstrates.

Success Story: Out of His Wheelchair With Alternative Medicine

Gerald, 45, was so severely affected by ankylosing spondylitis when he first came to see us that he was virtually wheelchair-bound. He walked, with great difficulty, with the assistance of two crutches. He also had severe fibromyalgia (SEE QUICK DEFINITION), chronic fatigue, and insomnia. He had spent many years trying to find help with his ailments, but had found no relief.

Gerald's health problems had started when he was a child. His diet was poor—lots of starches, meat, and sweets, very few fruits and vegetables—and he was constantly fatigued, had little energy, and complained of muscle pain. He received myriad doses of antibiotics for various ailments throughout his childhood. In his twenties, he began to notice stiffness in his lower back in addition to body-wide pain and inflammation. His diet was still poor at this time, consisting of large quantities of cola and chocolate (to artificially boost his energy levels), hamburgers, fast foods, and very few vegetables.

One morning, shortly after a severe bout of the flu, Gerald found he could not get out of bed because the stiffness and pain in his joints and muscles were so severe. He was 28 years old. As he continued to

The term *arthritis* is used loosely as if it encompassed one entity, although over 100 types of arthritis have been identified. It is an aggregate of illnesses whose common features include joint pain, stiffness, and inflammation. For millions, arthritis limits everyday movements such as walking, standing, or even holding a pencil.

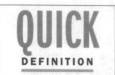

QUICK
DEFINITION

Fibromyalgia is multiple-symptom syndrome primarily involving widespread muscle pain (myalgia) that can be debilitating in its severity. The pain seems to be caused by the tightening and thickening of the myofascia, the thin film or tissue that holds the muscle together. Typical tender sites include the neck, upper back, rib cage, hips, and knees. Other symptoms include general fatigue and stiffness, insomnia and sleeping disorders, depression, mood swings, allergies, headaches, the sense of "hurting all over," tender skin, numbness, irritable bowel symptoms, and exercise intolerance. Post-traumatic fibromyalgia is believed to develop after a fall, whiplash, or back strain, whereas primary fibromyalgia has an uncertain origin.

For more **dietary recommendations for arthritis**, see Chapter 12: The Arthritis Diet, pp. 250-278. For **diagnostic tests for arthritis**, see Chapter 3: Diagnosing Arthritis, pp. 52-77.

try to function, Gerald had to get up earlier every morning, spending several hours to stretch and limber up his body enough to get to work.

Gerald consulted his family physician and specialists in rheumatology, but they were unable to provide a definitive diagnosis of his problem. He was given nonsteroidal, anti-inflammatory drugs (NSAIDs) to suppress the pain and sent home. He was even referred to a psychiatrist for his condition. Over the next several years, his health continued to decline. The stiffness and pain were made worse by inactivity and rest, which prevented him from sleeping more than two to three hours at a time. His hands and feet would stiffen up if he didn't continuously flex them and his back, shoulders, and muscles were so tight that he felt as if he was in "a cement suit." Simple tasks like shaving, bathing, and getting dressed became extremely difficult.

At age 39, Gerald was put on permanent disability leave from his job. He sought help from a string of rheumatologists and pain clinics. His condition was finally diagnosed as ankylosing spondylitis and fibromyalgia, but the therapies they offered—NSAIDs, psychotherapy, and exhausting physical therapy—provided no relief. It was in this state that Gerald came to the clinic.

The first thing we addressed was Gerald's diet. We put him on the "Arthritis Diet," a vegetarian, whole foods diet emphasizing fruits and vegetables, raw seeds and nuts, and whole grains. Gerald took vegetarian cooking classes and learned about juicing in order to help him with this transition. Almost immediately, he noticed a difference—less fatigue, more joint flexibility, and better sleep patterns.

We ran a stool analysis, blood tests, and food allergy test on Gerald to get a better picture of his condition. He was in an extreme state of dysbiosis (SEE QUICK DEFINITION), with tests indicating the absence of the friendly bacterial species *Lactobacillus* and *Bifidobacteria* in his intestinal tract. We did find two varieties of pathogenic bacteria, *Klebsiella* and *Streptococcus*, and a severe overgrowth of the yeast *Candida albicans*. *Klebsiella* is a factor in some ankylosing spondylitis cases because it is able to escape detection in the body due to a unique genetic marker. Gerald also had allergies to a large number of foods, including bananas, beans, chicken and turkey, clams, cheese and dairy products, eggs, oats and rye, salmon, wheat, and yeast (brewer's and baker's).

We started Gerald on a series of ten colonic irrigation treatments with Biocidin, an herbal antimicrobial formula, for the bacterial and yeast infections. He also received four additional (non-Biocidin) colonics containing probiotics to help repopulate his intestines with friendly bacteria. This therapy had a dramatic impact on Gerald: he had more energy, his inflammation would virtually disappear after each treatment, and he even lost weight. We also gave him *Streptococcinum* nosode (SEE QUICK DEFINITION), a homeopathic preparation, to decrease the abnormally high numbers of antibodies to this bacteria in his body.

To address his multiple underlying imbalances, Gerald began taking a number of remedies:

■ To combat the *Klebsiella* bacteria and yeast infection, we recommended Enterogenic Formula (3-4 tablets, four times daily, between meals), from

For more on colonic irrigation treatments, see Chapter 5: Detoxifying Specific Organs, pp. 102-129.

Thorne Research, which contains berberis and grapefruit seed extract, both powerful antimicrobials. We also prescribed Planti-Biotic, from Nature's Answer, a combination of botanicals to help kill the pathogenic organisms (two tablets with meals).

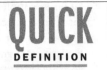

QUICK
DEFINITION

Intestinal dysbiosis refers to an imbalance of intestinal flora. Specifically, these flora are friendly, beneficial bacteria (probiotics), such as *Lactobacillus acidophilus* and *Bifidobacterium bifidum*, and unfriendly bacteria such as *Citrobacter spp. and Clostridium perfringens*. Dysbiosis is considered a primary cause or major cofactor in the development of many health problems, such as yeast overgrowth, chronic fatigue, depression, digestive disorders, food allergies, rheumatoid arthritis, and cancer.

A **homeopathic nosode** is a super-diluted remedy made as an energy imprint from a disease product, such as bacteria, tuberculosis, measles, influenza, and about 200 other substances. The nosode, which contains no physical trace of the disease, stimulates the body to remove all "taints" or residues it holds of a particular disease, whether it was inherited or contracted. Only qualified homeopaths may administer a nosode.

Circulating immune complexes (CICs) form in the body when poor digestion results in undigested food proteins "leaking" through the intestinal wall and into the bloodstream. The immune system treats these foreign substances or antigens as invaders, causing antibodies to form and couple with them. This antigen and antibody combination is known as a CIC. In a healthy person, CICs are neutralized, but in someone with a compromised immune system, they tend to accumulate in the blood where they burden the detoxification pathways or initiate an allergic reaction. If too many CICs accumulate, the kidneys and liver cannot excrete enough of them via the urine or stool. The CICs are then deposited in soft tissues, causing inflammation and bringing stress to the immune system. The overload can lead to a variety of chronic health conditions.

- To improve his digestion, we recommended a digestive enzyme supplement. This helped with Gerald's bacterial and yeast infections, because improving digestion in the upper part of the digestive tract will "starve" the pathogenic organisms in the bowel. Enzymes taken between meals also help dissolve circulating immune complexes (SEE QUICK DEFINITION), a factor in causing inflammation in the muscles and joints.

- For the chronic pain and inflammation, we gave Gerald Ananacur Powder (¼ tsp, four times daily, between meals), containing the enzyme bromelain (from organic pineapples) along with curcumin, both having excellent anti-inflammatory properties. We recommended Licorice Root Solid Extract (¼ tsp, four times daily on an empty stomach) as a tonic for his stressed adrenal glands. And we prescribed VT-2000, containing valerian root and white willow bark (four capsules, one hour prior to bedtime). We also gave him *Rhus Tox* 60C (three times daily), a homeopathic remedy specifically for muscular and rheumatic pain and stiffness that is made worse by inactivity.

- As antioxidant support, we recommended vitamin E (1,000 IU, three times daily with meals) and Free Radical Fighters (three tablets with each meal), from Twin Labs, to decrease the damage from free radicals. Gerald also took a fish oil supplement (three capsules with each meal), containing the omega-3 (SEE QUICK DEFINITION) essential fatty acids EPA and DHA.

- To support his liver as it processed the toxins out of his body, Gerald also took the herb milk thistle.

In just two months on this therapy regimen along with the dietary changes and colonics,

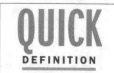

QUICK

DEFINITION

Omega-3 and omega-6 oils are the two principle types of essential fatty acids, which are unsaturated fats required in the diet. A balance of these oils in the diet is required for good health. The primary omega-3 oil is called alpha-linolenic acid (ALA) and is found in flaxseed, canola, pumpkin, walnuts, and soybeans. Fish oils, such as salmon, cod, and mackerel, contain the other important omega-3 oils, DHA (docosahexaenoic acid) and EPA (eicosapentaenoic acid). Omega-3 oils help reduce the risk of heart disease. Linoleic acid is the main omega-6 oil and is found in most plants and vegetable oils, including safflower, corn, peanut, and sesame. The most therapeutic form of omega-6 oil is gamma-linolenic acid (GLA), found in evening primrose, black currant, and borage oils. Once in the body, omega-3 and omega-6 are converted to prostaglandins, hormone-like substances that regulate many metabolic functions, particularly inflammatory processes.

For more information on **Biocidin**, contact: Bio-Botanical Research, Inc., 144 Pioneer Road, Corralitos, CA 95076; distributed by Wellness Health Pharmacy, 2800 South 18th Street, Homewood, AL 35209; tel: 800-227-2627. For **Enterogenic Formula** (available to licensed health-care practitioners only), contact: Thorne Research, P.O. Box 25, Dover, ID 83825; tel: 800-228-1966 or 208-263-1337; fax: 208-265-2488. For **PlantiBiotic**, contact: Nature's Answer, 320 Oser Avenue, Hauppauge, NY 11788; tel: 800-439-2324 or 516-231-7492; fax; 516-231-8391. For **Ananacur Powder** (licensed practitioners only) and **Licorice Root Solid Extract**, contact: Scientific Botanicals, P.O. Box 31131, Seattle, WA 98103; tel: 206-527-5521; fax: 206-526-7948. For **VT-2000**, contact: Karuna Labs, 42 Digital Drive, Suite 7, Novato, CA 94949; tel: 800-826-7225 or 415-382-0147; fax: 800-711-6740. For **Free Radical Fighters**, contact: Twin Labs, 2120 Smithtown Avenue, Ronkonkoma, NY 11779; tel: 800-645-5626 or 516-467-3140; fax: 516-467-3080.

Gerald made significant progress, moving from being 15% functional to 50% functional. A subsequent stool analysis showed that the *Klebsiella* had been eradicated and the friendly bacterial microflora were re-established. Gerald received regular massage therapy and chiropractic treatments to help with the pain and stiffness. He fasted on vegetable juice for seven days, which put an end to his pain. After the fast, he started incorporating "green" foods, such as spirulina and blue-green algae, into his diet. Green foods are important for detoxification and they helped improve Gerald's energy levels and sleep. Gerald also sought counseling to help with the emotional components of his arthritis.

For more information about **"green" foods**, see Chapter 4: General Detoxification, pp. 78-100. For more on **massage and other physical therapies for arthritis**, see Chapter 14: Exercises and Physical Therapies, pp. 314-339.

Since he embraced this holistic approach eight years ago, Gerald continues to improve. He shows no signs of ankylosing spondylitis through subjective and objective measurements and feels that he is almost completely functional again. He can now go out and engage in physical activities without having to endure days of pain and inflammation afterwards.

The Failure of Conventional Arthritis Treatment

As Gerald discovered, conventional medicine prescribes a whole "laundry list" of pharmaceutical drugs for arthritis. Many of these drugs block the symptoms of pain, often very quickly and with little effort on the part of the patients or doctors. While pain relief is important, these drugs merely hide the symptoms and ignore the underlying causes of the disease.

In addition, conventional drugs have side effects that cause daily discomfort and further remove the patient from an independent, symptom-free life. The first round of pharmaceutical drugs prescribed for most forms of arthritis include the NSAIDs aspirin, ibuprofen (Motrin), indomethacin (Indocin), and naproxen (Naprosyn). High dosages of NSAIDs may cause the following side effects: abdominal cramping or pain, gas, constipation, diarrhea, dizziness, fatigue, fluid retention and swelling, headaches, heartburn, loss of appetite, nausea, nervousness, rash, ringing in the ears, skin eruptions, stomach pain, or vomiting.[4]

NSAIDs also contribute to the continuation of degenerative changes by inhibiting the repair of cartilage (the structural support of

Conventional medicine prescribes a whole "laundry list" of pharmaceutical drugs for arthritis. While pain relief is important, conventional drugs merely hide the symptoms and ignore the underlying causes of the disease.

joints).[5] Studies have clearly illustrated that NSAIDs not only hinder the synthesis of cartilage's base materials, but actually accelerate the destruction of cartilage.[6] Furthermore, these drugs destroy the gastrointestinal lining, leading to the formation of ulcers and intestinal permeability, which are significant contributing factors to the onset of arthritis. Celebrex® and Rofecoxib® are NSAIDs that inhibit Cox II, mainly pro-inflammatory prostaglandins, but do not inhibit Cox I prostaglandins, which protect the gastrointestinal lining. Cox II inhibitors are therefore less destructive to the digestive system than other NSAIDs, but still have a long list of serious side effects (including diarrhea, nausea, edema, and kidney disorders, among others).[7]

Other drug treatments, such as injections of corticosteroids, control inflammation at a high price. Their side effects can alter the person's personality, causing psychotic behavior, severe depression, or mood swings. High doses cause fluid retention, particularly in the face; this is often referred to as "moon face." Prolonged use causes eye infections, weight gain, fragile skin, muscle weakness, brittle bones, or purplish stripe marks on the skin.

What Alternative Medicine Can Do for Arthritis

Alternative medicine offers arthritis sufferers lasting relief from pain and inflammation. According to the alternative medicine approach, arthritis is a disease that results from multiple causes, many of them with a less-than-obvious connection to the disease or not easily detectable. As you will discover in this book, a number of underlying imbalances, with accompanying physical, mental, and environmental factors, contribute to all forms of arthritis.

Specifically, arthritis develops as a result of a combination of: an accumulation of toxins in the body (from the environment, food, drugs, and other sources); bacterial and yeast infections (often due to excessive use of antibiotics); parasites; leaky gut syndrome; allergies (both food and environmental); nutrient deficiencies leading to slow repair of cartilage; biomechanical stress and imbalances; poor stress-coping abilities and other emotional factors; and immune dysfunction often resulting in an autoimmune reaction, in which the immune system attacks healthy tissues in the body, further worsening arthritic symptoms.

It is essential to understand the factors that went into creating arthritis in each person, because arthritis is never caused by one thing alone and no two people have exactly the same causal factors. Alternative medicine employs a battery of diagnostic tools—physical examination, dietary assessment, tests for immune, digestive, and detoxification function, and emotional evaluation—to build an individualized picture of the patient's condition. Skilled alternative practitioners take the time needed to find the root causes of arthritis and the patient also becomes actively involved in their treatment. Alternative medicine not only respects differences between individuals, but concentrates its diagnosis and treatment plan around this "customized" approach.

It draws upon a wide range of therapies to help treat—and even prevent— arthritis. The primary keys are proper diet and nutrition, detoxification, and stress reduction. Diet and nutrition can have a significant impact on pain and inflammation and special

Skilled alternative practitioners find the root causes of arthritis and the patient becomes actively involved in their treatment. Alternative medicine not only respects individual differences, but concentrates its diagnosis and treatment plan around this "customized" approach.

care should be taken to avoid substances that might cause allergic reactions in the body. Vitamins, minerals, herbs, and other natural supplements can provide effective relief without the side effects of conventional drugs.

Removing toxins from the body has shown to be remarkably therapeutic for our arthritis patients—alternative medicine offers a number of safe and effective detoxification strategies. Meditation, biofeedback, hypnotherapy, and other mind/body techniques can help reduce stress (another key factor in arthritis overlooked by conventional medicine). Skeletal and postural problems can also be addressed through a variety of other modalities, including bodywork, osseous manipulation, exercises and stretching, and yoga. With alternative medicine, health is restored to the whole patient, rather than simply providing superficial symptom relief. The goal is to help each person achieve a balance among physical healing and the emotional, mental, and even spiritual aspects of their life.

In the patient case history below, we explain the testing procedures, diagnosis of underlying causes, and therapies that enabled the patient Vanessa to reduce her joint pain and discontinue her use of conventional arthritis drugs that caused stomach upset and other gastrointestinal problems.

Success Story: A Holistic Approach Alleviates Arthritis

Vanessa, 63, had symptoms of both rheumatoid arthritis and osteoarthritis as well as the early stages of osteoporosis (bone loss). Her health survey revealed a number of other problems: diarrhea (which first occurred following a trip abroad), urinary incontinence, and other gastrointestinal difficulties, neurological disturbances, and migraine headaches. She was taking medications for her migraines and anti-inflammatory drugs for her arthritis, but she was concerned about possible side effects from prolonged use. As her conventional medical specialists had been unable to offer lasting relief for her health problems, Vanessa came to us for holistic evaluation.

A food profile showed that Vanessa's diet was diverse, consisting of tuna, chicken, eggs, oatmeal, yogurt, herbal teas, soups, and generous quantities of vegetables; she snacked on chocolate, nuts, and other salty snacks. But Vanessa also said that she had multiple food cravings, which alerted us to a possibility of food allergies. (People often crave the foods that trigger allergic reactions, which may include arthritis pain.) We ordered a test for potential food allergies and the results revealed sensitivities to wheat, white and brown rice, corn, broccoli, cucumbers, squash, cashews, black pepper, chocolate, coffee, and licorice.

A hair analysis for mineral deficiencies or heavy metal toxicity revealed high levels of calcium and magnesium, aluminum, and sodium and potassium. We interpreted the high calcium and magnesium levels to mean that these minerals were not being absorbed into her cells; deficiencies of calcium and magnesium are common in arthritis patients. The excess levels of aluminum, sodium, and potassium could have been contributing to Vanessa's neurological imbalances because they interfere with nerve signal transmissions. Her blood test revealed elevated liver enzymes, indicating a clogged and toxic liver, something we often find in arthritis patients. Her level of the hormone DHEA, a precursor of the sex hormones, was also low normal at 91 (the normal range is 80 to 160), which may be a natural result of aging or caused by chronic stress.

We also performed a darkfield microscopic analysis (SEE QUICK DEFINITION) of Vanessa's blood. We could see in the projected image of her blood many long, unidentified tubules, which we have found to correlate with the presence of parasites. The fact that her diarrhea had begun following foreign travel made us suspect parasites as well. Her red blood cells were oval-shaped, indicating heavy metals in her system and confirming the results of the hair analysis. Vanessa also had a high level of red and yellow crystals in her blood, which we associate with joint pain and swelling. Finally, the white blood cells called neutrophils were static, a sign of suppressed immune function.

Clearly, our treatment of Vanessa needed to employ multiple therapies (as is the case with all our arthritis patients), because of these underlying problems with parasites, nutritional deficiencies, and toxicity that contributed to her arthritis. In consultation with our nutritionist, Vanessa modified her diet to eliminate those foods that she was allergic to and we supported her with vitamins B6 and B12 as well as folic acid, which help with food allergies. We also wanted her to increase the amount of foods in her diet that contain omega-3 essential fatty acids. A deficiency in omega-3s often leads to inflammation (and even arthritis) in the body.

We also recommended a probiotic supplement containing the "friendly" intestinal bacteria (SEE QUICK DEFINITION) *L. acidophilus* and *B. bifidum*. In addition, we gave her a supplement containing fructo-oligosaccharides (FOS), which acts like an intestinal "fertilizer," selectively feeding the friendly microflora in the large intestine so that their numbers can usefully increase.

Vanessa was given two formulas developed by Serafina Corsello, M.D., of New York City: CV Antioxidant Formula (contains B vitamins, magnesium, selenium, potassium, taurine, and other antioxidant ingredients) and CFS Support Formula (contains antioxidants, choline and silymarin for liver support, shiitake mushroom, burdock, and licorice). We also suggested Dr. Corsello's vitamin C supplement C-Bioplex (one capsule with each meal) and

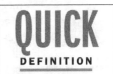

DEFINITION

Darkfield microscopy is a way of studying living whole blood cells under a specially adapted microscope that projects the dynamic image, magnified 1,400 times, onto a video screen. The skilled physician can detect early signs of illness in the form of microorganisms in the blood known to produce disease. Relevant technical features in the blood include color, variously shaped components (spicules, long tubules, and roulous), and the size and activity of certain immune cells. The amount of time the blood cells stay viable indicates the overall health of the individual. Darkfield microscopy reveals distortions of red blood cells (which indicate nutritional status), possible undesirable bacterial or fungal life forms, and blood ecology patterns indicative of health or illness.

Friendly bacteria, or probiotics, refer to beneficial microbes inhabiting the human gastrointestinal tract where they are essential for proper nutrient assimilation. The human body contains an estimated several trillion beneficial bacteria comprising over 400 species, all necessary for health. Among the more well known of these are *Lactobacillus acidophilus* and *Bifidobacterium bifidum*. Overly acidic bodily conditions, chronic constipation or diarrhea, dietary imbalances, consumption of highly processed foods, and the excessive use of antibiotics and hormonal drugs can interfere with probiotic function and even reduce the number of these microbes, setting up conditions for illness.

additional vitamin E (400 IU at breakfast and dinner). We had Vanessa start taking Essiac tea, an herbal tea created by holistic nurse Rene Caisse in the 1920s to treat cancer patients that is also good for blood cleansing and general detoxification. As additional liver support, we recommended Liverol, an herbal extract from milk thistle (silymarin).

For her digestive disturbances, Vanessa started on the herb cat's claw (uña de gato) and a glutonic acid supplement useful for soothing the intestines. To address her essential fatty acid deficiencies, we recommended Omega Balance, another Corsello formula, which provides omega-3s and omega-6s from black currant seed oil. Since we considered parasites to be a contributing factor to her digestive problems, we put her on an anti-parasitic formula called Parex, manufactured by Metagenics.

For more information on **herbs and nutrients for arthritis**, see Chapter 13: Supplements for Arthritis, pp. 280-313. For more on **fasting**, see Chapter 4: General Detoxification, pp. 78-100.

Vanessa also started on a fast to cleanse her gastrointestinal tract. For three days initially, we had her eat nothing but a watery soup made of cabbage and other vegetables rich in nutrients important for joint and bone structure. She also took UltraBalance, an intestinal-cleansing protein powder drink from Meta-genics, along with ground flax seeds as support during the fast. This moderate fast was a good way for Vanessa to give her toxic bowel a rest, begin to cleanse the liver, and allow her to experience some days free of joint pain. We normally recommend that patients continue this fast one day per week on an ongoing basis, but Vanessa had such good results that she decided to fast two days per week.

Additional therapeutic support included a weekly intravenous infusion of potassium chloride, magnesium sul-

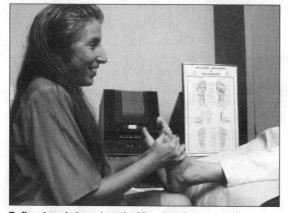

Reflexology is based on the idea that there are reflex areas in the hands and feet that correspond to every part of the body, including the organs and glands. By applying gentle but precise pressure to these reflex points, reflexologists release blockages that inhibit energy flow and cause pain and disease. Practitioners focus on breaking up lactic acid and calcium crystals accumulated around any of the 7,200 nerve endings in each foot. Eunice Ingham, a physiotherapist, pioneered the discipline in the late 1930s. He mapped out reflexes on the feet and developed techniques for inducing healing in those areas.

For more information about **Essiac**, contact: Essiac USA, Inc., 26 Union Street, Newburyport, MA 01950; tel: 508-462-4976; fax: 508-465-8214. For **UltraBalance**, contact: Metagenics, Inc., 971 Calle Negocio, San Clemente, CA 92673; tel: 800-692-9400; fax: 714-366-0818. For **Dr. Corsello's formulas**, contact: Global Nutrition, 175 E. Main Street, Huntington, NY 11743; tel: 888-461-0949. For **Parex**, contact: Metagenics, 166 Fernwood Avenue, Edison, NJ 08837; tel: 800-638-2848. For **cetyl myristoleate**, contact: EHP Products, Inc., P.O. Box 1306, Ashland, KY 41105; tel: 606-329-9339 or 888-EHP-0100; fax: 606-325-8569. For **homeopathic detoxosodes**, contact: HVS Labs, 3427 Exchange Avenue, Naples, FL 34104; tel: 800-521-7722. For **MSM**, contact: Jarrow Formulas Inc., 1824 S. Robertson Blvd., Los Angeles, CA 90035; tel: 800-726-0886 or 310-204-6936; fax: 310-204-2520. Futurebiotics, 145 Ricefield Lane, Hauppauge, NY 11788; tel. 800-645-1721 or 516-273-6300; fax: 516-273-1165; website: www.futurebiotics.com.

fate, manganese, zinc, vitamin B complex, vitamins B6 and B5, calcium, taurine, and glutathione. We also gave her two nutrients specifically to support her arthritic joints, cetyl myristoleate (a fatty acid) and MSM (methylsulfonylmethane, a sulfur compound), both useful for treating inflammation. For treatment of heavy metals, we recommended the homeopathic detoxosode program from HVS labs.

Vanessa started receiving monthly massage treatments from a massage therapist. We also encourage arthritis patients to go for regular chiropractic adjustments, although Vanessa opted not to do this. She also came with a friend to one of our reflexology classes, so that they could perform this specialized massage therapy for each other at no cost.

After three months on this program, Vanessa said that she felt much better and she continues on the program now after two years. Her rheumatologist discontinued her use of conventional pain medications, which in turn improved her gastrointestinal problems greatly. A subsequent bone density scan showed that she was no longer at high risk for developing osteoporosis. And her migraines have lessened in both frequency and intensity.

Most importantly, Vanessa feels that she is in control of her symptoms and that her quality of life has increased tremendously. Vanessa is now equipped with the tools to restore health. She knows which foods invoke arthritis pains and avoids these. Her diet is now tailored to support optimal joint function and prevent the further degenerative effects of aging. She plans to continue with the holistic approach to arthritis and stay away from conventional drug therapy and its adverse side effects.

Undoing Arthritis in Stages— The Scope of This Book

Vanessa's case demonstrates many common aspects of treating arthritis with alternative medicine therapies. She, like over 50% of arthritis patients, has a "mixed" disease process consisting of both osteoarthritis and rheumatoid arthritis. Clearly, no magic pill will correct what many may erroneously think is a natural part of aging. Instead several therapies are needed to reverse the underlying factors—nutritional deficiencies, infestation of parasites, and liver and digestive dysfunction, among others—that ultimately manifest themselves as arthritis.

When arthritis is viewed through alternative medicine, it becomes a correctable disease that requires adjustments to specific organ systems, diet, and lifestyle. This book will describe the tests that alternative medicine practitioners use to determine inadequacies or dysfunction, practical solutions to resolving underlying problems, and positive changes (diet, nutritional supplements, stress relief strategies, and exercises) that you can make to reverse or prevent the onset of arthritis.

Types and Causes—In the next chapter, Chapter 2: What is Arthritis?, we provide explanations of the various types of arthritis, their predominant symptoms, and their primary causes.

Testing—In order to start an effective treatment plan, you need to know all the components that are contributing to your arthritis. For Vanessa, we tested for nutritional deficiencies, food allergies, heavy metal toxicity, liver function, digestive capacity, and the infestation of parasites, viruses, or bacteria. Chapter 3: Diagnosing Arthritis covers these and other tests useful for pinpointing these underlying factors. Most of the testing involves simple blood, urine, and stool analyses that your conventional doctor may not be aware of.

Detoxifying the Body—Toxins from environmental and chemical pollutants, stress, poor diet, and food allergies can overwhelm and eventually exhaust the body's ability to process and eliminate harmful substances. These toxins can then accumulate in joint tissues and cause inflammation, free-radical damage, and arthritic degeneration. As seen in Vanessa's case, therapies such as fasting cleanse the body of accumulated toxins and relieve the liver of its toxic burden. Chapter 4: General Detoxification provides step-by-step instructions for all phases of fasting. Chapter 5: Detoxifying Specific Organs provides therapies to support and tone the organs involved in the detoxification process. Herbal therapies (such as the ones used to treat Vanessa), dietary recommendations, and other therapeutic methods lessen the body's toxic load, reduce joint pain, stop bone and joint deterioration, and boost the efficiency of vital organs.

Viruses, Infections, Candidiasis, and Parasites—Research and clinical evidence have shown that viruses, bacterial infections, candidiasis (infection with the yeast-like fungus *Candida albicans*), and parasites are often present in arthritis, particularly rheumatoid and infectious arthritis. As you will see in Chapter 6: Eradicating Bacteria and Yeast and Chapter 7: Eliminating Parasites, these factors both mimic arthritis-like symptoms and contribute to the toxic load in the body by eroding the lining of the intestines and escaping into the bloodstream.

Intestinal Permeability—Ninety percent of our arthritis patients have intestinal permeability, also known as "leaky gut syndrome." Viruses, disease-causing bacteria, *Candida*, parasites, and NSAIDs are the prime culprits of leaky gut. When inappropriate substances cross the intestinal barrier into the circulatory system, the immune system views them as invaders and sends antibodies to attach to the invaders, forming what are known as circulating immune complexes. These immune complexes can trigger collagen breakdown in the joints and autoimmune reactions, both factors in arthritis and joint disease. Chapter 8: Alleviating Leaky Gut Syndrome further explains the effects of intestinal permeability and how to correct it.

Underlying Allergies—Hidden allergies to foods may provoke arthritic symptoms of joint tenderness, inflammation, and swelling. Among the most common allergenic foods are wheat, dairy products, and the nightshade family of vegetables. The case of Vanessa demonstrates the role of food allergies in arthritis. The results of her allergy test revealed that she could not tolerate broccoli, coffee, wheat, white and brown rice, corn, cucumbers, squash, cashews, black pepper, chocolate, and licorice. Once these foods were eliminated from her diet, she experienced a decrease in joint pain. Chapter 9: Allergies and Arthritis describes other common sources of allergies, testing procedures, and simple therapies for reducing allergic reactions.

The Autoimmune Response—The autoimmune diseases (rheumatoid arthritis, ankylosing spondylitis, juvenile rheumatoid arthritis, and lupus) involve destruction of healthy cells by the body's own defensive mechanism, the immune system. Normal cartilage cells that line the joints and ensure smooth motion become the target of repeated attacks by the immune system. In effect, the body has become allergic to its own tissues, causing joint deformities and disabilities. In Chapter 10: Desensitizing the Autoimmune Reaction, we discuss safe and effective methods to quell the immune system's aggressive behavior without suppression of its normal activities.

Healing the Psychological Side of Arthritis—A constant state of stress can lead to a number of adverse physiological consequences that can directly affect the severity of your arthritis. Psychological evaluations of our arthritis patients have also defined a specific "arthritis personality," a kind of mental predisposition for arthritis. In Chapter 11: Mind/Body Approaches to Arthritis, you will learn how stress, suppressed emotions, and lifestyle choices can contribute to arthritis, how to undo damaging thoughts, and how to incorporate habits for relaxation and increased confidence into your life.

Eating Away Arthritis—It is an old concept, but "food as medicine" is a powerful tool accessible to all. The dietary recommendations in Chapter 12: The Arthritis Diet show you the foods needed in a daily diet to prevent inflammation and improve overall health, the foods that will exacerbate arthritis symptoms, and recipes for making delicious healthy meals.

Nutrients and Natural Supplements for Arthritis—Like most arthritis sufferers, Vanessa had multiple nutritional deficiencies resulting from age—as we grow older, our nutritional reserves decline—and from an infestation of parasites. Eliminating the parasites and improving her digestion made it possible to focus on boosting levels of nutrients needed to synthesize cartilage and connective tissue (to rebuild her joints) and to fight the damaging effects of free radicals. Chapter 13: Supplements for Arthritis details the nutrients commonly deficient in arthritis sufferers as well as those nutrients useful in promoting joint health. In addition, Chapter 13 offers a compendium of Chinese and Western herbs used to decrease inflammation and relieve pain.

Exercises and Physical Therapies—While daily exercise and physical activity are both important components of a healthy lifestyle, they are an absolute necessity for people who suffer from arthritis. Regular exercise improves energy levels, provides nourishment for muscles and connective tissues, and maintains a healthy weight. By keeping muscles toned and fit so that they can adequately support joints, exercise helps reduce pain and stiffness and halt the progression of the disease. Daily exercise can be further augmented by massage, acupressure, or other physical therapies to promote relaxation and improve

For **detailed treatment protocols for each type of arthritis,** see Appendix, pp. 340-358.

the circulation of blood and lymphatic fluid. Therapeutic baths, showers, and other water treatments can improve circulation, clear the body of toxins, and initiate healing of internal organs. In Chapter 14: Exercises and Physical Therapies, we discuss some of the most widely available physical therapies so that you and your health-care professional can determine which one would be most beneficial for you.

2

What is Arthritis?

AMONG THE MOST common types of arthritis are osteoarthritis (degenerative joint disease), rheumatoid arthritis (an autoimmune disease), and gout (usually affecting small joints in the hands and feet). Other types of arthritis include psoriatic arthritis (associated with the skin condition psoriasis), ankylosing spondylitis, and infectious arthritis (caused by bacterial or viral infections). Arthritis is a manifestation of similar underlying imbalances that overload the body and impair the normal process of cartilage repair. Specifically, these causes include intestinal imbalances (dysbiosis or parasites), food allergies, heavy metal toxicity, nutritional deficiencies, improper intake of dietary fats, and emotional, psychological, and biomechanical stressors.

Osteoarthritis

Osteoarthritis (OA) causes the breakdown of cartilage, the smooth, gelatinous tissue that protects the ends of bones from rubbing against each other. Healthy cartilage shields bones against being worn down by friction, but in OA, the cartilage is worn away, allowing bone ends to make direct contact. As the disease progresses, direct contact creates bone spurs and abnormal bone hardening, and leads to inflammation and severe pain as bones continue to rub together without proper cushioning. As a result, bones may become more brittle and subject to fracture. There are over 300,000 knee and hip replacements in the U.S. annually, usually due to osteoarthritis.

In This Chapter

- Osteoarthritis
- Rheumatoid Arthritis
- Gout
- Less Prevalent Joint Diseases (Ankylosing Spondylitis, Psoriatic Arthritis, and Infectious Arthritis)

There are two types of osteoarthritis: primary and secondary. Primary OA is considered "wear and tear" arthritis due to an unhealthy aging process. It most commonly develops over the age of 45 and affects the weight-bearing joints in the hips, lower back, knees, and feet, as well as the neck and fingers. It occurs when joints are placed under excessive long-term stress from supporting too much weight (as seen in obese people with arthritic knees) or from normal weight demands placed on weak, unhealthy joints. Heredity also plays a role. According to a *Science News* report, as many as six million osteoarthritis sufferers can trace their aches and pains to DNA—meaning that a genetic propensity for the disease runs in families.[1]

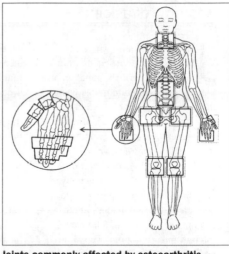

Joints commonly affected by osteoarthritis.

Secondary osteoarthritis is the less common of the two types but has a more apparent, direct cause: trauma, injury, previous inflammation (even from rheumatoid arthritis), congenital joint misalignment, infection, surgery, or prolonged use of medications.[2] It often appears before the age of 40 and is most commonly caused by sudden or recurring (chronic) trauma. A fall from a ladder is an example of sudden trauma. Chronic trauma results from repetitive impact on a particular joint; for example, the shoulder joint of a baseball pitcher that eventually wears down from years of repeated-motion stress. Joe Namath, the retired New York Jets quarterback, now suffers from arthritis in his knees, which were repeatedly assaulted by defensive players. Other examples of secondary OA include an arthritic wrist joint of a construction worker or worn joints in the feet of a tap dancer. Over time, repeated motion can lead to a breakdown of cartilage and that degeneration often leads to bone deformity.

Osteoarthritis Symptoms

The onset of primary OA is gradual as the disease usually progresses over the course of many years. It most frequently starts with mild pain and stiffness, which can lead to a narrowing of the joint, limited joint

Anatomy of a Joint

Joints are the area where two bones meet or articulate (that is, move together). The function of the joint is to facilitate mobility and flexibility. The joints of the body are classified into three types, of which arthritis usually affects two, the cartilaginous and synovial joints.

Cartilaginous joints allow only slight movement. The space between each vertebra in the spine is an example of a cartilaginous joint. Another example of this type of joint allows the pelvis of a pregnant woman to expand. As the name suggests, cartilaginous joints cushion the intersection of two bones with cartilage, a sponge-like buffer.

Synovial joints are the freely movable joints in the fingers, arms, legs, hips, and wrists. Their names describe their structure, such as the ball-and-socket joint (which connects the upper leg with the pelvis) or the hinge joint in the elbow and the knee. The wrist joint is called an ellipsoidal joint because it moves in the shape of an ellipse or oval. And the thumb, or cellar joint, is flexible and gives humans and some primates the ability to use tools. Synovial joints experience more wear and tear than other types of joints.

Synovial joints are made up of numerous components:

■ Synovial membrane lines the joint capsule, enclosing all the components of the joint. It is dense with nerves and is the source of much of the pain that patients with arthritis experience. The synovial membrane also produces one of the most important substances of the joint, known as synovial fluid.

■ Synovial fluid or synovium coats the joints much like a lubricant coats the parts of a car's engine. It also carries nutrients to the cartilage and removes waste products. The synovial fluid is usually clear, colorless, or pale yellow, resembling blood plasma or serum.

■ Cartilage covers the ends of bones at joints, serving to buffer the bones from rubbing together. Cartilage is one of the smoothest surfaces known to man—it is rubbery, gel-like, tough, flexible, and slippery. There are two types of cartilage: articular (or moving cartilage) and meniscus (or cushioning cartilage). Both types are very compliant and also act as shock absorbers thanks to their high water content—cartilage is 65%-80% water.

Cartilage does not contain blood or lymphatic vessels or nerves. It is nourished entirely through a process which involves contraction and expansion. When pressure is applied to the joints, the cartilaginous structures are compressed; as movement stops or the body relaxes, the cartilage re-expands. This compression and relaxation allows the nutrient-bearing synovial fluid to circulate freely in and out of the joint. When we are moving, we're actually feeding our joints. And conversely, when we stop moving, we begin to starve our joints by shutting down the flow of nutrients. Without synovial fluid, the articular cartilage in joints would begin to wear away like the parts of a car engine that are not adequately lubricated.

■ Joints are surrounded by soft tissue: tendons, which attach muscles to the bone; ligaments, which connect bone to bone with extremely tough, fibrous tissue known as elastin; and muscles, which make the different parts move as one. To reduce friction during motion, tendons are covered by tendon sheaths, which use a lubricating substance called hyaluronan. To absorb shock during motion, bursa (small sacs filled with synovial fluid) are strategically placed throughout the joints. You may be familiar with the condition called bursitis or "tennis elbow," which involve inflammation of the bursa.

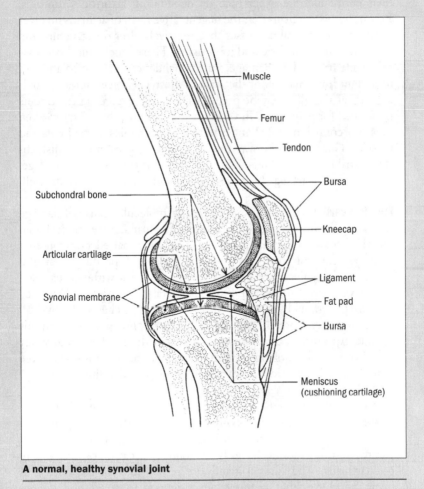

A normal, healthy synovial joint

mobility, and sometimes a grating sensation and grinding sound called "crepitus." This additional stress can lead to the development of bone spurs (osteophytes), which, in turn, cause more friction, further joint breakdown, and pain.[3]

Causes of Osteoarthritis

Although a lifetime of "wear and tear" on the joints is commonly considered the cause of osteoarthritis, studies have shown that constant use of the joints by itself doesn't cause bone and cartilage to erode.[4] Many elderly men and women who have been physically active over their entire lifetime experience no debilitating arthritic symptoms. Research now confirms that the degenerative form of arthritis involves ongoing biochemical processes that negatively alter the structure and regeneration of cartilage and joint tissue. These biochemical processes include free-radical damage, nutritional deficiencies, imbalances of important hormones, poor dietary and lifestyle choices, food or environmental allergies, genetic predisposition, and even drug treatments prescribed for pain relief. In various combinations, these factors often cause (or contribute to) changes in the biomechanics of the joints and muscles. Changes in the way the joints and muscles interact disturbs the distribution of fluids and nutrients in tissues and cartilage. Consequently, cartilage becomes injured and is unable to repair itself.

Free Radicals—Free radicals are the major molecular cause of damage to healthy connective tissue in all kinds of arthritis. A free radical is an unstable, toxic molecule of oxygen with an unpaired electron that steals an electron from another molecule and produces harmful effects. Free radicals are formed when molecules within cells react with oxygen (oxidize) as part of normal metabolic processes. Free radicals are generated by any type of stress, including chemical, physical, biochemical, emotional, and mental. Other sources of free radicals include exposure to environmental toxins in the food, air, and water and also through smoking cigarettes. By the time arthritis sets in, free radicals have been oxidizing cartilage for an extended time.

Imbalanced Hormones—Researchers have investigated the role of hormones, the regulators of bodily functions, in the development of osteoarthritis. Specifically, imbalances of adrenal, thyroid, and parathyroid hormones have been found to cause or exacerbate osteoarthritis. The adrenal glands are responsible for the release of many hormones that regulate our reactions to stress and energy metabolism. These hormones include DHEA, pregnenolone, cortisol, and adrenaline. When the body is under chronic stress, the adrenals produce high levels of steroid hormones (adrenaline and cortisol) instead of DHEA (the precursor of estrogen and testosterone). The result of prolonged exposure to steroid hormones is an increase in bone degeneration, muscle breakdown, accumulation of fat, and an imbalance of important mineral ratios.

Because women experience OA at a rate three times greater than men, estrogen and progesterone imbalances have been investigated as one of the many potential causative factors. In fact, estrogen has been shown to accelerate osteoarthritis in experimental studies.[5] Excess levels of estrogen (and decreased levels of progesterone) can cause deficiencies in zinc, magnesium, and the B vitamins, which are involved in hormone maintenance and bone and tissue health. Osteoarthritis sufferers may benefit from using natural substances which help to balance estrogen and progesterone levels.

The thyroid gland secretes hormones that regulate body temperature, energy use, and organ function. Along with many other hormones, the thyroid secretes calcitonin, a hormone required for calcium metabolism, which influences bone and cartilage development. Thyroid deficiency is involved in up to 64 common ailments, including osteoarthritis. Patients with hypothyroidism (low thyroid function) have been shown to have an increased rate of osteoarthritis compared with the general population.[6]

Nutrient Deficiencies—As people age, their levels of many nutrients involved in the synthesis of cartilage become deficient. Although these deficiencies may not directly cause OA, studies have shown that supplementation can often bring pain relief. Vitamin E helps to increase the production of the building-blocks of cartilage, as well as to decrease cartilage breakdown and joint pain.[7] Vitamin C levels are often low in OA patients and this vitamin is vital for joint repair and building collagen.[8] Vitamin B3 (niacinamide) has demonstrated good results when used to treat joint pain and stiffness associated with OA.[9] International studies have noted that high levels of OA are found in areas where the mineral boron is deficient in the soil and food supply. Boron supplementation is regularly used for OA patients in Germany and significant improvement in OA after boron supplementation has been documented.[10]

Diet and Food Allergies—When comparisons are made of particular cultural groups, evidence points to the Standard American Diet (which is high in processed, refined foods, fat, and sugar) as a major contributing factor to the development of OA. OA is a very rare disease in Japan, where the diet is high in fish and sea vegetables. But an interesting phenomenon occurs when Japanese individuals begin to adopt a Standard American Diet (SAD): there is a marked increase in the development of OA, as well as many other degenerative diseases, after this diet has been consumed for a number of years.

Food allergies, often a result of poor dietary choices, are also implicated as a causative factor in many cases of arthritis. A common allergy is to plants in the nightshade family, including tomatoes, green peppers, eggplant, potatoes, and tobacco. About one third of the arthritis sufferers who remove all nightshades from their diet will experience some relief of symptoms.

Dietary intake of fats affects the composition of cell membranes and the degree of inflammation and pain that a person experiences. Although most of the research on fats and their role in joint pain has been done on rheumatoid arthritis, patients with OA can also vastly benefit from increasing the essential fatty acids, and decreasing the pro-inflammatory fats, in their diet.[11]

Other Contributing Factors—Researchers at Jefferson Medical College in Philadelphia, Pennsylvania, have identified a possible genetic correlation in osteoarthritis. In some individuals, they have discovered a defect in the gene that instructs cartilage cells to manufacture collagen (the structural protein of the connective tissue), so the collagen is more likely to break down, leading to degeneration of joints.[12]

Patients with osteoarthritis often display insulin resistance or deficiency. Insulin resistance, often considered a precursor to adult-onset diabetes, is a blood sugar disorder that occurs when the body fails to "recognize" the effects of insulin in the blood. This makes it more difficult for the body to use sugar (glucose) for energy. The body then begins to break down protein as an alternative energy source, which negatively affects the connective tissue and leads to further destruction within the joints. Diets high in carbohydrates, including sugars and wheat products, tend to increase insulin resistance, reducing the person's blood sugar levels even more.

To contact **Peter Zilahy, D.C.**: 35 Candee Hill Road, Watertown, CT 06795; tel: 860-274-9641.

Biomechanical Changes—According to Dr. Peter Zilahy, a chiropractic orthopedist in Watertown, Connecticut, osteoarthritis develops as joints lose their full range of motion. Compromised mobility decreases the flow of oxygen and nutrients to the surrounding cartilage, and leads to cartilage breakdown. Cartilage can obtain nourishment, repair itself, and get rid of wastes through balanced motion. When a joint is compressed—for example, each time you step forward you compress your knee joint—synovial fluid in the cartilage between the knee bones is pumped out of the area; this is called "on-loading." As the knee comes to rest, the joint expands, and fluid rushes back in carrying a fresh supply of oxygen and essential nutrients; this is called "off-loading." This exchange of nutrients and waste products is dependent upon balanced (full range), frequent motion. Stress, injury, or lack of activity causes a series of imbalances that alter the interactions of ligaments, tendons, bones, and muscles. As a result, balanced motion is hindered and the surrounding cartilage starves as the on-loading and off-loading exhange of substances is compromised.

The body also responds to joint and muscle biomechanical imbalances by sending calcium to weak or impaired areas to stabilize the weak joint. This response results in hard, inflexible deposits of calcium where once there were smooth, elastic ligaments, tendons, and even muscle. The joint stiffness that arthritis patients frequently experience is caused by these calcium deposits. Eventually

The density of calcium spurs can be gauged from the following example: while treating a woman with OA in her neck and shoulder, we inserted an acupuncture needle into the front muscle of the neck and hit one of these calcium deposits; the deposit was so impenetrable that it actually bent the needle.

these calcium deposits form spurs that protrude from the joints much like stalactites found inside caves, and the joint ultimately can fuse.

Fibrosis (an excess accumulation of fibrous tissue) can also set in as waste products build up in the muscle and joint area and further restrict motion. These impediments deprive joints of key nutrients needed to build new cartilage as old cells die. As a result, cartilage physically wears away exposing bone and leading to the onset of arthritis. Arthritis can actually be transferred to neighboring joints when surrounding muscles and cartilage attempt to compensate for the weakened joint's immobility.[13]

Traumatic injury to cartilage caused by sports, accidents, or any other means can initiate the development of OA. The injury site may remain slightly sensitive and then develop OA many years later. Trauma has been associated with the onset of OA in young individuals, especially those who participate in contact sports. Rapid compres-

Arthritis: The Breaking Down of Cartilage

The kinds, symptoms, and causes of arthritis are numerous and almost too varied to be grouped under one term. But the commonality of the various arthritic diseases is the erosion of cartilage (the elastic buffer protecting bones). Under healthy conditions, old or damaged cartilage is replaced by new cartilage constructed by chondrocytes, a specialized cell.

Chondrocytes make the constituent parts of cartilage, collagen and proteoglycans. The quality or type of cartilage replaced is a function of the raw materials—vitamins, minerals, proteins, amino acids, and GAGs (glycosaminoglycans)—available to the chondrocytes and the stresses being placed on the joints. This stress can be physical, toxic, immunological, emotional, or any other type that produces biochemical inflammants and free radicals that attack joints.

Collagen is the structural protein of cartilage and forms the "scaffolding" of the body, a major part of bone, skin, ligaments, tendons, and all tissues and organs giving us shape and form. It has elastic band-like qualities and is strong and resilient. When the molecular components of collagen are changed—due to the aging process, increased free-radical production, or poor nutrition—the collagen protein becomes less structured and begins to sag. The structure of the collagen molecule, normally a triple-helix shape, begins to unwind. This is when we begin to wrinkle. As the degeneration of collagen progresses, the molecular bonds that create strong connective tissue begin to weaken and dissolve, a process that can lead to arthritis.

Proteoglycans are attached to and cover the framework of collagen fibers. Proteoglycans have the consistency of gelatin and tend to swell up and absorb water like a sponge. They fill in the gaps between collagen molecules. Under a

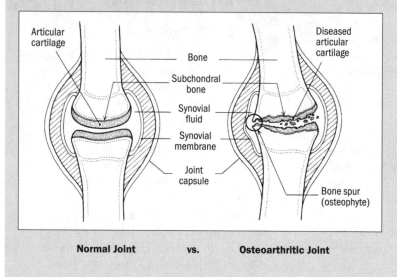

Articular cartilage
Diseased articular cartilage
Bone
Subchondral bone
Synovial fluid
Synovial membrane
Joint capsule
Bone spur (osteophyte)

Normal Joint　　vs.　　**Osteoarthritic Joint**

microscope, they look like a long-handled brush used to clean bottles: their long protein core resembles the handle of the bottle brush and the chains of sugar that radiate out from the core resemble the bristles of the brush.

Proteoglycans maintain the content and direct the flow of fluids circulating throughout the cartilage as well as in the joints.[14] The sulfur found in proteogly-cans has a negative charge, so that, like a magnet, sulfur attracts water molecules to the cartilage, giving the cartilage a cushion to protect the ends of the bones from premature wearing. But the bonds between water and cartilage tend to be weak and easily broken by stress or shock. When these bonds are broken, the water (and cushioning) flows out of the cartilage.

sion and excessive torque can tear or damage cartilage or bone, leaving a weakened area that may later develop into arthritis. Ligaments, tendons, and muscles that are damaged can cause either hyper- or hypomobility of the joints. Repetitive impact loading is a specific type of trauma we often see in major league baseball pitchers. We also see it in other occupations involving repetitive motion, like carpenters or jackhammer operators. Repetitive motion causes an accumulation of microtraumas and subsequent calcifications that, over a long span of time, can contribute to OA.

Rheumatoid Arthritis

Rheumatoid arthritis (RA) is an inflammatory disease in which the body's immune system attacks its own healthy tissues. This is called an autoimmune response. The disorder affects many organs throughout the body, but is most noted for its significant disability, deformity, and inflammation of the joints and other structures comprised of connective tissue (supports and binds together other tissues and forms ligaments and tendons). RA can lead to crippling.

Symptoms of Rheumatoid Arthritis

The onset of RA symptoms can be slow with mild discomfort in the joints, morning stiffness, low-grade fevers systemically or in the affected joints, and a gradual increase of symptoms. People can also develop rheumatoid arthritis seemingly overnight. The onset of symptoms can be so rapid and debilitating that one day a patient of ours went bike riding and the next day she could not get out of bed because the inflammation and pain in her joints were so severe. We have found that rheumatoid arthritis sets in more

For **detailed treatment protocols for each type of arthritis**, see Appendix, pp. 340-358.

Rheumatoid arthritis is an inflammatory disease in which the body's immune system attacks its own healthy tissues. This is called an autoimmune response. The disorder affects many organs throughout the body, but is most noted for its significant disability, deformity, and inflammation of the joints.

quickly if there are multiple causative factors, such as infections, nutritional deficiencies, and heavy metal toxicity.

In the early stages of the disease, the synovial membrane (which secretes synovial fluid, the lubricant in joints) swells and begins to grow rapidly (it can increase over 100-fold in weight).[15] As a result, the entire joint swells and at times can feel inflamed; this is called "feverish" joints. RA may sometimes affect only one side of the body, but typically it is found in both sides. It is common for RA to strike the same joints on both sides of the body simultaneously—in the elbows, for instance. Other symptoms include chronic aches, stiffness, loss of appetite and weight loss, muscle weakness, fatigue, fever, and depression.

Later in the development of the disease, the affected joints become thicker and deformed. The deformity usually comes from contraction of the muscles and tendons that causes them to deviate from their normal shape and pattern. Joint linings become inflamed and in that chronic state they thicken and eventually infiltrate cartilage and other local connective tissue (ligaments and tendons). For reasons yet unknown, the synovial cells in patients with rheumatoid arthritis become altered in such a way that they begin to produce large amounts of destructive enzymes, which contribute to the destruction of healthy tissues and leads to joint fusion.

Underlying Causes of Inflammation in Rheumatoid Arthritis

In various combinations and severity, food allergies, nutritional deficiencies, toxicity, intestinal permeability, and microorganisms cause inflammation in the body. For someone who has rheumatoid arthritis, inflammation (the immune system's attack on foreign substances) amplifies and becomes the more destructive autoimmune response, in which the immune system begins to attack healthy tissues.

See Chapter 6: Eradicating Bacteria and Yeast, pp. 130-151, for more information about **diagnosing and eradicating bacterial infections**.

Viruses and Bacteria—Many symptoms of viral diseases are almost identical to rheumatoid arthritis. Mumps, viral hepatitis, rubella, and viral-like organisms such as mycoplasmas are capable of creating an arthritis-like syndrome. In addition,

Symptomatic Differences Between Osteoarthritis and Rheumatoid Arthritis

OSTEOARTHRITIS	RHEUMATOID ARTHRITIS
Usually affects the elderly	Can affect anyone, even children
Metabolic deficiencies or traumatic injuries are attributable origins	Unproven origin, but infections, particularly bacterial, have been indicated in many cases
Gradual onset of symptoms with mild pain and swelling; mild heat and redness in affected joints	Rapid onset with moderate to extreme pain and swelling; moderate to extreme heat and redness in affected joints
Stiffness from joint damage	Stiffness from swelling
Increased bone density	Loss of bone density

Source: Robert Bingham, M.D. *Fight Back Against Arthritis* (Desert Hot Springs, CA: Desert Arthritis Medical Clinic, 1994).

there are cases of direct viral infection of the joints. Mounting evidence points more convincingly to the role of bacterial infections in RA's autoimmune response. Bacteria, such as *Streptococcus*, *Gonococcus*, *Pneumococcus*, *Propiobacterium*, *Salmonella*, *Staphylococcus*, and *Burgdorferi* (the spirochete that has been implicated in Lyme disease), can cause illnesses which are similar to rheumatoid arthritis.

Intestinal Permeability—Many scientific studies have documented that there is increased permeability in the walls of the intestines in over 90% of patients with autoimmune disease and arthritis.[16] Due to the use of alcohol, drugs, NSAIDs (nonsteroidal, anti-inflammatory drugs), imbalance of intestinal microorganisms, allergens, and lectins (SEE QUICK DEFINITION), the intestinal lining becomes inflamed. During inflammation, chemicals are released that actually dissolve the barrier-like membrane of the intestines, allowing undigested proteins and intestinal microorganisms to enter the general blood circulation. Here, they trigger more inflammation throughout the body.

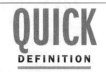

QUICK DEFINITION

Lectins are protein fragments of incompletely digested foods that bind with specific sugars on the surface of all cells of the body. They tend to stick like Velcro® to the lining of the gastrointestinal tract, where they irritate the tissues and can destroy cell membranes. Most dietary lectins come from the indigestible fractions of plant products, often deriving from beans, grains, soy and wheat. Lectins can lead to food allergy and toxic reactions at the mucosal membranes in the intestines. In particular, soybean and wheat lectins can produce an increase in permeability in the cells they bind to, often leading to cell death. Further, lectins can cause the intestinal villi (the finger-like projections that afford the intestines its absorptive surface area) to atrophy.

Food Allergies—Studies conducted by rheumatologists document the positive effect of removing food allergens from the diet of arthritis patients.[17] The top foods that are known to trigger rheumatoid symptoms include milk, yeast (both brewer's and baker's), wheat, nightshade vegetables (tomatoes, eggplant, peppers, and potatoes), corn, and eggs. We have found that patients who eliminate these foods for three weeks (without other supportive treatments) and then reintroduce them one at a time will often develop their arthritis symptoms again, although they may have improved during the elimination period.

Fatty Acid Imbalance—Under healthy conditions, the chemical agents that cause inflammation in the body are balanced in precise ratio with agents that suppress inflammation. In arthritis and autoimmune ailments, however, this ratio abnormally favors pro-inflammatory substances and results in too much inflammation. This imbalance is partially caused by diet: the raw ingredients needed to manufacture inflammatory chemicals are typically derived from different types of fats. Prostaglandins, for example, are hormone-like substances involved in both causing and controlling inflammation. When the diet is rich in essential fatty acids (EFAs—SEE QUICK DEFINITION), especially omega-3 oils, prostaglandins that stop inflammation are manufactured in the body. Eating large servings of commercial meat products on a regular basis introduces chemicals (known as arachidonic acids) that are converted by the body into inflammation-causing prostaglandins and leukotrienes.

Patients with rheumatoid arthritis and other rheumatoid diseases have high levels of arachidonic acid in their tissues. A special enzyme converts arachidonic acid into prostaglandins that worsen swelling and sensitize tissues to painful stimuli. Elevated concentrations of pro-inflammatory prostaglandins have been found in fluids and tissue samples taken from people with arthritis, especially rheumatoid arthritis.

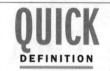

DEFINITION

The two principal types of **essential fatty acids** are omega-3 and omega-6 oils. The primary omega-3 oil is alpha-linolenic acid (ALA), found in flaxseed and canola oils, as well as pumpkin, walnuts, and soybeans. Fish oils, such as salmon, cod, and mackerel, contain the other important omega-3 oils, DHA (docosahexaenoic acid) and EPA (eicosapentaenoic acid). Linoleic acid is the main omega-6 oil and is found in most vegetable oils, including safflower, corn, peanut, and sesame. The most therapeutic form of omega-6 oil is gamma-linolenic acid (GLA), found in evening primrose, black currant, and borage oils. Once in the body, omega-3 and omega-6 are converted to prostaglandins, hormone-like substances that regulate many metabolic functions, particularly inflammatory processes.

Other Causes—The work of clinical ecologist William Rea, M.D., director of the Environmental Health Center in Dallas, Texas, has demonstrated that chronic exposure to certain chemicals, such as formaldehyde and benzene, can elicit symptoms similar to those of rheumatoid arthritis. Low levels of antioxidants have been found in rheumatoid arthritis patients; without the protection of antioxidants, the body is more susceptible to damage from free radicals. Free radicals have been implicated in the destruction of tissue in rheumatoid arthritis. Many free radicals are produced by the body during an inflammatory response. Normally antioxidants are released by surrounding cells to quench the effects of free radicals, but the chronic inflammation that many rheumatoid arthritis patients suffer quickly consumes their stores of antioxidants, leaving surrounding tissue vulnerable to attack.[18]

Causes of the Autoimmune Response

The underlying causes addressed above work in various combinations to trigger inflammation, which is a normal ocurrence in the body. It helps mend damaged cells, remove toxins, and attack invading microorganisms. During a normal inflammatory response, pro inflammatory agents (leukotrienes and prostaglandins) dilate blood vessels, which facilitates the transportation of white blood cells to the injury. Increased blood flow to an area is what causes swelling, redness, and heat. The second wave of pro-inflammatories (or chemotactic factors) are released to activate white blood cells so they can begin digesting immune complexes and damaged cells, and attacking pathogens. White blood cells destroy pathogens through oxidizing chemicals that can also affect surrounding cells.[19] As the disease-causing agents are destroyed and their cell fragments removed, the pro-inflammatory chemicals are soon suppressed by anti-inflammatory chemicals (secreted by neighboring cells). The inflammatory response subsides: the production of antibodies ceases, blood vessels return to normal size, and the repair process begins to mend damaged tissues.

But in patients with rheumatoid arthritis and other types of autoimmune disorders, this return to normalcy never occurs. The immune system resists attempts to suppress itself and begins to produce antibodies that attack the body's own cells, called autoantibodies ("against self"). The destruction of healthy cells can trigger a further autoimmune response. When cell membranes are torn apart, the cell's internal components leak out. Since the immune system is only familiar with the body's outer cell membranes, these internal components are viewed as foreign bodies and attacked.

We have already explored the causes of inflammation—intestinal permeability, viral or bacterial infections, toxicity—involved in rheumatoid arthritis. But these factors do not explain why the immune system seemingly loses control and begins to attack the body's normal cells. Below are several theories that account for the immune system's chaotic and aggressive behavior.

Cell Wall Deficient Bacteria—The observation of live blood samples has identified an evolutionary trick of ordinary bacteria: they can change the shape of their cell wall to escape detection by the immune system. Known as "stealth pathogens" by microbiologists, these masked bacteria can then gain access to sensitive tissues and organs where the immune system has difficulty differentiating healthy cells from the disguised bacteria.

The cell wall or membrane, composed of fats and proteins, regulates the passage of materials into and out of the cell. Stealth pathogens do not have cell walls, which enables them to assume the "identity" of the surrounding cells. "These organisms are clandestine, almost unrecognizable, and omnipresent," says Lida Holmes Mattman, Ph.D., professor emeritus in biology at Wayne State University. Dr. Mattman explains that these types of bacteria can exchange DNA with other cells, change shape, and increase their own growth rate. They can work their way into "all aspects of microbe participation in life" and create a myriad of new forms so that the body's immune system cannot recognize and efficiently eliminate them.

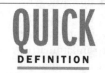

In the case of rheumatoid arthritis, Philip Hoekstra, Ph.D., a student of Dr. Mattman's and director of ThermaScan, Inc., a blood-imaging and specialty diagnostic company in Huntington Woods, Michigan, has found that virtually all the patients he has studied have had significant amounts of a bacteria called *Propioni bacterium acnes*, a common bacteria that is in an altered state—its cell wall is missing and it can "hide" from the immune system. In our practice, we have observed what Dr. Hoekstra has described. After years of performing darkfield (SEE QUICK DEFINITION) microscopic analysis on patients with arthritis, we have documented the presence of several microorganisms that appear as a cross between bacilli, cocci, spirochetal, and fungal forms.

Dr. Mattman proved the causal relationship between *P. acnes* and rheumatoid arthritis in laboratory tests. She extracted bacteria from the synovial fluid of arthritis patients and injected it into chicken embryos. The chicks, soon after hatching, began exhibiting symptoms of rheumatoid arthritis. When she treated the chicks with antibiotics known to disable *P. acnes*, the disease disappeared. The *P. acnes* bacteria is passed from mother to fetus during pregnancy and this may be responsible for the occurrence of rheumatoid arthritis in multiple generations. The prevalence of this bacteria in arthritis patients is not clear; however, some researchers suggest that the overuse of antibiotics may be a factor in encouraging its growth and increasing the number of new forms.[20]

To contact **Philip Hoekstra, Ph.D.**: Therma-Scan, Inc., 26711 Woodward Avenue, Suite 203, Huntington Woods, MI 48070; tel: 810-544-7500. Hematologic-Physiologic Research Institute, P.O. Box 1850, Royal Oak, MI 48068.

The autoimmune response is triggered when the immune system detects and attacks the camouflaged microorganisms. Nearby normal cells that are damaged during the attack, then "leak" internal cellular material that is not recognized by the immune system. As a result, the immune system initiates an attack against any cells, including the healthy cells that the pathogenic organisms mimicked. This response becomes a self-perpetuating autoimmune cycle.

Homotoxins—One of the most comprehensive theories about the cause of the autoimmune response in rheumatoid arthritis was synthesized by Dr. Hans-Heinrich Reckeweg, a German physician who founded HEEL Homeopathic Manufacturing Company in 1936. Dr. Reckeweg theorized that the connective tissue is one of the most important detoxification pathways in the body, the area where the body neutralizes toxins that were not broken down by the liver or kidneys. Reckeweg and other researchers discovered that the connective tissue had a diurnal (or daily) rhythm, similar to the ebb and flow of the ocean tides. At certain times of this 24-hour "tide," the connective tissue eliminated toxins from the body.

Beginning at 3 a.m., the acidic stage begins. Inflammation in the connective tissues increases, the lymphatic system swells, the metabolic rate increases, and body temperature rises. Dr. Reckeweg explained that this is when homotoxins (toxins that cause disease) are combusted and destroyed. Certain enzymes (such as histamine) cause the connective tissue to dissolve into a gelatinous state, which increases the pain and stiffness experienced by many arthritis sufferers in the morning. At 3 p.m., the tide reverses and the alkaloid stage becomes dominant. The connective tissue is gradually reorganized and anti-inflammatory substances begin to take control. All results of the acidic stage are slowly reversed. In our clinical studies, we have observed that patients' pain and inflammation occurs at predictable times—worsening of symptoms in the morning and improvement in the evening—coinciding with Dr. Reckeweg's theory.

Dr. Reckeweg felt that conventional medications (such as NSAIDs, cortisone, or antibiotics) inhibited the alkaloid stage, during which tissues are reconstituted after the destruction of homotoxins. Conventionally prescribed drugs trapped incompletely broken-down homotoxins inside of the tissues. Reckeweg termed these "wild peptides," which are "foreign molecules of bacterial endotoxins, chemicals, and allopathic drugs, coupled with our own tissue albumin to create an alien protein."[21] The immune system then assaults this alien protein with antibodies and aggressively hunts and destroys any similarly structured tissue in the body. An autoimmune response is now underway.

Autoimmune diseases, including arthritis, according to Dr. Reckeweg, are the body's attempt to establish a state of balance, or homeostasis. Inflammation is the outward sign of the body's attempts to re-dissolve the tissues so it can free up and remove the homotoxins that have been trapped for eventual destruction. The re-dissolving process, however, involves bathing the joint and connective tissue with powerful enzymes that act by dissolving all tissues and membranes, both healthy and diseased tissue. This process is even more damaging if antioxidant levels are low in the cells, which is often the case in arthritis patients.[22]

Theory of Defective Immunoregulation—The theories above postulate that the immune system has lost control over itself while attacking foreign substances. But this theory maintains that a faulty immune system, not invading microorganisms, produce an autoimmune response. The immune system, according to this theory, is so defective that it does not produce normal, healthy antibodies that can discriminate between cells. In addition, cells that control antibodies fail to stop the overzealous B-lymphocytes (cells that make antibodies) and the disease spirals out of control.

Rheumatoid Factor Theory—Rheumatoid factor (RF) is a specialized protein called an immunoglobulin or antibody, usually of the IgM type, that is programmed to attack IgG circulating immune complexes (CICs—SEE QUICK DEFINITION) or altered IgG molecules. When RF attacks a CIC, it perceives it as being alien to the body, even though 50% of the molecule is foreign and 50% is your own protein (the antibody). The immune system then begins to attack the body's own tissues. RF is usually present in 70% of cases of rheumatoid arthritis, and it also appears in the blood of patients with tuberculosis, parasitic infections, leukemia, or other connective tissue disorders. RF is measured through a blood test and is often, but not always, high in patients who are complaining of joint pain and stiffness. If the RF level is high, it is considered one of the factors leading to a definitive diagnosis of rheumatoid arthritis.

Gout

In gout, a buildup of uric acid (a waste product of the urine cycle) causes razor-sharp crystals to be deposited in the joint spaces between bones, rather than eliminated by the kidneys. These dagger-like crystals often find their way to the first joint of the big toe, but also attack the wrists, knees, elbows, and ankles. Heat, swelling and stiffness result. Gout usually strikes suddenly, with a rapid onset. A person once afflicted will often have recurring bouts, although it can be an isolated occurrence. Raised bumps (caused by urate crystal deposits) can often be seen on the affected joints, as well as other areas of the body, notably the ear lobes. Gout is characterized by episodes of excruciating pain, redness, inflammation, severe discomfort upon moving the joints, and intermittent fever and fatigue.

> **QUICK**
> **DEFINITION**
>
> **Circulating immune complexes (CICs)** form in the body when poor digestion results in undigested food proteins "leaking" through the intestinal wall and into the bloodstream. The immune system treats these foreign substances or antigens as invaders, causing antibodies to form and couple with them. This antigen and antibody combination is known as a CIC. In a healthy person, CICs are neutralized, but in someone with a compromised immune system, they tend to accumulate in the blood where they burden the detoxification pathways or initiate an allergic reaction. If too many CICs accumulate, the kidneys and liver cannot excrete enough of them via the urine or stool. The CICs are then stored in soft tissues, causing inflammation and bringing stress to the immune system. The overload can lead to a variety of chronic health conditions.

The main cause of gout is high levels of uric acid (hyperuricemia) in the fluids of the body (however, not everyone with elevated uric acid develops gout). This can occur due to genetic factors, biochemical abnormalities, underlying kidney disease, or poor diet. The body's fluids, including synovial fluid, become saturated with more uric acid than can be efficiently excreted through the kidneys, and uric acid crystallizes into urate crystals, which accumulate in the joints. These crystals are sharp and act like microscopic needles. We have often observed uric acid crystals floating in patients' blood samples while performing the darkfield microscope examination.

The crystals irritate the surrounding tissues and the body responds by sending in white blood cells, which flood the area and increase swelling and inflammation. Enzymes used by the white blood cells during the inflammatory response damage surrounding cartilage and cell membranes as well as the irritating uric acid crystals. Active neutrophils also release lactic acid, increasing the acidity of the fluid, which causes more crystals to form. As the white blood cells are destroyed, they release an alarm chemical that calls even more white blood cells to the area and an inflammatory cascade ensues.

Although most people initiate a gout attack through poor lifestyle choices (obesity, rich foods, alcohol), 10%-15% of gout patients have attacks due to a metabolic problem, such as a deficiency of enzymes (xanthine oxidase) that break down purines or too much purine production by the body. Purines come from certain foods, but are also normally present in the protein portion, such as DNA and RNA, of our own body cells. Purines are broken down into uric acid, which is then normally excreted through the urine. Purine content in body fluids is increased by alcohol consumption (especially beer), obesity, and foods high in purines (meat products, especially liver and other organ meats, sausages and other processed meats, anchovies, crab, shrimp, milk, eggs, and many types of beans, including soy).

Research has confirmed that alcohol increases the incidence of gout and beer stands out as the worst offender. It is interesting to note that in the 18th century, port was stored in lead-lined casks, and probably caused low-level lead poisoning. Lead accumulates in the kidneys and depletes their ability to break down toxins, including uric acid. This may partially explain the high incidence of gout among port drinkers.[23] Lead-induced gout is called Saturnine gout.[24] Medications, including aspirin and diuretics, can cause gout by putting extra stress on the kidneys; 25% of new gout cases are caused by these drugs. Kidney stones and other kidney problems are present in 90% of gout sufferers, because urate crystals also accumulate in the kidneys.

Less Prevalent Joint Diseases

There are a number of less well-known types of joint or arthritic conditions, among them ankylosing spondylitis, psoriatic arthritis, infectious arthritis, and Lyme disease.

Ankylosing Spondylitis (AS)

Most common in young men, ankylosing spondylitis is an inflammatory disease that bends or fuses spinal vertebrae; the spine, over time, stiffens. AS also inflames sacroiliac joints where the spine meets the pelvis in the lower back. Symptoms include lower back pain, chest pain when inhaling (as the disease spreads upward), weight loss, fatigue, and inflexibility. In its advanced stage, AS causes the severe stooping posture sometimes observed in elderly men, the result of a permanently bent spine. Ankylosing spondylitis patients suffer increased stiffness and pain in the back, spine, and buttocks, particularly of the low back in the morning. Chronic inflammation in this region of the body leads to the development of bone bridges (osteophytes); eventually these can take an otherwise mobile joint and "ankylose" or fuse it. AS strikes one in 1,000 people under age 40 and is most common in males between the ages of 16 and 35. The disease is found almost exclusively in men who have the HLA-B27 gene; only 20% of men with that gene, however, actually develop the illness. Researchers are now investigating whether certain infections trigger AS.

Psoriatic Arthritis (PSA)

Psoriatic arthritis occurs in one out of ten patients who have psoriasis, a skin disease that causes red, scaly patches most frequently on the knees, neck, and elbows. Golden-brown pitting in the fingernails is also a common symptom.[25] The disease usually begins ten to twenty years after the onset of psoriasis and includes swelling in many joints, but particularly in the end joints of the fingers and toes. While the disease is chronic, it is usually not disabling, except for 5% of PSA sufferers who develop hand deformities.[26]

We have also found that there are underlying factors that contribute to the onset of psoriasis. These include improper bowel and liver function as a result of an overgrowth of the yeast *Candida* or infestations of other pathogenic organisms in the microflora of the bowels. Pathogenic microflora cause increased levels of toxins to enter the bloodstream. Research has revealed that patients with psoriasis or psoriatic arthritis have very high levels of circulating endotoxins (toxic substances resulting from the bowel flora) as well as circulating immune complexes in the blood.[27] Studies have shown that the amount of essential fatty acids in the blood of patients with psoriasis and psoriatic arthritis is inadequate.[28] Researchers have also looked at the fatty acid content of the skin lesions in patients with psoriasis. They found that in these patients, there is a predominance of fats that are derived from arachidonic acid (SEE QUICK DEFINITION).[29] Copper toxicity is also a very important underlying pathologic problem in patients with psoriatic arthritis. High levels of

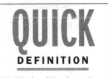

QUICK DEFINITION

Arachidonic acid is a fatty acid obtained from consumption of animal products (shellfish, meats, and dairy). In psoriasis, arachidonic acid is deposited into the cell membrane and, through the action of the enzyme lipoxygenase, is turned into inflammatory compounds, causing pain and redness.

copper decrease levels of zinc, which is important for skin health. Zinc has been found to be very low in patients with psoriasis.[30]

Infectious Arthritis

Viruses, bacteria, and fungi can cause infectious arthritis, which most often inflames the knee joint and is characterized by fever and stiffness. Conventional medicine has spent an enormous amount of time and research money searching for a particular microorganism as a cause of arthritis. As a result, many microorganisms have been linked to arthritis, but a direct causal relationship to any one species has never been established.[31] There are two basic kinds of infectious arthritis: septic arthritis, in which microorganisms directly infect the joints; and reactive arthritis, in which no microorganisms are found in the joints, but an inflammation reaction is triggered by microorganisms found elsewhere in the body. Lyme disease is another type of infectious arthritis.

In septic arthritis, the microorganisms directly invade the synovial membrane that surrounds the joint and the synovial fluid. Patients who suffer from chronic rheumatoid arthritis are more susceptible to the further complication of septic arthritis if they are taking oral corticosteroid drugs, have had cortisone injected directly into a joint, or experience a weakness in small blood vessels as is common in joints affected by RA. These weakened vessels can be more easily invaded by opportunistic microorganisms.[32] This kind of arthritis usually affects an isolated joint and is characterized by sudden onset, redness, heat, swelling, and pain.

Reactive arthritis is an immunological disorder triggered by the presence of an infection systemic to the body. Immune complexes are formed which throw the body into an autoimmune reaction. In reactive arthritis, there is no direct infestation of the joint by microorganisms, but the microbe itself or cell fragments of the microorganism are involved in triggering the immune system. Antibodies attach to the microbial substance and form circulating immune complexes, which lead to the arthritis.[33] Reactive arthritis, once initiated, may continue for years after the initial systemic infection clears up.[34] Reactive arthritis includes rheumatic fever and Reiter's syndrome, a type of arthritis that usually affects the eyes and urinary tract as well as the joints.[35]

Lyme disease was first identified in 1976 and named after the town of Old Lyme, Connecticut, where the first cases appeared. By 1991, the number of cases had increased by 200 times, affecting people in most parts of the U.S. but concentrated mainly in New York, New

Jersey, Connecticut, Pennsylvania, Mass-achusetts, and Rhode Island. Since 1982, over 180,000 cases have been reported in the U.S., with nearly 16,000 new cases in 1998 alone.[36] Lyme disease is presumed to be caused by a spirochete bacterium called *Borrelia burgdorferi* (similar to the spirochete that causes syphilis) and carried by a deer tick or black-legged tick. The incubation period can be lengthy, with initial exposure commonly ocurring during the summer and symptoms developing weeks or months later.

Lyme disease is a multi-system inflammatory disease affecting the skin in characteristic rashes at first, then spreading to the joints and nervous system later. The Lyme spirochetes have an affinity for nerve cells and, once they enter the nervous system, attack brain tissue and spinal cells. In our clinical experience, people with a long-term Lyme infection exhibit the blank expression, shuffling movement, and stiffness associated with syphilis. Symptoms are variable, including skin lesions or rashes, fatigue, flu like symptoms, sleeping difficulties, muscle pains and weakness, headache, back pain, fever, chills, nausea or vomiting, facial paralysis, enlargement of the lymph glands or spleen, irregular heartbeat, seizures, blurry vision, moodiness, memory loss, dementia, and joint pains similar to arthritis.

The Difficulty of Diagnosing Arthritis

The distinctions between different types of arthritis, at times, can become quite vague. Their symptoms often overlap and many patients can have more than one type of arthritis, according to a recent survey. Of 119 arthritis patients at the Desert Arthritis Medical Clinic in Desert Hot Springs, California, 70 had symptoms of two or more types of arthritis. The most common combinations were:

- osteoarthritis coupled with osteoporosis or less prevalent joint diseases such as bursitis or gout
- bursitis coupled with degenerative or intervertebral disc disease, infectious arthritis, gout, or osteoarthritis.

One type of arthritis can also develop into another type. For example, a patient may not recover completely from a joint infection or the infection may damage the blood supply to the joint, resulting in degenerative changes and osteoarthritis.[37] This makes it difficult to accurately diagnose the type of arthritis.

CHAPTER
3

Diagnosing Arthritis

DIAGNOSIS OF ARTHRITIS begins with a patient's visit to a health-care practitioner because of joint pain and stiffness. Both conventional and holistic practitioners will perform several types of assessments to determine if the patient has arthritis and, if so, what kind of arthritis. Most patients will not need every test listed in this chapter. Osteoarthritis, for instance, is fairly easy to diagnose from its symptoms; X rays can help diagnose the bone changes in later stages of osteoarthritis. However, a positive diagnosis of rheumatoid arthritis requires more extensive laboratory tests. Gout, infectious arthritis, and Lyme disease all have specific tests as well.

An in-depth patient history and complete physical will help the practitioner determine the possibility of a genetic propensity towards arthritis. Most doctors will draw a sample of blood for analysis according to the tests described below. Synovial fluid (transparent fluid secreted by membranes in joint cavities, bursae, and tendon sheaths) may also be drawn from joints for analysis. X rays may be taken of the painful areas of the body, but bone changes visible on X ray will only appear in more advanced stages of disease. X rays are not a useful tool in early diagnosis. MRIs (Magnetic Resonance Imaging) can be more helpful in determining actual changes in cartilage, ligaments, tendons, and other soft tissues.

Standard Laboratory Tests

For more on the **different kinds of arthritis and their symptoms and causes,** see Chapter 2: What is Arthritis?, pp. 30-51.

The different types of arthritis are often difficult to diagnose using only conventional tests. Patient symptoms and blood tests are most often used to attempt to confirm an arthritis diagnosis.

Osteoarthritis

Osteoarthritis is most often diagnosed by evaluating the patient's symptoms, which usually include pain in one or more joints combined with diminished joint mobility and grip strength. Diagnosis is confirmed by X ray. However, the degree of pain a person experiences does not always correlate to the amount of bone changes seen on X rays. A severely arthritic joint may cause no pain, while a mildly affected joint may be very stiff and painful. The X ray can reveal the degeneration of the cartilage (elastic tissue) that covers the end of the bone.

Rheumatoid Arthritis

It is difficult to reach a conclusive diagnosis of rheumatoid arthritis (RA) when the disease is in its early stages. Usually, the patient must have certain characteristic symptoms for at least six weeks to rule out the possibility of infectious arthritis (see "Symptoms of Rheumatoid Arthritis" p. 53). Tests on blood and synovial fluid may be performed to determine both the probability of rheumatoid arthritis and the extent of damage to joints and surrounding tissues that has already occurred at the time of diagnosis.

Blood Tests for Rheumatoid Arthritis—
The following blood tests assess inflammatory conditions and other indicators of rheumatoid arthritis:

Symptoms of Rheumatoid Arthritis

The diagnostic criteria for rheumatoid arthritis, as outlined by the American Rheumatism Association, requires that seven of the following symptoms be continuous for at least six weeks; failure to meet these criteria may mean that the disease is still in its early stages:

1) Morning stiffness

2) Pain on motion or tenderness in at least one joint

3) Swelling (soft tissue thickening or fluid, not bony overgrowth alone) in at least one joint

4) Swelling of at least one other joint

5) Symmetric joint swelling (simultaneous involvement of the same joint on both sides of the body)

6) Nodules over a bony prominence; nodules are small rounded lumps of a mineral or mineral aggregate that typically appear on fingers, elbows, or knees

7) X-ray changes typical of rheumatoid arthritis, including loss of bone calcium localized to the joints

8) Positive rheumatoid factor (confirmed by blood tests)

9) Synovial fluid with a high white blood cell count

10) Elevated sedimentation or C-reactive protein, a biological marker indicating inflammatory activity in the blood

■ Anemia: the number of red blood cells is lower than normal, causing diminished cellular oxygenation and slow toxin removal; 80% of RA patients are considered anemic.

- Erythrocyte Sedimentation Rate (ESR): refers to how quickly red blood cells settle to the bottom of a special tube. An elevated ESR indicates inflammation; 90% of RA patients have elevated ESR.[1]
- Rheumatoid Factor (RF): antiglobulin antibodies usually present in 70% of cases of rheumatoid arthritis, but not specific to this illness.[2] An antiglobulin antibody is a specialized IgM immune protein that works against circulating immune complexes. An attack enhances the degree of joint inflammation, thus rendering joints more susceptible to damage by other immune cells.
- Elevated C-Reactive Protein: a non-specific marker of inflammation, it refers to a protein produced in the liver which activates the immune system and increases white blood cell activity. It is often elevated in RA patients.
- Homocysteine: an amino acid and normal by-product of protein metabolism; specifically, of the amino acid methionine, which is found in red meat and milk products. In the body, methionine undergoes a two-phase conversion—first it is converted into homocysteine and then into cystationine, another amino acid. But in some individuals, the conversion stalls at the homocysteine phase and abnormally high levels of this amino acid begin to accumulate. Elevated homocysteine levels are present in many disease processes, including rheumatoid arthritis and heart disease.[3]
- Hyaluronic Acid: found in the skin and in ligaments of the joints; it acts as a sponge, retaining water and moisture within these structures. Elevated levels of hyaluronic acid mean that the joint is retaining excess water. Elevated blood levels of hyaluronic acid is actually more indicative than C-reactive protein or ESR for RA.[4]
- Anti-Nuclear Antibodies (ANAs): antibodies that attack the nucleus of one's own cells that are often present in autoimmune or "self-attack" diseases. Under the microscope, a blood sample will have a speckled pattern of ANAs if rheumatoid arthritis is present.[5]
- Genetic testing screens for specific, physical patterns on the blood cells: the presence of Human Leukocyte A (HLA)-DR4 and HLA-B27 genetic markers indicates a predisposition for RA. The absence of protective genetic alleles (alternative forms of a gene) is also possible.[6]

Synovial Fluid Biopsy—The physician draws fluid from swollen joints. If RA is present, the synovial fluid is usually thick and opaque and contains a high white blood cell count and elevated rheumatoid factor. The fluid is cultured for the presence of bacteria or other microorganisms. The synovial fluid can also be examined microscopically for the presence of parasites and bacteria.

■ Collagen Metabolism: Collagen is the fundamental component of the intracellular "glue" or connective tissue that holds the cells of the body together. The amount of collagen that has been broken down is present in the synovial fluids of patients with RA and can help determine the progression of the disease. Elevated levels may indicate a breakdown in joint structure.[7]

Gout and Other Types of Arthritis

The diagnosis of gout is based on several factors. Blood levels of uric acid will be elevated (although many people have elevated blood levels of uric acid, but don't have gout). Aspiration of fluid from the affected joint is viewed under a microscope to examine for uric acid crystals.[8] A 24-hour urine collection is often performed when treating chronic gout to determine if the patient is producing too much uric acid (over 800 mg) or not excreting enough uric acid (under 800 mg).[9]

Conventional doctors sometimes use the drug colchicine diagnostically. Since this drug is specific for gout, if the symptoms are relieved by taking colchicine, it is considered a confirmation of the diagnosis of gout. However, colchicine can be quite toxic, causing nausea, cramps, vomiting, diarrhea, hair loss, fatigue, bone marrow suppression, anemia, leukopenia, bruising, numbness, and liver damage.

From a holistic point of view, arthritis and other illnesses are an accumulation of problems that stem from layers of toxicity, malnutrition, and dysfunction.

Streptozyme titer checks for the presence of antibodies to *Streptococcus* bacteria (commonly referred to as strep), which may help to diagnose infectious arthritis. Lyme titer checks for antibodies to *Borrelia burgdorferi*, the organism that causes Lyme disease.

Alternative Medicine Diagnostic Tests

A holistic diagnostic approach to arthritis is less concerned with "diagnosis" and more interested in determining the underlying causes. We survey the body's organ systems to build a complete picture of the patient's illness. This helps us to assess the phases of the body's breakdown that precipitated the onset of arthritis. From a holistic point of view, arthritis and other illnesses are an accumulation of problems that stem from layers of toxicity, malnutrition, and dysfunction. This is why holistic doctors will investigate the functioning of a patient's digestive,

Alternative Medicine Diagnostic Tests

- Electrodermal Screening
- Digestive Function Tests
  - Comprehensive Digestive Stool Test
  - Urine Analysis
- Liver Function Tests
  - Functional Liver Detoxification Profile
- Immune System Tests
  - Darkfield Microscopic Blood Analysis
  - Herbal Crystallization Analysis
- Hormone Tests
  - Adrenal Stress Index
  - TRH Thyroid Test
- Allergy Tests
  - Applied Kinesiology
  - IgG ELISA Test
  - Blood Typing
  - Skin Testing
- Tests for Nutrient Deficiencies
  - Pantox Antioxidant Profile
  - Functional Intracellular Analysis (FIA)
  - Nutricheck USA
  - Cell Membrane Lipid Profile
  - Organic Acid Analysis
- Tests for Parasites
- Tests for Heavy Metal Toxicity
  - Hair Analysis
  - ToxMet Screen
  - EDTA Lead Versonate Test

immune, and detoxification systems. A psycho-social profile can help ascertain any mental and emotional stressors, which can contribute to the dysfunction of the endocrine glands and immune system and the resultant illness. Personality and psychological profiles can reveal the negative or unresolved emotions that may perpetuate a cycle of illness. In some cases, a patient's joint pain may be the body's attempt to resolve mental suffering.

Of course, even in holistic medicine, serious bone and tissue deformities cannot be reversed. However, the quality of life can be vastly improved with freedom from pain and increased mobility. Holistic physicians understand that pain and inflammation are due to a complex interplay of dynamic factors in the body and will use additional testing procedures to obtain a more individualized picture of the patient as well as the pathology.

Electrodermal Screening (EDS)

We use electrodermal screening to determine where to start the protocol of intervention for the arthritis patient. Since arthritis is a multifaceted illness, we cannot begin to change every aspect of the person's life at once—it would be too overwhelming. Instead, we use EDS testing to prioritize which system in the patient's body needs attention first.

By quickly pinpointing problems, EDS can indicate the degree of stress that is affecting an organ and prevent unnecessary guesswork testing. As a cross-reference, specific blood, urine, and stool analyses can then be ordered to confirm electrodermal results. For example, if

EDS indicates that a person has a specific type of parasite, a stool analysis for that parasite eliminates the trial-and-error of the process of testing for parasites. EDS can also help to select an individualized treatment protocol for each person based on their sensitivities to certain natural medicines or supplements.

In EDS, a blunt, noninvasive electric probe is placed at specific points on the patient's hands, face, or feet, corresponding to acupuncture points at the beginning or end of energy meridians. Minute electrical discharges from these points serve as information signals about the condition of the body's organs and systems. The key idea with EDS is that it is a "data acquisition process" in which the trained practitioner conducts an "interview" with the patient's organs and tissues,

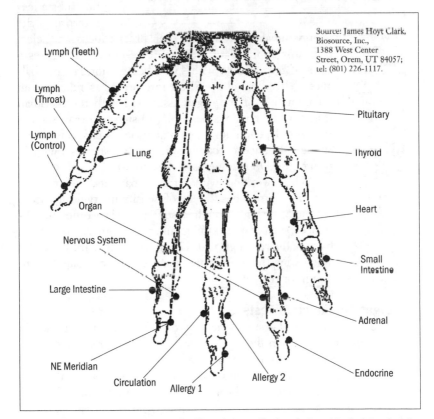

Source: James Hoyt Clark, Biosource, Inc., 1388 West Center Street, Orem, UT 84057; tel: (801) 226-1117.

Electrodermal screening probes specific points on the hands (see black dots above) to gather information about the health, function, or possible toxicity of organs and body systems. These points are part of acupuncture meridians.

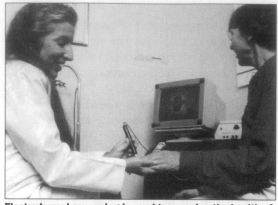

Electrodermal screening is used to examine the health of a patient.

For more on **electrodermal screening**, contact: James Hoyt Clark, Biosource Inc., 1388 West Center Street, Orem, UT 84057; tel: 801-226-1117.

For more information on **digestive imbalances and arthritis**, see Chapter 6: Eradicating Bacteria and Yeast, pp. 130-151, and Chapter 8: Alleviating Leaky Gut Syndrome, pp. 172-190.

gathering information about the basic functional status of those systems and their energy pathways. As such, EDS is an investigational, not diagnostic, device because it requires the practitioner's knowledge of acupuncture, physiology, and therapeutic substances to interpret the energy imbalances, establish their precise focus, and select the most appropriate therapeutic response. EDS uses a scale of zero to 100, with 45-55 being "normal" or "balanced." Readings above 55 are interpreted as indicating an inflammation of the organ associated with the meridian tested, while readings below 45-50 suggest organ stagnation and degeneration. The practitioner's task is to find a single substance or combination of substances that will bring the EDS reading back close to 50.

When working with arthritis patients, we measure painful joints. These areas of sensitivity typically score around 85 or higher on the test. Then we try different substances, such as glucosamine sulfate and other nutrients, to balance the reading to 50. The nutrients that are successful at lowering the reading are then used in future supplementation for the patient.

Digestive Function Tests

The health of the digestive system is of paramount importance in arthritis. Imbalances in the digestive system have far-reaching effects on the body and contribute to the development of serious illness. The development of arthritic symptoms, such as joint pain and inflammation, can often be linked to chronic digestive inflammation.[10] Chronic gastrointestinal problems (irritable bowel syndrome, gas, bloating, diarrhea, or indigestion) frequently lead to intestinal permeability, or leaky gut syndrome, in which the intestinal mucosa (lining) breaks down, allowing undigested food matter and other toxins access to the

A Primer on Digestion

Digestion begins in the mouth—if you adequately chew your food—with digestive enzymes secreted by the salivary glands. From the mouth, food travels to the stomach where more enzymes work to break down carbohydrates, fats, and proteins into their absorbable molecular components. In the stomach, food is also mixed with hydrochloric acid (HCl), which sterilizes the stomach so that bacteria can not grow. HCl also lowers the pH of the pre-digested food so that it is more acidic and can pass into the lower stomach for the next phase of digestion. Adequate HCl is required to activate pepsin, which digests protein in the lower stomach.

In the next stage of digestion, the partially digested food moves to the upper part of the small intestine. Here, enzymes (produced by the pancreas), bile, and an alkalizing substance (bicar-

bonate) mediate the activity of enzymes. Bicarbonate neutralizes the stomach acids to a more alkaline pH, which is required for this stage of digestion and activation of additional enzymes. Digestion continues in the next section of the intestine (jejunum) where sugar-digesting enzymes are secreted (if the jejunum is healthy). From the small intestine, the majority of nutrients from digested food are absorbed into the blood. The large intestine's primary function is to absorb water (about one liter a day). This is also where soluble fiber, starch, and undigested carbohydrates are acted upon by intestinal microflora to produce short-chain fatty acids, an energy source for colon cells. This undigested material is then stored until it can be excreted by the body through the anus.

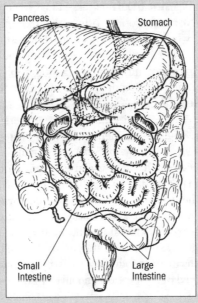

Pancreas · Stomach · Small Intestine · Large Intestine

bloodstream. Once in the bloodstream, toxins initiate a cascade effect that can ultimately weaken the immune system and put stress on the liver. Bacteria and parasites that escape through the permeable intestinal wall can gain access to vital organs and connective tissue. Synovial fluid taken from the joints of arthritis patients have shown high levels of intestinal bacteria and parasites. These pathogens play an important role in triggering the autoimmune response of rheumatoid arthritis. Malabsorption of nutrients also sets the stage for deficiencies of critical nutrients, like antioxidants, that quell joint inflammation and pain. Since digestion has many phases (see "A Primer on Digestion," p. 59), there are many abnormalities that can occur to jeopardize the process. Stool and urine samples serve as a "window" into digestive inadequacies.

Comprehensive Digestive Stool Analysis—The Great Smokies Laboratory in Asheville, North Carolina, offers the Comprehensive Digestive Stool Analysis, which consists of 18 tests. The test reviews the patient's overall gastrointestinal health by investigating the following areas:

Colonic Environment—To give a better picture of the overall colonic environment, the stool analysis measures the following indicators of dysbiosis:

■ Dysbiosis Index: intestinal dysbiosis refers to an imbalance of intestinal flora. These flora include friendly bacteria called probiotics (for example, *Lactobacillus acidophilus*) and harmful or unfriendly bacteria. At times, especially after the use of antibiotics, the balance of intestinal flora is skewed allowing "unfriendly" or pathogenic bacteria to flourish. These harmful bacteria include *Pseudomonas aeruginosa*, *Proteus vulgaris*, and *Klebsiella pneumoniae*, which are particularly important in arthritis. When the colonic environment favors unfriendly bacteria, known as a state of dysbiosis, the pathogenic bacteria begin to ferment, producing toxic by-products, which interfere with the intestinal pH, digestion and absorption, and the normal elimination cycle.

■ *Lactobacillus* and *Bifidobacteria*: friendly bacteria that are involved in vitamin synthesis, the detoxification of pro-carcinogens (substances that become carcinogenic or cancer-causing), and supporting the immune system. Deficiencies of *Lactobacillus* have been linked with a higher risk for many chronic diseases.

■ *Candida*: the intestinal tract normally contains small amounts of *Candida albicans*, a yeast-like fungus, and other species of yeast. In some cases, wide use of antibiotics, birth control pills, and a high carbohydrate diet may cause an overgrowth of *Candida*, a condition known as candidiasis. Overgrowth of *Candida albicans* and other intestinal yeast has been linked to joint inflammation, food allergies, migraines, irritable bowel syndrome, indigestion, and asthma.

■ Fecal pH: reflection of the acid/alkaline balance in the colon. The preferred range is 6.0 (mildly acidic) to 7.2 (mildly alkaline). A

The stool analysis provides information about the health of the intestines and their function, particularly the levels of friendly and pathogenic bacteria, the degree of digestive dysfunction, and how well nutrients are being aborbed.

fecal pH that is too alkaline suggests dysbiosis as pathogenic bacteria thrive in an alkaline environment.

■ Short-Chain Fatty Acids (SCFAs): elevated levels of any of the four SCFAs can indicate poor nutrient absorption in the colon or bacterial overgrowth. Decreased levels suggest lack of dietary fiber, unbalanced metabolic processes, or dysbiosis. The key factor here is the ratio among the four SCFAs, which usually remains relatively constant in healthy individuals, but can shift noticeably when metabolism becomes disordered.

■ Beta-Glucuronidase: this is an enzyme produced by various bacteria in the colon. Elevated levels may result from bacterial overgrowth and abnormal intestinal pH, too much dietary fat (especially from meat), or low levels of beneficial bacteria.

■ Macroscopic: another indicator of intestinal health is the color of the stool. Yellow to green stools may indicate diarrhea and a bowel that has been sterilized by antibiotics. Black or red may reflect bleeding in the gastrointestinal tract. Tan or gray can indicate a blockage of the common bile duct; mucus or pus can point to irritable bowel syndrome, polyps, diverticulitis, or intestinal wall inflammation; and occult (hidden) blood might result from eating too much red meat, hemorrhoids, or possibly colon cancer.

Digestive Abnormalities—Maldigestion, or incomplete digestion, is a common problem for many Americans, especially people over 60. As people grow older or due to an overgrowth of pathogenic bacteria, the production of HCl (hydrochloric acid) decreases, altering the stomach's pH and the release of digestive enzymes. Enzymes are necessary for the digestion of carbohydrates, fats, and proteins. Without enzymes, these nutrients pass through the gastrointestinal tract undigested. Improper digestion affects the body's ability to absorb nutrients (malabsorption) and gives pathogenic bowel bacteria fodder to multiply and crowd out the beneficial species. Different nutrients (fats, carbohydrates, and proteins) depend upon different digestive processes and it is common for an individual to have malabsorption of one nutrient while adequately absorbing other nutrients.

The stool analysis measures the presence of the following markers to determine how well fats, carbohydrates, proteins, and other nutrients are being digested and absorbed:

■ Triglycerides: most dietary fats are triglycerides, a term that denotes their chemical structure. During digestion, lipase, a pancreatic enzyme, breaks down triglycerides into glycerol and free fatty acids. Elevated fecal triglyceride levels indicate incomplete fat digestion and possible problems in the pancreas.

■ Chymotrypsin: relative levels of this digestive enzyme, produced in the intestines, can indicate the patient's enzyme status and activity. Decreased levels mean the pancreas is not releasing enough enzymes and/or that the stomach is low on digestive acids, which are needed to activate chymotrypsin. Elevated levels suggest a rapid transit time (the speed at which fecal matter moves through the intestines). When material moves through the intestines too quickly, the body can not adequately absorb nutrients.

■ Valerate and Iso-butyrate: valerate and iso-butyrate are short-chain fatty acids produced when intestinal bacteria ferment protein. Elevated levels indicate that the protein was not digested properly in the stomach and intestines. This can be due to many factors, including not enough time spent chewing, a diet that is too high in meat, a deficiency of hydrochloric acid, or a deficiency of pancreatic digestive enzymes.

■ Meat and Vegetable Fibers: these are crude microscopic markers for digestive function. Elevated levels may indicate inadequate chewing, stomach acid, or digestive enzymes.

■ Long-Chain Fatty Acids (LCFAs): under healthy conditions, LCFAs are absorbed directly by intestinal mucosa. Elevated levels reflect malabsorption of fats, a result of maldigestion or inflammation of the lining of the small intestine.

■ Cholesterol: cholesterol in the feces comes from either dietary fats or the breakdown of the cells lining the intestines. Generally, fecal cholesterol remains stable, despite dietary intake. Elevated fecal levels suggest malabsorption or irritation of the mucosal lining.

■ Total Fecal Fat: this represents the sum of all fats or lipids except for SCFAs, and can indicate either maldigestion or malabsorption.

To order a **Comprehensive Digestive Stool Analysis**, contact: Great Smokies Diagnostic Laboratory, 63 Zillicoa Street, Asheville, NC 28801; tel: 704-253-0621 or 800-522-4762; fax: 704-252-9303. For information about receiving a **urine analysis**, contact: Lita Lee, Ph.D., P.O. Box 516, Lowell, OR 97452; tel: 541-937-1123; fax: 541-963-1132. 21st Century Nutrition, 6421 Enterprise Lane, Madison, WI 53719; tel: 800-662-2630; fax: 608-273-8110.

Integrity of Immune System—The largest part of the immune system is located just outside of the intestinal wall. Known as the secretory IgA, these antibody proteins act as sentries against escaping food particles or other inappropriate substances. A stool analysis can determine the levels at which the secretory IgA is functioning. Low levels of fecal IgA mean an increased susceptibility to infection and food allergies, while high levels indicate normal activity or an active infectious process.

Urine Analysis—Many alternative health-care professionals rely on urine analysis to assess a patient's digestive function and enzyme status. The urinalysis provides information on what a person cannot digest, absorb, or assimilate, along with any nutritional deficiencies one might have. A urinalysis can also reveal kidney function, levels of bowel toxicity, and pH, and how the body is handling proteins, fats, carbohydrates, vitamin C, and other essential nutrients. This test is prognostic rather than diagnostic, except for the identification of substances, such as glucose, not normally found in the urine, which would indicate disease conditions (this is the focus of standard urine tests). In other words, it predicts what lies ahead if you do not clean up your diet and digestion.

An individual's total urine output over a 24-hour period must be collected, not just periodic samples. This enables a physician to see how the concentrations of various substances in the urine change over time.[11] The fluctuations are then averaged to give a complete picture of digestive problems. Looking at a 24-hour urinalysis is a way of peeking at the blood. The health of the blood takes precedence in the body and cells will sacrifice nutrients in the service of maintaining the blood's relatively narrow pH range of 7.35 to 7.45 as well as its supply of electrolytes, protein, and other nutrients. Thus, the blood takes what it needs from the cells to achieve its necessary balance, or homeostasis.

The following specific values are measured in urine analysis:

■ Volume: the total urine output, either excessive (polyuria) or minimal (oliguria), in relation to the specific gravity (see below). This indicates how well the kidneys are functioning.

■ Indican (Obermeyer test): indican comes from putrefying proteins in the large intestine, is extremely toxic, and may cause inflammation, among other symptoms. Indican levels in the urine indicate the degree of toxicity, putrefaction, gas, and fermentation in the intestines. The higher the level, the greater the intestinal toxemia or inflammation in the digestive tract.

■ Calcium phosphate: indicates the status of carbohydrate digestion; a reading of 0.5 is normal.

■ pH: this value indicates the degree of urine acidity versus alkalinity on a scale of zero to 14, with urine pH usually ranging from 4.5 to 8.0 and with 7.0 being neutral.

■ Chloride: these are salt residues in the urine and the values here give information on salt intake and assimilation. Too much or too little natural salt intake can influence inflammation in arthritis.

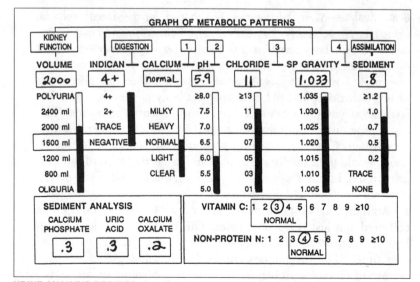

URINE ANALYSIS RESULTS. A patient's total urine output is collected over a 24-hour period, then analyzed in a laboratory for the status of key biochemical factors.

■ Specific (SP) Gravity : measures the weight of total dissolved substances in the urine against an equal amount of water, such that a normal reading of 1.020 means that the urine is 20% heavier than water. Specific gravity shows the general water content (hydration) of the body. Values can typically range from 1.005 to 1.030; a high reading indicates solute concentrations and possible kidney stress. Levels that are too low may indicate that the body is maintaining too much fluid.

■ Total Sediment Analysis: this indicates the amount of dissolved organic and mineral substances remaining in the urine after digestion; an optimal total reading for the three sediment categories is 0.5. High sediment readings may indicate the accumulation of sediment crystals in body fluids. These crystals are ultimately deposited in joint tissues, leading to pain and inflammation. The three sediment categories are calcium phosphate, uric acid, and calcium oxalate. Calcium phosphate indicates the status of carbohydrate digestion. Uric acid is a by-product of the breakdown of purines, a kind of protein, mostly excreted by the kidneys; a high reading of uric acid may indicate gout. Calcium oxalate indicates the status of fat digestion; a reading of zero signifies optimum fat digestion.

■ Vitamin C: levels of vitamin C indicate body reserves of this key nutrient; a reading of 1 is high, 2-5 is normal, and 6-10 is deficient.

Liver Function Tests

The liver is the body's main filter of blood and lymphatic fluid; it neutralizes and eliminates antigens (foreign substances that provoke an immune response), metabolic wastes, and cholesterol from the body. But exposure to toxic chemicals or abnormalities in the digestive system (such as intestinal permeability) can overburden the liver and its detoxification functions. This can lead to an increase in free-radical production and accumulation of toxins in the bloodstream, organ tissues, and connective tissues. Undischarged toxins can contribute to autoimmune reactions associated with rheumatoid arthritis.

Functional Liver Detoxification Profile—This test can identify abnormal liver function earlier than standard liver tests, which only measure levels of enzymes. Early detection of liver dysfunction can prevent irreversable damage to the liver. The liver detoxification profile tests the liver's ability to detoxify various substances. The patient swallows tablets of aspirin, acetaminophen (Tylenol®), and caffeine,

For information about the **Functional Liver Detoxification Profile**, contact: Great Smokies Diagnostic Laboratory, 63 Zillicoa Street, Asheville, NC 28801; tel: 704-253-0621 or 800-522-4762; fax: 704-252-9303.

which are common substances detoxified by the liver. Then urine and saliva samples are collected at specific time intervals and sent to the laboratory for analysis. The analysis reveals the liver's ability to detoxify the body, as well as where specific irregularities are occurring in the detoxification system. In addition, blood can be drawn and examined for the presence of free radical metabolites and antioxidants, especially glutathione, a key component in liver detoxification. This can help to guide the practitioner on the correct course of action for the individual patient.

Immune System Tests

We use two tests to assess overall immune system function, darkfield microscopy and herbal crystallization analysis.

Darkfield Microscopic Blood Analysis—Darkfield microscopy is a way of studying living whole blood cells under a specially adapted microscope that projects the dynamic image, magnified 1,400 times, onto a video screen. For arthritis patients, darkfield testing can be particularly useful for viewing the distortions of red blood cells, which can indicate fatty acid deficiencies. We also look for crystalline substances that can lead to joint pain and inflammation. Immune system analysis can be done by looking at the size, shape, and motility of the white blood cells. Allergic status can be ascertained by the activity of the basophils (the white blood cells that release histamines). Darkfield analysis is a particularly useful tool because it helps patients visualize what is happening in their blood during the disease process; it also gives them immediate feedback on their efforts to improve their health.

Herbal Crystallization Analysis—Rudolf Steiner, Ph.D., the Austrian philosopher and scientist, noticed that by looking at crystallized saliva samples, he could recognize specific states of illness and disease as well as determine which herbal and homeopathic treatments would be most useful for that patient. The Herbal Crystallization Analysis test is a simple saliva test that is analyzed under a microscope and compared with known herbal patterns. It reveals exactly which herbs the body may require and in what amounts. The result is a personalized combination of herbs that help to enhance the vitality and well-being of the individual. Botanist George Benner, inspired by Steiner's work, delineated over 800 species-specific herbal crystal patterns in the 1980s. He was surprised to find that the crystalline pattern in a person's saliva was a clue to the herbs they need. His first discovery

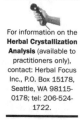

For information on the **Herbal Crystallization Analysis** (available to practitioners only), contact: Herbal Focus Inc., P.O. Box 15178, Seattle, WA 98115-0178; tel: 206-524-1722.

involved a colleague whose saliva crystallized in the pattern of juniper berries, an herb known to tonify the kidneys. Upon questioning him, Benner learned that the man had been taking diuretics until recently for weak kidneys.

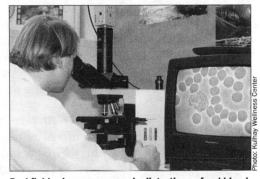

The saliva crystalline test is done in a practitioner's office and the dried saliva sample (on a slide) is mailed to the laboratory for analysis. The results

Darkfield microscopy reveals distortions of red blood cells (which indicate nutritional status), possible undesirable bacterial or fungal life forms, and blood ecology patterns indicative of health or illness.

are returned to the practitioner within two weeks. There are usually several patterns that appear on the slide, which are all evaluated for levels of importance or need. After receiving the results of the Herbal Crystallization Analysis, we prepare an herbal formula mixed in the exact proportions indicated by the test. Our patients' response to these individualized herbal mixtures is usually excellent.

Hormone Tests

Hormone imbalances are commonly associated with arthritis. The stress hormones DHEA, cortisol (SEE QUICK DEFINITION), and adrenaline are frequently implicated in the symptoms of fatigue and muscle and joint pain. These and other hormones are secreted by the adrenal glands (located above the kidneys), which play a central role in maintaining the body's energy levels. Abnormal adrenal rhythms (the cyclical release of hormones) are known to compromise tissue healing. Reduced tissue repair and increased tissue breakdown leads to muscle and joint injury, chronic pain, and arthritis. An underactive thyroid (see "The Thyroid," p. 69), a condition known as hypothyroidism, causes the adrenal glands to work overtime to compensate for the malfunctioning of the thyroid gland.

Adrenal Stress Index (ASI)—A simple, noninvasive test, ASI can pinpoint whether an imbalance in the production of hormones by the adrenals may be contributing to arthritis. The adrenal glands do not secrete their hormones at a constant level throughout the day; instead, hormones are released in a cyclical nature, the highest volume in the morn-

QUICK
DEFINITION

ing and the lowest at night, following a 24-hour cycle (circadian rhythm). Four saliva samples are taken at intervals throughout the day to plot the adrenal rhythm and determine if the main adrenal hormones (DHEA, cortisol, and adrenaline) are being secreted in proper proportion, amounts, and at the appropriate times.

TRH (Thyrotrophin-Releasing Hormone) Test—

Conventional testing often misses malfunction of the thyroid gland because the tests are not sensitive enough to identify hypothyroidism, but the TRH test will often be able to detect an inactive or underactive thyroid. The TRH test measures abnormal function levels, while standard blood tests only measure extreme pathology. Although this test is slightly cumbersome and time consuming, it is important for correctly evaluating thyroid function. This test can also be used to monitor the effectiveness of thyroid hormone supplementation.

First, through a simple blood test, the healthcare practitioner measures the patient's level of TSH (thyroid-stimulating hormone), an indicator of thyroid functioning. The practitioner then gives the patient an injection of TRH (a completely harmless synthetic hormone) that stimulates the pituitary gland to produce TSH. After 25 minutes, blood is drawn again to re-measure TSH levels. The results can determine if the thyroid gland is functioning properly. In arthritis and other degenerative diseases, the thyroid is usually underactive, even if conventional testing does not indicate it.

A simple at-home temperature test can also be used to determine thyroid function. A basal thermometer (available in most drug stores), several small disposable cups, and graph paper are the materials needed. In the morning, catch some urine in the cup and place the thermometer in the urine

For more information on the **Adrenal Stress Index**, contact: Diagnos-Tech, Inc., 6620 South 192nd Place, J-104, Kent, WA 98032; tel: 800-878-3787 or 425-251-0596; fax: 425-251-0637.

The Thyroid

The thyroid gland, the largest of the body's seven endocrine glands, is located just below the larynx in the throat. The thyroid is the body's metabolic thermostat, controlling body temperature, energy use, and, for children, the body's growth rate. It affects the operation of all body processes and organs.

Hypothyroidism is a condition of low or underactive thyroid gland function that can produce numerous symptoms. Among the 47 clinically recognized symptoms are: fatigue, depression, lethargy, weakness, weight gain, low body temperature, chills, cold extremities, general oversensitivity to cold, infertility, rheumatic pain, menstrual disorders (excessive flow, cramps), repeated infections, colds, upper respiratory infections, skin problems (eczema, psoriasis, acne, skin pallor, and dry, coarse, scaly skin), memory disturbances, concentration difficulties, paranoia, migraines, muscle aches and weakness, anemia, constipation, brittle nails, and poor vision.

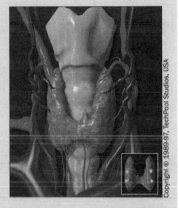

and record the temperature on the graph paper; repeat the test every day for one month. At the end of the month, calculate your average daily temperature. An average temperature of less than 97.8° F usually indicates an underactive thyroid, although it can indicate low adrenal function as well.

Allergy Tests

Unhealthy eating habits and food sensitivities (allergies) are primary factors in joint pain.[12] The "gold standard" of food allergy testing is accomplished by fasting and then challenging the body by introducing one new food at a time. Although most accurate, this method may be impractical due to time considerations. Other effective and more convenient tests for identifying allergens, or allergy-causing substances, include applied kinesiology, electrodermal screening, the IgG ELISA test, blood typing, and skin testing.

Applied Kinesiology—We use the basic techniques of applied kinesiology (SEE QUICK DEFINITION) to test for food allergies. To isolate the allergy-inducing substances, we ask our patients to provide small samples of their regular diet. While holding one food sample in their hand, we apply pressure to a specific muscle. If the muscle can resist the pressure, then the tested food does not cause allergic reactions in the patients. But if the muscle cannot withstand the applied pressure, then the tested food causes an allergic response. We continue this process until the most common foods in their diet have been tested. This technique is so easy and noninvasive that we even teach it to our patients, so they can test themselves at home. Their results aren't always precise, but it gives them a feeling of control over their food allergies.

Another method that uses kinesiology to detect food allergies is the Nambudripad Allergy Elimination Technique (NAET). Developed by Devi Nambudripad, D.C., L.Ac., R.N., Ph.D., this method also eliminates allergies by using acupuncture (or acupressure) and chiropractic. After determining the allergy-inducing substances through muscle testing, the patient again holds the offending substance while the NAET practitioner uses acupuncture or acupressure to reprogram the way the body responds to the substance, thereby removing the allergic charge.

Electrodermal Screening (EDS)—Electrodermal screening is widely used by holistic practitioners in Europe and the United States to screen for a wide range of allergens, including food and environmental substances. It determines what remedies to use to properly neutralize allergic reactions as well as monitors the success of prescribed remedies. However, it is not always accurate.

IgG ELISA Test— Most allergy tests only measure the presence of a certain antibody, IgE or immunoglobulin E (SEE QUICK DEFINITION). IgE allergies cause immediate reactions that patients can usually recognize soon after eating the offending food. However, some allergies are more difficult to identify because they result in delayed reactions, 48-72 hours after ingestion of the offending food. Delayed food allergies involve another type of antibody known as IgG. The IgG ELISA (enzyme-linked immunoabsorbent assay) test is the only commercially available test of its kind for delayed food allergies. The IgG ELISA test involves computer analysis of a blood sample for the presence of IgG antibodies in response to over 100 foods. The test can be done through the mail, as long as samples reach the lab within 72 hours after the blood is drawn. James Braly, M.D., medical director of Immuno Laboratories in Fort Lauderdale, Florida, explains, "We know that one of the fundamental causes behind food allergies is the penetration of undigested or partially digested food from the digestive tract into the bloodstream. With the IgG ELISA test, we can measure the presence of specific foods and their specific IgG antibodies in the blood to precisely determine which foods a person is allergic to."

Blood Typing—A simple blood test, also referred to as a lectin serotype test, can determine a patient's blood type (A, B, AB, or O). This is necessary information because each blood type, according to Peter D'Adamo, N.D., is allergic to certain foods. In his book *Eat Right 4 Your Type* (G.P. Putnam's Sons, 1996), Dr. D'Adamo delineates the foods that are good and bad for one's blood type. He also developed the D'Adamo Serotyping Profile, a test that determines more specific genetic information within the blood type. These results are then correlated with specific dietary lectins (SEE QUICK DEFINITION) that may aggravate a patient's symptoms.

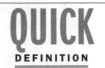

QUICK
DEFINITION

An **immunoglobulin** is one of a class of five specially designed antibody proteins produced in the spleen, bone marrow, or lymph tissue and involved in the immune system's defense response to foreign substances. The main types of immunoglobulins, grouped according to their concentration in the blood, are: IgG (805), IgA (10-15%), IgM (5-10%), IgD (less than 0.1%), and IgE (less than .001%).

Lectins are protein fragments of incompletely digested foods that bind with specific sugars on the surface of all cells of the body. They tend to stick like Velcro® to the lining of the gastrointestinal tract, where they irritate the tissues and can destroy cell membranes. Most dietary lectins come from the indigestible fractions of plant products, often deriving from beans, grains, soy and wheat. Lectins cause food allergy and toxic reactions at the mucosal membranes in the intestines. In particular, soybean and wheat lectins can produce an increase in permeability in the cells they bind to, often leading to cell death. Further, lectins can cause the intestinal villi, the finger-like projections that afford the intestines its absorptive surface area, to atrophy.

Skin Testing—There are two types of skin tests used to determine allergies to molds, dusts, pollen, and other environmental factors. The Serial Endpoint Titration (SET), also called the Lee-Miller Neutralization Test, is far more accurate than the commonly used scratch test. During a SET test, a diluted form of a potential food allergen is injected just under the skin. The body immediately reacts to the introduction of this foreign substance by forming a wheal about 4 mm (millimeters) in diameter. After ten minutes another measurement is taken. The wheal will grow according to the severity of the immune reaction. A 5-mm diameter wheal indicates no allergic reaction, while a 7-mm wheal (or larger) indicates an allergic response. If the test shows a positive result, the process is then repeated with increasingly diluted forms of the same allergen to evaluate the degree of sensitivity. After the offending foods (or environmental allergens) are determined, a formula is created specifically for the patient. Each allergic substance is combined in a vial in the exact titration needed to help neutralize the allergic effect. The patient still needs to avoid those foods to which they are highly allergic, but the "do at home" injections help rebuild the immune system and lessen the overall allergic response.

Tests for Nutrient Deficiencies

Deficiencies and imbalances in various vitamins and other nutrients are well documented in arthritis patients.[13] Specifically, arthritis patients tend to be deficient in vitamins A and E and beta carotene. In people with arthritis, imbalances also exist in fatty-acid composition, which is involved in inflammatory reactions. Deficiencies can be due to poor diet, stress, impaired digestion, environmental toxins, or a combination of these factors.

Pantox Antioxidant Profile—Using a small blood sample, this diagnostic screen measures the status of more than 20 nutritional factors as a way of determining the body's antioxidant defense system. Specifically, the screen reports on lipoproteins (cholesterol, triglycerides), fat-soluble antioxidants (vitamins A and E, carotenoids, coenzyme Q10), water-soluble antioxidants (vitamin C, uric acid, bilirubin), and iron balance. It then compares the results against a database of 7,000 healthy profiles to determine if the patient is getting the right antioxidants in the correct amounts. The Pantox Profile is displayed in bar graphs with accompanying explanatory medical text, which tells the patient the specific nutrient deficiencies, and if this poses a health risk.

Functional Intracellular Analysis (FIA)—The Functional Intracellular Analysis is a group of tests that measure the cellular function of key vitamins, minerals, antioxidants, amino acids, fatty acids, and metabolites (choline, inositol). Rather than simply measuring the levels of micronutrients in the blood (which may or may not provide useful information about actual cell metabolism), the FIA test measures how these micronutrients are actually functioning within the activities of living white blood cells. More specifically, FIA assesses the amount of cell growth for metabolically active lymphocytes, a type of white blood cell, as a way of identifying micronutrient defi-

For more information on **nutrients for arthritis relief**, see Chapter 13: Supplements for Arthritis, pp. 280-313.

ciencies that are known to interfere with growth or immune function in the cell. These tests also assess the status of carbohydrate metabolism in terms of insulin function and fructose intolerance.

Nutricheck USA—The Nutricheck USA test helps to identify specific nutrient imbalances. The patient fills out a questionnaire that includes 110 questions indicative of various nutritional deficiencies. The results are returned with a bargraph printout indicating probable nutritional deficiencies. This test is noninvasive, easy-to-use, and inexpensive. Along with other diagnostic assessments, it is an invaluable tool in putting together an accurate and appropriate nutrition and supplementation program. The questions address physical, psychological, and emotional parameters, which provide further insight.

Cell Membrane Lipid Profile—This blood test screens for adequate levels of essential fatty acids (SEE QUICK DEFINITION) by analyzing red blood cell membranes. The correct formation of cell membranes is dependent upon essential fatty acids. The test measures levels of omega-3 and omega-6 fatty acids that inhibit inflammation as well as toxic pro-inflammatory fatty acids. Correct fatty-acid content in the body is extremely important in arthritis and other inflammatory processes. Dietary supplementation to correct fatty-acid imbalances can be accurately monitored through this profile.

Organic Acid Analysis—The levels at which organic acids (intermediate compounds of metabolism) appear in the blood or urine help determine how well energy production, enzyme reactions, and other chemical operations are functioning. Organic acid analysis allows you to peer into the energy cycles of the cell (also called the Krebs cycle) and pinpoint nutritional deficiencies as well as the presence of toxic chemicals. Low or high levels of a particular organic acid suggests a deficiency in a specific amino acid, vitamin, or mineral needed to "start" its corresponding biochemical reaction. This

For information on the **Pantox Antioxidant Profile** (available only to a licensed health-care practitioner), contact: Pantox Laboratories, 4622 Sante Fe Street, San Diego, CA 92109; tel: 888-726-8698 or 619-272-3885. For the **Functional Intracellular Analysis**, contact: SpectraCell, 515 Post Oak Blvd., Suite 830, Houston, TX 77027; tel: 713-621-3101 or 800-227-5227. For **Nutricheck USA**, contact: Nutricheck USA, 11312 200th Street Fast, Graham, WA, 98338-8812; tel: 800-771-7926. For the **Cell Membrane Lipid Profile**, contact: MetaMetrix Medical Laboratory, 5000 Peachtree Blvd., Suite 110, Norcross, GA 30071; tel: 800-221-4640 or 770-446-5483; fax: 770-441-2237.

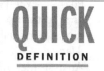

QUICK

DEFINITION

Essential fatty acids are unsaturated fats required in the diet. These fatty acids are converted into prostaglandins, hormone-like substances, that regulate inflammatory processes. Omega-3 and omega-6 oils are the two principal types of essential fatty acids. The primary omega-3 oil is alpha-linolenic acid, found in flaxseed, pumpkins, walnuts, and soybeans. Fish oils, such as salmon, cod, and mackerel, contain the other important omega-3 oils. Linoleic acid is the main omega-6 oil and is found in most vegetable oils, including safflower, corn, peanut, sesame, and borage.

information can be of assistance in developing therapeutic programs of avoidance and nutritional support.

Tests for Parasites

The presence of parasites in the body, mostly in the intestines, is a little-appreciated but major health problem, according to nutrition educator Ann Louise Gittlemen, M.S., C.N.S., of Bozeman, Montana, author of *Guess What Came to Dinner*. Many people assume that they are vulnerable to parasites only when traveling in tropical countries, but the United States has an undiagnosed parasitic epidemic. One estimate contends that 25% of New York City residents have parasites and that, by the year 2025, 50% of the world's population will have parasitic infections as well.

Parasites tend to reside in the intestines, but in various stages of their life cycle can migrate to the blood, lymph, heart, liver, and other vital organs. Parasites are a very common problem in arthritis. Infestations of some types of parasites cause symptoms strikingly similar to arthritis, such as inflammation and pain in joints and destruction of cartilage. They can destroy cells faster than they can be regenerated and, over time, they can exhaust the immune system.

According to Martin Lee, Ph.D., director of Great Smokies Diagnostic Laboratory, many doctors, hospitals, and laboratories fail to diagnose parasitic infections because they rarely allow the time for careful analysis or multiple procedures using stool specimens collected over several days. Dr. Lee suggests that if you suspect you may have an intestinal parasite, make sure your physician, hospital, or lab follows the guidelines set by the U.S. Centers for Disease Control in the *Manual of Clinical Microbiology*. The Comprehensive Digestive Stool Analysis (described above) provides useful indications of general parasitic activity, but a simple stool test is not sufficient to determine the presence of parasites. Immunofluorescent staining is another method used to detect parasites. This technique uses antibodies against parasites tagged with fluorescent dyes, which makes them highly visible under the microscope. As they attack specific parasites, the antibodies will show up only where there is a parasite presence. We often use darkfield microscopy to analyze a patient's blood sample for long tubules. The presence of such tubules typically correlates with an infestation of parasites.

Tests for Heavy Metal Toxicity

Chronic low-level exposure to a variety of toxic heavy metals (such as aluminum, lead, copper, and mercury) poses serious health dangers to the body. These toxins are commonly found in our food, water, and air, as well as auto exhaust, tobacco smoke, many of the building materials and fabrics in our work and living environment, and dental materials in our teeth (mercury fillings). Exposure to toxic materials and accumulation in the body of toxic chemicals can wreak havoc on a person's immune system function and their level of wellness. The presence of toxic chemicals, such as benzene, PCBs (polychlorinated biphenols), PBBs (polybrominated biphenols), and organic pesticide residues, among others, is highly implicated as a possible cause of arthritis.

High levels of copper, mercury, cadmium, and aluminum are found in many arthritis patients. Excess copper along with iron depletes vitamin C (which is needed to build connective tissue) and zinc (an antioxidant important for protein and cartilage synthesis); it also creates free radicals that attack and erode joint cartilage. Physical and emotional stress as well as adrenal exhaustion and thyroid imbalances have been linked to toxic levels of copper.[14]

Imbalances in important minerals (such as boron, selenium, manganese, molybdenum, zinc, and calcium) can result from heavy metal toxicity. Often the ratio of one mineral to another is even more important than the levels of the individual minerals. Sodium and potassium must exist in a strict balance in the body to ensure the proper functioning of the adrenal glands. When sodium levels are higher than potassium, the body becomes more inclined towards inflammation. Additional problems ensue when potassium levels are higher than sodium. This ratio typically indicates a degenerative condition accompanied by adrenal exhaustion due to high cortisol (an adrenal stress hormone) levels. In the first stages of arthritis, many patients exhibit high sodium to potassium levels. But as the disease progresses, and after prolonged use of conventional cortisone treatments, they will exhibit low sodium to potassium levels.[15]

Calcium may be displaced by heavy metals (such as aluminum and copper) and begin accumulating in muscles, tendons, and ligaments rather than in bones. Calcium accumulation in tissue leads to hardening of areas in the muscles and joints, which can alter the way the joint moves, leading to arthritis. Calcium can also be lost due to deficiencies of magnesium, manganese, and boron.

Testing for heavy metal toxicity can identify which metals are present and in what amount. On the basis of this information, a practitioner can develop an individualized detoxification and nutritional prescription program both to eliminate the toxic metals from the system and to restore depleted essential nutrients.

Hair Analysis—Hair trace mineral analysis allows you to measure critical mineral and toxic metal levels in the body's tissues. Hair is a soft tissue of the body; testing the hair is obtaining the equivalent of a soft-tissue biopsy, without any surgery. Although hair is technically dead, the minerals present in the hair cell during its formation are locked within the hair structure. Minerals as well as toxic metals in the hair are in higher concentration than in the blood, making these elements easier to measure through hair analysis.

Hair analysis is an average reading over a several-month period; it gives a larger picture over time of the body's metabolic changes. A one-gram sample of hair (hair cannot be dyed, permed, bleached, or treated; pubic hair can be substituted) is cut and sent to the laboratory by the health practitioner. The laboratory then burns the hair and the elements are viewed and quantified via atomic spectroscopy. The results are then returned to the practitioner for interpretation. Hair analysis and its diagnostic value were once considered controversial, but due to stricter standards within the industry and better handling of samples, accuracy and reliability are now excellent. The U.S. Environmental Protection Agency states that hair analysis is an accurate, inexpensive screening tool for heavy metal toxicity.

ToxMet Screen—The ToxMet Screen is an inexpensive but detailed analysis of the levels of specific heavy metals in the body, based on a urine sample. Levels of four highly toxic metals—arsenic, cadmium, lead, and mercury—are tested, as well as ten potentially toxic elements, such as aluminum, bismuth, boron, nickel, and strontium. Finally, information is gathered on the levels of 14 essential metals and minerals, such as copper, calcium, chromium, molybdenum, selenium, and vanadium. When test results exceed limits believed to be safe, the report indicates a "high" concentration.

EDTA Lead Versonate 24-Hour Urine Collection Test—This test must be administered by a physician. EDTA (ethylene-diamine-tetra-acetic acid), a chemical that chelates or binds with heavy metals, is administered intravenously. EDTA pulls heavy metals out of the patient's

For more on **hair analysis**, contact: Analytical Research Labs, Inc., 8650 North 22nd Avenue, P.O. Box 37964, Phoenix, AZ 85069-7964. 602-995-1580. For the **ToxMet Screen** and **Organic Acid tests**, contact: MetaMetrix Medical Laboratory, 5000 Peachtree Blvd., Suite 110, Norcross, GA 30071; tel: 800-221-4640 or 770-446-5483; fax: 770-441-2237. To find a **physician in your area who can perform the EDTA Lead Versonate 24-Hour Urine Collection**, contact: American College for Advancement in Medicine, 23121 Verdugo Drive, Suite 204, Laguna Hills, CA 92653; tel: 800-532-3688 or 714-583-7666.

system. The patient's urine is then collected over a 24-hour period and analyzed by the laboratory for proportions of heavy metals present in the urine.

CHAPTER

4

General Detoxification

ARTHRITIS IS NOT CAUSED by a single factor. More often it results from a gradual degeneration of internal organs and tissues that is brought about by a variety of stressors and imbalances, including environmental and dietary pollutants. Toxic chemicals that accumulate in the body contribute significantly to this problem. These toxins can impair or effectively shut down the organs and related systems (intestines, liver, lymphatic system, and skin) involved in neutralizing harmful substances. When these organs are overloaded and working improperly, the toxins they normally process are not fully eliminated from the body. Referred to as undischarged toxicity, this residue can cause damage directly related to arthritis, such as joint degeneration and inflammation. Undischarged toxicity may, in fact, be the prime factor contributing to arthritis in many men and women.

Alternative medicine offers ways to begin "cleaning house" through safe and effective methods of detoxification. Detoxification flushes out toxins circulating in the bloodstream, embedded in soft tissues, and clogging important organs, so that healing and wellness can flourish. Detoxification therapies can target the body in general or specific organs (covered in the next chapter). Our most effective general detoxification program includes physician-supervised fasts: we have seen patients make remarkable improvements in reversing all types of arthritis due to an individualized fasting program. Fasting and similar therapies cleanse the body of detrimental substances, heal the gastrointestinal tract, put an end to allergies, and help quell excessive inflammation.

In This Chapter

- Success Story: Detoxifying Relieves Painful Hips
- The Toxic Load
- Sources of Toxins
- Basic Detoxification Strategies
- Therapies for General Detoxification

Success Story: Detoxifying Relieves Painful Hips

Maggie, 48, complained of pain in both of her hips. Her orthopedic physician had diagnosed her with osteoarthritis, told her to stop exercising, and placed her on anti-inflammatory medications. He also said there was no other treatment for osteoarthritis and that Maggie could expect her condition to progressively grow worse. Maggie, not willing to accept this, came to us looking for another option.

In our initial exam, we found that, in addition to osteoarthritis, Maggie had chemical sensitivities, seasonal allergies, and occasional PMS (pre-menstrual syndrome) symptoms. An examination of her blood using a darkfield microscope (SEE QUICK DEFINITION) revealed a high level of spicules, which can indicate liver dysfunction, and elevated levels of red and yellow crystals, which correlate to joint pain. Her white blood cells were overactive, something often seen in autoimmune conditions (when the immune system attacks the body's own tissues). We also saw increased numbers of basophils, an immune cell associated with allergic reactions, and eosinophils, which may indicate a parasite infestation. In addition, she had an elevated level of *Candida* yeast.

A blood test, which showed elevated levels of anti-*Candida* antibodies, confirmed the yeast infection. Maggie's blood test revealed several other factors that were contributing to her arthritis. We found low magnesium and high protein levels as well as a slightly elevated cholesterol count at 220 (normal is 135-200) and triglycerides. These results indicated that Maggie's diet would need to be improved dramatically. An organic, mostly vegetarian diet high in omega-3 oils would decrease cholesterol and triglycerides and give the body higher levels of minerals, such as magnesium, needed to help reverse the arthritis. Elevated levels of

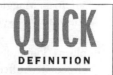

DEFINITION

Darkfield microscopy is a way of studying living whole blood cells under a specially adapted microscope that projects the dynamic image, magnified 1,400 times, onto a video screen. The skilled physician can detect early signs of illness in the form of microorganisms in the blood known to produce disease. Relevant technical features in the blood include color, variously shaped components (such as spicules, long tubules, and roulаux), and the size of certain immune cells. The amount of time the blood cell stays viable and alive indicates the overall health of the individual. Specifically, darkfield microscopy reveals distortions of red blood cells (which indicate nutritional status), possible undesirable bacterial or fungal life forms, and blood ecology patterns indicative of health or illness.

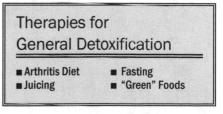

Therapies for General Detoxification

- Arthritis Diet
- Juicing
- Fasting
- "Green" Foods

Arthritis is not caused by a single factor. More often it results from a gradual degeneration of internal organs and tissues that is brought about by a variety of stressors and imbalances, including environmental and dietary pollutants.

For more information on the **24-hour urinalysis** and the **IgG ELISA food allergy tests**, see Chapter 3: Diagnosing Arthritis, pp. 52-77.

Epstein-Barr antibodies were also detected, indicating a past infection with this virus.

A 24-hour urinalysis revealed that Maggie's creatinine clearance was low at 41 (normal range is 80-110). The creatinine clearance test shows the patient's level of kidney function and this result clearly indicated that Maggie's kidneys were underfunctioning. The urinalysis also showed some heavy metal toxicity, with high levels of aluminum and copper.

A food allergy (IgG ELISA) test revealed a multitude of food sensitivities. Maggie was allergic to barley, buckwheat, rice, cabbage, carrots, cauliflower, celery, cucumber, lettuce, onion, squash, string beans, tomatoes, cantaloupe, grapefruit, oranges, peaches, pineapple, plums, kidney beans, lentils, peanuts (high sensitivity), black pepper, chocolate, coffee, and licorice.

Odd as it may sound, Maggie was actually delighted that we had run so many tests while investigating the source of her hip pain, particularly since her conventional physician had simply X-rayed her hips and put her on medications. What these tests told us was that her joint degeneration had multiple causes that needed to be addressed in treatment, including food allergies, environmental sensitivities (Maggie complained of chemical and seasonal allergies), and past or present viral infections, among other factors.

Our initial treatment was designed to detoxify her colon and large intestine. We started Maggie on a cleansing product (developed by Serafina Corsello, M.D., of New York City) called FiberMax, a combination of apple pectin, flaxseed powder, and psyllium (fiber sources for intestinal cleansing), along with herbal cleansers such as red clover, dandelion, yellowdock, burdock root, fenugreek seed, ginger, and cascara sagrada bark. We also started her on supplements of the "good" fats, including flaxseed oil and powder along with omega-3 oils (SEE QUICK DEFINITION) from both vegetable and fish oils.

Maggie also began a rotational diet to alleviate her food allergies—total avoidance of her most highly allergenic foods and eating lower-level allergenic foods only once every four days. As extra support, we also gave her C-Bioplex, a multivitamin/mineral formula along with extra vitamin E (400 IU). She also took an *acidophilus* (beneficial intestinal bacteria) supplement to help address the yeast infection. We gave her another Corsello formula, Super Garlic Glutathione, to help support her liver function (one capsule per day). Specifically to support Maggie's hip joints, we gave her Dr. Corsello's Bone Plus Formula (two capsules twice daily), containing calcium, magnesium, boron, and vitamin D, along with microcrystalline calcium (one capsule daily) and glucosamine sulfate (500 mg, three times daily).

After two weeks on this dietary and supplement program, Maggie reported that her joint pain had improved to some degree. We advised her to begin an exercise program, being careful to avoid any exercises that put direct stress on her hip joints. She began a yoga stretching and breathing program and she started swimming at her local pool once a week. She also started getting weekly physical therapy in the form of chiropractic adjustments and massage therapy. After two more weeks, she reported that her hip pain had definitely lessened.

A stool analysis (from Great Smokies Diagnostic Laboratory) revealed that Maggie had a parasite infection, including cysts of *Giardia lamblia*. The test also indicated that her liver's ability to detoxify the body was compromised. We were already addressing her liver function with glutathione supplements. To further alleviate her allergies, we started her on a special desensitization program. We prepared a vial of her allergenic substances in dilution which she was instructed to inject every other day. This is different from getting a conventional allergy shot—it is an individualized treatment to address the patient's specific allergies.

After six months, we repeated the initial tests. The darkfield tests showed reduced levels of red and yellow crystals (indicating joint pain had decreased), the movement and number of her white blood cells now appeared normal, and the visible yeast forms were greatly reduced. We began at this point to deal with her parasite infection, using homeopathic preparations as well as herbal preparations containing the anti-parasitic substances *Artemisia annua* and citrus seed extract.

After five days, Maggie called to say that both her hips were very tender to the touch and that other joints in her body were also sore. This exacerbation of symptoms is not unusual while going through

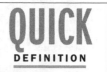

QUICK

DEFINITION

Omega-3 and omega-6 oils are the two principle types of essential fatty acids, which are unsaturated fats required in the diet. A balance of these oils in the diet is required for good health. The primary omega-3 oil is called alpha-linolenic acid (ALA) and is found in flaxseed, canola, pumpkin, walnuts, and soybeans. Fish oils, such as salmon, cod, and mackerel, contain the other important omega-3 oils, DHA (docosahexaenoic acid) and EPA (eicosapentaenoic acid). Linoleic acid is the main omega-6 oil and is found in most vegetable oils, including safflower, corn, peanut, and sesame. The most therapeutic form of omega-6 oil is gamma-linolenic acid (GLA), found in evening primrose, black currant, and borage oils. Once in the body, omega-3 and omega-6 are converted to prostaglandins, hormone-like substances that regulate many metabolic functions, particularly inflammatory processes.

For more information on **Dr. Corsello's formulas**, contact: Global Nutrition, 175 E. Main Street, Huntington, NY 11743; tel: 888-461-0949. For **homeopathic parasite formulas**, contact: HVS Labs, 3427 Exchange Avenue, Naples, FL 34104; tel: 800-521-7722 or 941-643-4636. For **herbal preparations for parasites**, contact: Metagenics, 166 Fernwood Avenue, Edison, NJ 08837; tel: 800-638-2848 or 732-417-0972.

a detoxification program. It's a sign, in fact, that the program is working and that the body is trying to rid itself of toxins. To deal with these uncomfortable symptoms, we encouraged Maggie to see a colon therapist for colonics to help speed the cleansing of her system. We also advised her to drink more vegetable juice containing yellowdock root, escarole, kale, and other bitters, along with carrots and ginger to aid in the removal of toxins.

Two weeks later, Maggie said that the exacerbation of symptoms was completely resolved. In fact, she said that her yoga stretches seemed easier now and that she could move her joints more easily than before the parasite cleanse. Recently, after a year and a half on our program, Maggie reported that all symptoms of her osteoarthritis were completely gone.

The Toxic Load

An analogy may help to exemplify the negative cumulative effects of undischarged toxicity: our body accumulates and releases toxins on a sustained basis like a barrel collecting rainwater. But as the proportion of toxins being absorbed slowly exceeds the toxins eliminated, the barrel overflows. Once that happens, internal poisons are no longer entirely eliminated from the body, but circulate throughout the system, progressively damaging organs and tissues and creating numerous acute or chronic problems, much as the overflowing rainwater may damage the foundation of a house. If the foundation of your health is damaged by toxins, it can lead to allergies, immune system breakdown, and chronic degenerative conditions such as arthritis.

While our bodies are designed to handle a certain level of toxins, our stressful lives, overly polluted environment, and poor dietary choices can overtax the system. Another useful analogy is to think of toxicity in terms of the image of a funnel: numerous dietary, environmental, and emotional poisons spill into the body through the wide mouth of the funnel, but when they get to its narrow neck—representing our body's detoxification capacity—this toxic stream becomes overwhelming. Biopsies of fat samples taken from patients with environmental poisoning and toxicity found over 300 foreign chemicals had accumulated in the body, concentrated most notably in the brain, the nervous system, and in human breast milk.[1] The result is ill health.

The Loading Theory of Toxicity

The loading theory of toxicity, according to its formulator, Serafina Corsello, M.D., director of the Corsello Centers for Nutritional Complementary Medicine in New York City and Huntington, New York, states that no single factor causes a disease. Rather, the *cumulative load* of multiple poisons creates an illness like arthritis. People don't get most diseases—they develop them, Dr. Corsello explains.

In Dr. Corsello's view, multiple stressors weigh down the immune system and eventually throw it out of balance. Among the typical stressors are toxic metals (mercury leaching from dental fillings, copper, and aluminum), petrochemical residues (pesticides and fertilizers), chemical pollutants in the water and air, electromagnetic pollution (power lines), inappropriate foods (trans-fatty acids—SEE QUICK DEFINITION—in many cooking oils and other foods), undiagnosed food allergies, nutritional deficiencies, biochemical imbalances, insufficient exercise, and emotional stress (family, job, and personal). These factors impinge on the immune system's natural vitality to resist the downhill slide into illness. Dr. Corsello explains that "these stressors may be accumulating for years, over a lifetime, before they send the system into disrepair. One injurious effect is to lower the body's threshold of resistance to illness."

No single factor causes a disease, says Serafina Corsello, M.D. Rather, the cumulative load of multiple poisons creates an illness like arthritis.

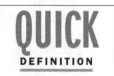

QUICK

DEFINITION

A **trans-fatty acid (TFA)** is a chemically and structurally altered hydrogenated vegetable oil (such as margarine). It is estimated that Americans consume over 600 million pounds annually of TFAs in the form of frying fats. TFAs can increase the risk of heart disease by 27% when consumed as at least 12% of the total fat intake

How Toxins Become Harmful

While our emotional and physiological systems are remarkably resilient and adaptable by nature, they need to be maintained to adequately defend against outside contamination. When we undergo prolonged psychological stress without taking measures to alleviate it or expose ourselves involuntarily to pollution, when we eat foods that lack nutritional value on a regular basis or neglect to exercise and resign ourselves to chronic constipation, we essentially invite toxins to gain an upper hand. Once inside the body, toxins may roam free, creating or worsening a variety of negative conditions that contribute to the development of acute and chronic illnesses, including arthritis.

Studies by environmental scientists and physicians indicate that pollutants play a role in the creation of all types of arthritis and

When we undergo prolonged psychological stress or expose ourselves to pollution, when we eat foods that lack nutritional value or neglect to exercise, we essentially invite toxins to gain an upper hand. Once inside the body, toxins may roam free, creating or worsening a variety of negative conditions that contribute to the development of chronic illnesses, including arthritis.

autoimmune illnesses.[2] According to William Rea, M.D., an environmental physician in Dallas, Texas, key detoxification organs, such as the intestines, liver, and the lymphatic system, become unable to fully detoxify themselves or the body. A pattern of chronic allergies may develop in which the immune system attacks its own unprocessed toxic load; this state of heightened allergic reactivity keeps the immune system on full alert and, eventually, makes it hyperactive. The constant circulation of toxins in the body taxes the immune system, which must continually strive to destroy them. Again, one common result is inflammation of joints and tissues.

The Damaging Effects of Free Radicals—Free radicals create oxidation, which is why iron turns to rust and the exposed surfaces of sliced apples turn brown. They are "free" in the sense of being unattached: molecular loose cannons that combine with oxygen in the air to initiate the process of spoilage. Internally, the same sort of deterioration occurs. Free radicals attack cell membranes, often in a matter of minutes. To counter the effects of free radicals, our bodies manufacture or rely on outside sources of antioxidants (SEE QUICK DEFINITION), whose purpose is to scavenge for free radicals, bind with them, and eliminate them before they contaminate healthy cells. Toxins, however, impede this process by creating too many free radicals, which quickly deplete the body's reserve of antioxidant nutrients.

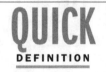

QUICK DEFINITION

An **antioxidant** (meaning "against oxidation") is a natural biochemical substance that protects living cells against harmful free radicals. They react readily with oxygen breakdown products and neutralize them before damage occurs. Numerous sources include vitamins A, C, and E, beta carotene and selenium. Herbal antioxidants, such as those found in green tea, grape seeds, and milk thistle, are the most potent.

Sources of Toxins

We are exposed to toxins every day of our lives, from chemicals and pesticide residues in the foods we eat, mercury amalgam dental fillings, biological contaminants such as pollen and parasites, and genetically altered foods, among other sources. Even our own bodies can produce toxins, called endobiotics, which can prove harmful to us if not properly controlled.

Toxins in the Environment

Toxins emanate from a variety of noxious sources, but chiefly from environmental pollution. Unavoidably, many of us carry around an internal "chemical cocktail" derived from absorbing industrial by-products (coal tar or fuel exhaust), pesticides, herbicides, household contaminants (found in cleaners, paints, plastics, and solvents), and biological contaminants (pollens, molds, dust mites, and parasites). We are also exposed to toxins from processed or genetically altered foods, alcohol or tap water (which usually contains heavy metals), and even the newspaper (from the inks used in printing).

Since the 1980s, physicians began using the term *sick building syndrome* (SBS) to refer to a host of symptoms produced by low-grade toxic environmental conditions found in living or office spaces. SBS symptoms include respiratory, eye, and skin diseases, headaches, memory loss, fatigue, lethargy, temporary weight loss, infections, irritability, and impaired balance. All of these suppress the immune system, rendering the individual susceptible to long-term chronic illness.

Office workers are exposed to toxic air that is continuously recycled throughout sealed buildings. According to William Lee Cowden, M.D., a clinical researcher in Richardson, Texas, the air inside most modern buildings is five to 100 times more toxic than the outside air.[3] Since most people in industrialized nations spend more than 90% of the time indoors, these indoor concentrations of pollutants can lead to a permanent chronic exposure to toxic factors. This hazard received national publicity when CBS's *60 Minutes* disclosed that the head office of the Environmental Protection Agency in Washington, D.C., was environmentally unsafe for its workers. In most cases, problems with a building's engineering, construction, and ventilation system are the causes. Add to this the toxic vapors and fumes produced by construction materials and bio-electromagnetic pollution, and the result is new, seemingly inexplicable illnesses that affect neurological and biochemical processes.

Xenobiotics or environmental estrogens (SEE QUICK DEFINITION) have been linked to endocrine disruption and to severe breakdown of the integrity of the digestive system, which can lead to arthritis.[4] Each year, an estimated 1,000 new synthetic chemicals enter the world market, swelling the planetary total to well over 100,000. All of these are completely foreign and potentially harmful to the function of the digestive system and endocrine glands (SEE QUICK DEFINITION). Evidence is accumulating that these chemicals, even at very low concentrations and exposures, cause "hormone havoc"—autoimmune diseases, clinical depression, and reproductive system disorders, among others.

Toxins can also enter the body in ways other than through breathing or swallowing—in particular, through the skin's pores. (Those same pores, of course, also facilitate the elimination of toxic chemicals.) Approximately 70% of the toxins from tap water enter the body through the skin; the remaining 30% of the toxins enter via ingestion. Tap water in the United States contains chlorine, aluminum, pesticides, lead, copper, and other toxic substances.[5]

Harmful Metals and Chemicals

Conventional dental amalgams or "silver" fillings are actually made of tin, copper, silver, nickel, zinc, and the toxic metal mercury. These fillings disintegrate over time, and have been shown in some instances to release these toxic metals into the body, affecting the bones, the joints, and the central nervous system and brain. Evidence now shows that mercury amalgams are the major source of mercury exposure for the general public, at rates six times higher than those found in fish and seafood.[6] Symptoms of mercury toxicity include some of the hallmarks of arthritis, such as joint aches and pains, as well as immune dysfunction. Mercury and other toxic metals increase free radicals, which attack cell membranes and initiate swelling and inflammation.

Copper-lined pipes in plumbing systems can be another source of toxicity. A greenish-brown ring around the tub, sink, or toilet can indicate that your water is contaminated with copper, which is toxic at high levels. Extremely high levels can have a destructive effect upon protein structures, such as joint cartilage. According to Paul C. Eck, Ph.D., and Larry Wilson, M.D., of the Eck Institute of Applied Nutrition and Bioenergetics in Phoenix, Arizona, many of the most prevalent metabolic dysfunctions of our time are in some way related to a copper imbalance and/or copper toxicity. Copper toxicity can cause liver problems, adrenal fatigue, allergies, and osteoarthritis.[7]

Copper in high levels also displaces calcium from the bones and into the muscles. High calcium in the muscles contributes to fibromyalgia and muscle pain syndromes as well as the formation of bone spurs or osteophytes. The synovial fluid (joint-lubricating fluid) in rheumatoid arthritis patients has been noted to have three times the normal level of copper and, in some cases, people with arthritis often have a high tissue copper level.[8] Individuals who drink unfiltered water, as well as welders, metal and construction workers, plumbers, and auto mechanics can be exposed to potentially toxic levels of copper. Other sources of copper include birth control pills and intrauterine devices, and many fungicides and pesticides—all of which contain copper as a main ingredient. A thorough analysis from a health-care practitioner, including nutritional and heavy-metal assessment, can determine whether copper detoxification or supplementation is needed.

Chemicals found in dry-cleaning fluids (trichloroethyl ene), paint solvents (toluene), municipal water supplies (phenol and chlorine), carpets and flooring (formaldehyde), and some imported produce (DDT pesticide residues) are also potentially harmful, depending on your level of susceptibility. Studies have proven that these chemicals can interfere with proper nerve and muscle function, cause skeletal and muscular changes, and alter mental functioning.[9] Often only a very small dose of these toxic agents is required to produce injurious effects, according to Dr. Rea. In a double-blind study, Dr. Rea compared ambient doses of the chemicals cited above versus a placebo inhaled by patients with rheumatoid arthritis. Dr. Rea found that minute amounts were sufficient to exacerbate arthritic symptoms and that certain chemicals, such as formaldehyde, phenol, various insecticides, chlorine, and petroleum products, can induce rheumatoid disease.[10]

See Chapter 3: Diagnosing Arthritis, pp. 52-57, for information about the following tests for determining possible mercury toxicity: **hair mineral analysis** and the **EDTA Lead Versonate 24-Hour Urine Collection Test** (checks for mercury, along with lead, cadmium, aluminum and copper).

Only in high levels is copper potentially dangerous. At its correct levels and in balance with other minerals, copper benefits the body by assisting in the repair of connective tissue. See Chapter 13: Supplements for Arthritis, pp. 280-313, for more information about **supplementing with copper.**

Inner Toxins

Environmental toxins are only one layer of the toxic load that our bodies must process. Endobiotics—toxins produced within the body—are also present and are potentially dangerous if not efficiently eliminated. Endobiotics include uric and lactic acid, homocysteine, nitric oxide, intestinal toxins, and cellular debris from dead microorganisms. These are normal by-products of metabolic processes that are typically broken down by the liver and excreted from the body. But in someone with a compromised immune system, they tend to accumulate in the blood where they burden the detoxification pathways or initiate an

QUICK
DEFINITION

allergic reaction. The immune system views these substances as a threat and sends antibodies (SEE QUICK DEFINITION) to form circulating immune complexes (SEE QUICK DEFINITION). If too many immune complexes accumulate, the kidneys cannot excrete enough of them via the urine. They are then stored in soft tissues, triggering inflammation and bringing stress to the immune system, potentially leading to arthritic conditions.

For example, arginine and ornithine (important amino acids) enter the body in the course of a normal diet, but if your system is unable to digest them, they undergo unfavorable chemical changes. Ornithine is converted by bowel bacteria into a toxic substance called putrescine, which in turn, degrades into polyamines, such as spermadine, spermine, and cadaverine (literally meaning "the essence of dead cadavers"). The endotoxins putrescine and cadaverine tend to be high in individuals with psoriasis, psoriatic arthritis, and other forms of arthritis.

Basic Detoxification Strategies

A detoxification program should be tailored to the individual's specific condition, including disease state, toxic burden, and the functional capacity of their major detoxifying organs (intestines, liver, and lymphatic system, among others). In arthritis, patients are often too toxic or too deficient in functional capacity to aggressively and rapidly attempt to rid the body of toxins (see "Testing Your Detoxification Capabilities," p. 89). The process must progress at a rate that the body can handle without causing greater injury.

During detoxification, many people experience a "healing crisis" or brief worsening of symptoms immediately followed by significant improvement. Although the healing crisis is uncomfortable, it usually indicates that toxins are being effectively removed from the body. However, a health-care professional should be alerted when symptoms worsen during detoxification to avoid complications or unintended injury. Efforts must be made to increase the production of antioxidants prior to any detoxification program to avert or diminish a healing crisis.

Testing Your Detoxification Capabilities

Determining how efficiently the body can detoxify itself is especially useful for arthritis sufferers. Here are two laboratory tests that can help.

Functional Liver Detoxification Profile—If your liver is unable to adequately detoxify your body's store of toxins and waste products, this situation may contribute significantly to the emergence and continuation of your arthritis. Excess free radicals and by-products of incomplete metabolism resulting from poor detoxification can create problems in the cells. Specifically, they can interfere with the movement of substances across the cell membrane and induce damage to the mitochondria, the cells' "energy factories." The Detoxification Profile helps to identify places where your system is impaired in its ability to detoxify. It looks at the liver's ability to convert potentially dangerous toxins into harmless substances

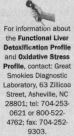

For information about the **Functional Liver Detoxification Profile** and **Oxidative Stress Profile**, contact: Great Smokies Diagnostic Laboratory, 63 Zillicoa Street, Asheville, NC 28801; tel: 704-253-0621 or 800-522-4762; fax: 704-252-9303.

that can then be eliminated by the body; this conversion process occurs in two major chemical reactions referred to as Phase I and Phase II. The Detoxification Profile determines the presence of enzymes needed to start the conversion process and the rate at which Phase I and II detoxification are operating.

Oxidative Stress Profile—When your ability to detoxify is impaired and/or you are deficient in antioxidants, free radicals run unchallenged throughout the body, damaging cells. They tend to affect the immune, endocrine, and nervous systems, damaging mitochondria, interrupting communication among cells, and depleting key nutrients and antioxidants. This is called oxidative stress. The Oxidative Stress Profile assesses the degree of free-radical damage in the body and it measures the body's levels of glutathione, an amino acid–complex central to detoxification.

Before getting started on a detoxification program, it is important to make fundamental lifestyle and dietary changes so that you do not reintroduce more toxins for your body to process. Here are some basic steps that you can take to reduce your toxic load:

Use Only Organically Raised Foods—Take this recommendation as a mandatory general guideline in your food choices. Eat foods that are grown and certified organic. They will be free of the contaminants, synthetic pesticides and herbicides, hormones, preservatives, dyes, artificial colorings, and antibiotics found in conventionally raised foods. Many health food and grocery stores offer organic produce and meat as do some farmers markets.

Maintain a Toxic Chemical-Free Household—Remove chemical contaminants and toxic household cleansers from your home, or at least limit your exposure to them. Substitute natural cleaning products, such as distilled white vinegar, baking soda, Borax, lemon juice, citrus cleaners (non-petroleum-based), Castille soaps, and safe commercial products, for the toxic ones. These products are available in many health food stores or through mail-order services provided by environmentally concerned companies.

Get the Poisons Off Your Vegetables—Since the U.S. Food and Drug Administration tests only about 1% of produce for pesticide residues, cleaning your food is the only way to ensure that you are not eating agricultural poisons. Even organic foods may have residues of potentially harmful substances. The solution to this problem may be naturally derived produce washes, now available to consumers concerned about preventing food-borne illnesses.

Breathe Clean Air—As the average late-20th-century American spends most of their time indoors, the quality of indoor air becomes crucial. Unfortunately, indoor air ranks near the top of the list of polluted environments. Toxic substances such as pollens, dust mites, mold spores, tobacco smoke residues, benzene, chloroform, chemical gases, and formaldehyde are now commonly found in tightly-sealed indoor environments.

In nature, a thunderstorm can clean up the stagnant air in a local environment by way of ionization and ozone release. Alpine Industries says it has devised a way to imitate the refreshed air quality of the thunderstorm with an indoor air purification device called Living Air®. The unit uses ozone to reduce the amount of most of the common indoor airborne pollutants. Ozone burns up many of the organic polluting materials and odors in the air. The device also uses a fan to distribute negative and positive ions. The ions (produced by a pulsating negative/positive ion field generator) help remove particulate matter from the air and create an environment that Alpine Industries says "feels like" or has a rejuvenating energy similar to the perky quality of a mountain top, ocean breeze, or waterfall.

Common houseplants can be used as filters to remove pollution from indoor air, an idea that first came out of NASA space research in the 1970s. Scientists discovered that not only could plants recycle oxygen, but they seemed to be able to remove air pollutants too.

Common plants include English ivy, spider plants, peace lily, snake plant, pothos, philodendrons, palms, mums, and ferns.

Filter Your Household Water—Tap water is a major source of the toxic chemicals that the liver is required to process. The practical solution is to get a water filter for the home and office, or at least to start using commercially purified and bottled water.

Therapies for General Detoxification

Detoxification strategies can help arthritis patients reverse the accumulation of toxins that otherwise promote the destruction of joint tissues and other degenerative conditions. Several methods of detoxification are currently available, including fasting, juicing, and specific diets. Related therapies for detoxification incorporate colon- and bowel-cleansing therapies, renal (kidney) cleansing, homeopathic remedies, bodywork, lymphatic drainage, aromatherapy, antioxidant defense support, and nutrient and herbal support to bolster the organs of detoxification. Any program of detoxification must include specific techniques for the mind to foster positive emotions, thoughts, and feelings. The mind/body connection cannot be overlooked in arthritis, because hormones released by stress directly and adversely affect the immune system.

> Detoxification strategies can help arthritis patients reverse the accumulation of toxins that otherwise promote the destruction of joint tissues and other degenerative conditions.

The first step in most detoxification protocols is a general body cleanse, including such methods as nutrient-specific diets, fasting, and juicing. These methods are the cornerstone of detoxification therapy and are critical in the successful treatment of arthritis. Avoiding solid foods and ingesting only liquids or teas allows the

---

For a **mail-order source of organic foods**, contact: Walnut Acres Organic Farms, Walnut Acres Road, Penns Creek, PA 17862; tel: 800-433-3998 or 570-837-0601. For **environmentally friendly cleaning products**, contact: Seventh Generation, One Mill Street, Box A-26, Burlington, VT 05401-1530; tel: 800-456-1191 or 802-658-3773; fax: 802-658-1771. For **natural fruit and vegetable washes**, contact: Organiclean™, 10877 Wilshire Blvd., 12th Floor, Los Angeles, CA 90024; tel: 888-VEG-WASH or 310-824-2508; website: www.organiclean.com. EarthSafe™, GrowMore, 15600 New Century Drive, Gardena, CA 90248; tel: 310-515-1700; fax: 310-527-9963. VegiWash™, Consumer Health Research, P.O. Box 1884, Bandon, OR 97411; tel: 800-282-WASH or 609-645-1110; fax: 609-645-8881; website: www.vegiwash.com. For **air filtration devices**, contact: The Fresh Air Company, 1181 North Hollywood Drive, Reedley, CA 93654; tel: 800-860-4244 or 209-638-7908; fax: 619-723-0603. Environmental Detoxification Consultants, 413 Grassy Hill Road, Woodbury, CT 06798-3129; tel/fax: 203-263-2970.

body to focus on cleansing and breaking down circulating toxins and decreasing their adverse effects.

Scandinavian researchers have documented decreased joint stiffness in patients with arthritis after a program of fasting and a follow-up vegetarian, arthritis-friendly diet.[11] Physical symptoms of inflammation and the biological indicators (SED rate and C-reactive protein) used to measure inflammation tend to decrease after a fast.[12] Other researchers have found that fasting reduces the release of pro-inflammatory immune cells, such as leukotrienes and eosinophils (a type of white blood cell commonly elevated in allergic reactions or parasitic infections).[13] These findings have profound implications for patients with arthritis, since these changes indicate more tolerant immunological activity and an overall cessation of the inflammatory response. Fasting and similar therapies are also credited with improving energy levels, reducing allergies and acne, losing weight, and sharpening mental acuity.

The Arthritis Diet

An overwhelming number of arthritis sufferers will note partial to complete relief of symptoms after a month of strict adherence to a primarily vegetarian, arthritis-friendly diet. The basis of the diet is that it eliminates refined, canned, and frozen foods, processed oils and rancid fats, alcohol, caffeine, refined sugars, animal products, and foods which tend to cause food allergies and toxic reactions. Additional foods to avoid include yeast, wheat and other high-gluten grains, cow's milk and dairy products, refined or concentrated natural sugars (even fruit juices), corn, and nightshade vegetables (tomatoes, green peppers, eggplant, and potatoes). Organic vegetables and fruits should be incorporated into a daily diet. We have found that arthritis patients suffer relapses of symptoms when they deviate from this diet. Typically we prescribe the Arthritis Diet for one month during which we carefully monitor the patient for nutritional status, inflammatory markers, and digestive function. Based on the results of these tests, the diet can be tailored to meet the individual's needs.

Fasting

For more on **stress and arthritis**, see Chapter 11: Mind/Body Approaches to Arthritis, pp. 226-249.

Each cell needs a constant supply of nourishment in the form of oxygen, proteins, glucose, amino acids, fatty acids, vitamins, minerals, and trace elements. Equally important to the cells is waste removal. Metabolic wastes are poisonous and must be carried away from the cells by the lymphatic system, the "garbage disposal" of the cells. When nutritional deficiencies, sluggish metabolism, lymphatic stagnation, and environmental and internal toxins have "choked" the cells, fasting is a necessity. True fasting is done by consuming only filtered water and/or herbal teas, with zero caloric intake. Fasting on water causes rapid release of internal and external toxins in the body, where they have been buried in the fat for long periods of time.

Incorporating vegetable or fruit juices and "green" foods into the regime is less aggressive than a true, water-only fast and is better tolerated by most people with borderline hypoglycemia (low blood sugar). For many people, fasting on water can create health problems if the body is not adequately prepared for this shock. While we feel water fasting is the best method of detoxification, especially for arthritis, it should be done only under the guidance of a health-care practitioner who has experience in supervising fasts of this type. It is our recommendation that water fasts should *always* follow a healing, nutrient-dense detoxification diet. We emphasize a wide range of antioxidants and lipotropic nutrients preceding a water fast in order to support the kidneys and other eliminative organs; toxins can reach high concentrations in the stool, lymph, blood, urine, and breath during fasting.

Preparing for the Fast

Fasting traditionally starts at the beginning of a new season (typically autumn or spring), but can be undertaken at any point during the year. For several weeks before a fast, follow the Arthritis Diet (see Chapter 12: The Arthritis Diet) and incorporate into your daily diet two glasses of "Rainbow Feather Veggie Juice," Detox Tea, and the supplements recommended below.

Rainbow Feather Veggie Juice

1 lemon, juiced	½ beet root
3-5 beet greens	1 cucumber
½" slice of ginger	1-3 carrots
2 stalks celery	½ fennel stalk
1 bunch parsley and/or cilantro	
2"-4" burdock and or yellow dock root	

Use organic vegetables only. Juice ingredients in a juicer and add one teaspoon of spirulina, chlorella, or any of the organic green food combinations available in health food stores. Dilute by 50% with filtered or purified water.

For the **full program of the arthritis-friend-ly diet**, see Chapter 12: The Arthritis Diet, pp. 250-278.

Mucus-Cleansing Diet

Mucus is naturally created by the body to trap toxins or disease-causing organisms circulating in the sinus cavity and gastrointestinal tract. Certain foods can also trigger the release of mucus and, in turn, cause a buildup that stagnates waste elimination and other processes. This diet consists of foods and beverages that are used to thin and dislodge mucus. The mucus-cleansing diet should be followed for three to five days to be effective for conditions such as obstinate sinusitis, asthma, hay fever, or other allergies. It is also very beneficial for arthritis and to prepare for a fast.

An excellent combination to start with is "The Lemonade Special," which contains a freshly juiced lemon. Lemons help loosen mucus and cleanse the liver. Make an 8-12 ounce glass of this drink in the morning and drink it throughout the day.

- Juice a whole organic lemon into a quart glass jar
- Fill the jar with filtered water
- Add 1 tsp of honey (or substitute the herb stevia, a natural sweetener)
- Add 1 pinch of powdered cayenne pepper (or a little fresh grated horseradish)

Drink this mixture, water, and an herbal tea consisting of peppermint, spearmint, fenugreek, eucalyptus, ginger, and licorice. These herbs have mucus-removing properties and can be mixed in equal proportions for a tea that should be consumed five or more times a day.

A potassium broth can also be enjoyed throughout the day. Simmer about one cup each of cut-up pieces of celery, carrots, beets, onions, garlic, parsley, kale, and parsnips (use only organically grown produce) in filtered water for 45 minutes; you can add sea salt and/or Bragg's Liquid Aminos™ (containing soybeans and filtered water). Drain and store the stock in the refrigerator; consume over the next day or two. Steamed carrots, mustard greens, onions, and garlic should be eaten throughout the day as an accompaniment. Horseradish (fresh, not pickled) can be grated on top.

Bragg's Liquid Aminos is available in most health food stores. For more information, contact: Live Food Products, Box 7, Santa Barbara, CA 93102; tel: 800-446-1990 or 805-968-1020.

⚠CAUTION

When calories are restricted, toxins embedded in fatty tissues are liberated and can be flushed out of the body. Care must be taken to decide how rapidly to mobilize the pollutants in the body. It is imperative to consult with a health-care practitioner before starting any detoxification therapy.

Detox Tea

Drink six or more cups of this tea per day one month prior to a fasting period. In a tea strainer or empty tea bag, mix together equal parts of the following herbs: dandelion, burdock, red clover, peppermint, and green tea.

Daily Supplements

Boosting your nutritional reserves with supplements is also necessary before beginning a fast. For one month prior to starting the

fast, take the following supplements:
- Multivitamin without copper: 2-3 tablets with each meal
- Multiple antioxidant: 2-3 tablets with each meal
- Lipotropic factors: three tablets, two times a day
- Joint Food (contains plant bioflavonoids and nutrients useful for connective tissue): ¼ tsp, three times a day, between meals

The Fifteen-Day Fast

It is best to ease into a fast over a three-day period. The fast itself lasts for five days. Then, we recommend a full week to slowly re-introduce healthy foods back into your diet.

Day 1: Eliminate beans and whole grains. Eat only fruits, vegetables (raw or cooked), tofu, nuts and seeds, and juices. *Always* dilute juices by 50%-75% with purified water. Drink at least eight glasses of water. Drink Detox Tea (see recipe above) and use stevia to sweeten, if desired. Take the nutritional supplements discussed above for the duration of the fast.

Day 2: Consume only raw or steamed vegetables and fruits. Eliminate tofu, nuts, and seeds. Limit portions of meals to decrease the capacity of the stomach.

Day 3: Eat only raw vegetables and fruits. Chew the food thoroughly. Discontinue the fruits.

Days 4-8: Eliminate all solid foods. Drink unlimited quantities of warm herb tea throughout the day. Consume liberal quantities of water—water will dilute and flush the lymphatic, circulatory, and urinary systems; urine must stay diluted so it does not damage the kidneys. Water should be filtered through a solid block carbon filter, or through reverse osmosis and then a solid block of carbon. Bottled water, spring water, or distilled water are not acceptable.

Take the following supplements to support the organs of detoxification and minimize any temporary worsening of symptoms (healing crisis): the antioxidants milk thistle (80% standardized of silymarin, 450 mg, three times a day) and artichoke root (5% standardized cynar-

For more information about **antioxidant products**, contact: NF Formulas (PhytoPhenols and Oxystat; for licensed professionals only), 9775 SW Commerce Circle, C-5, Wilsonville, OR 97070; tel: 800-547-4891; website: www.nfformulas.com. Iwin Labs, 2120 Smithtown Avenue, Ronkonkoma, NY 11779; tel: 800-645-5626 or 516-467-3140; fax: 516-467-3080. For **lipotropic products**, contact: Tyler Encapsulations (Lipotropic Complex; for licensed physicians only), 2204-8 NW Birdsdale, Gresham, OR 97030; tel: 800-869-9705; fax: 503-666-4913). NF Formulas (SLF Forte; for licensed physicians only), 9775 SW Commerce Circle, C-5, Wilsonville, OR 97070; tel: 800-547-4891; website: www.nfformulas.com. Prevail (Metabolic Liver Formula; for consumers), 2204-8 NW Birdsdale, Gresham, OR 97030; tel: 800-248-0885 or 503-667-5527; fax: 503-667-4790. For **Joint Food**, contact: Nature's Answer, 320 Oser Avenue, Hauppauge, NY 11788; tel: 800-439-2324 or 516-231-7492; fax: 516-231-8391.

in, 300 mg, three times a day), the amino acids SAMe (S-adenosylme-thionine, 500 mg, twice daily), NAC (N-acetyl-cysteine, 500 mg, twice daily), and glutathione (150 mg, twice daily). L-glutamine (4 g daily), an amino acid that supports the regeneration of the gastrointestinal barrier, is particularly useful during a fast.

Day 9: Take a full week to ease into your healthy diet again. On the first day of eating solids, consume only one light meal of steamed or baked vegetables, such as squash, sweet potatoes, or carrots. Eat only one type of vegetable; don't mix. Take one to three capsules per meal of digestive enzymes or bromelain (an enzyme from pineapples) tablets to help support the digestive system, which has now been inactive for an extended time period.

Day 10: The following day, the diet can be supplemented with more varieties of cooked foods and a raw salad (with a dressing of flaxseed oil, lemon juice, and sea salt) can be consumed. Look for reactions to foods as you re-introduce them into your diet. Work with a practitioner to determine the extent of your hidden food allergies and sensitivities.

Day 11-13: Re-introduce into your diet easily digestible proteins (such as organic tofu) and whole grains, such as brown rice, millet, quinoa, amaranth, and buckwheat. Avoid highly glutenous foods, such as wheat, spelt, rye, barley, and oats.

Day 14-15: Now you can return to following the Arthritis Diet. At this point, you have successfully completed the fast.

Activity During the Fast—Proper rest and energy preservation during fasting are important. Vigorous exercise is discouraged because of the increased physiological need for glucose, which will come from either fat or muscle protein if you push yourself too hard. Light aerobic exercises, such as walking, swimming, stretching, yoga, or *tai chi* are encouraged. Stress, whether physiologic or psychological, hampers your healing and even promotes toxemia through the production of stress hormones and free radicals. Focus on reducing these negative emotions through creative endeavors, such as journal writing or meditation. Good strategies to deal with potential food obsessions or excessive hunger during fasting is light exercise, sleep, or avoidance of situations where food is prominent. Avoid being around food as much as possible—have someone else prepare meals for the family if this is one of your responsibilities. We recommend taking days off from your job or normal routine during the fast.

Bathing and Bowel Detoxification While Fasting—About one-third of all body impurities are eliminated through the skin, commonly referred to as the "third kidney." The sweat and sebaceous secretions during a fast will contain higher concentrations of fat-soluble pollutants, heavy metals, and salts. Shower or bathe three times per day during the fast to prevent reabsorbing these toxins. Bathing in Epsom salts, baking soda, sea salt, diluted hydrogen peroxide, ginger root, bentonite clay, and/or burdock root help remove toxins more quickly than regular bath water. To encourage drainage of the lymphatic fluid through the skin, use a loofah sponge or soft brush on dry skin. Taking showers or baths in which the temperature of the water alternates between hot and cold aids in detoxification and flushes the lymphatic system.

The fat-soluble toxins present in the body, made up primarily of bile formed by the liver, will be flushed out through the stool. The stool of an individual fasting typically contains more toxins than normal. For this reason, it is important to avoid constipation and encourage elimination through colonics, enemas, and herbal support (see Chapter 5: Detoxifying Specific Organs, for recommendations).

For more information on **solid block carbon water filters**, contact: Environmental Detoxification Consultants, 413 Grassy Hill Road, Woodbury, CT 06798-3129; tel/fax: 203-263-2970.

For information on **detoxifying baths**, see the hydrotherapy section in Chapter 14: Exercises and Physical Therapies, pp. 314-339.

Experiences During a Fast—People report a spectrum of feelings as they proceed through a fast. Most encounter physiological and psychological withdrawal effects during days one through three and, in some cases, for longer periods. The more prepared your body is, the fewer and less intense the side effects. Transient headaches, energy fluctuations, hypoglycemia, halitosis (bad breath), increased body odor, constipation, nausea, rectal mucus discharge, acne, and a temporary aggravation of many conditions are common.

Serious side effects are very rare, especially in those who have adhered to the pre-fasting program previously outlined, and usually occur in people on long fasts, who should be under medical supervision. Symptoms can include fainting/dizziness, dangerously low blood pressure, cardiac arrhythmias, severe vomiting or diarrhea, renal problems, and gouty "attacks." As we've emphasized before, it is important to consult with a practitioner skilled in fasting before you execute this vital aspect of detoxification.

Support Therapies for Detoxification

Specific nutrients, particularly the so-called green foods, along with fresh juices can help nutritionally support the body during an intensive fast. They are also useful to promote cleansing on a daily basis.

Shorter Fasts

■ **Two-Day Fast:** For two days, drink the Rainbow Feather Juice (see recipe above), UltraBalance Protein Powder (two drinks a day), and Detox Tea.

■ **Three- to Five-Day Fast:** Follow the guidelines for the Two-Day Fast. Add to this fast the following organic vegetable soup: one head of cabbage, two carrots, one onion, two cloves of garlic, one bunch of parsley, and two stalks of celery. Cut up the vegetables into bite-size pieces and place in a soup pot with one gallon of water; simmer for one hour. Add Bragg's Liquid Aminos™ (available in most health food stores) to taste.

■ **Three- to Five-Day Mono Diet:** For those who find it difficult to complete a liquid fast, try eating only one type of non-allergenic food for several days. The proper food to consume on your mono diet can be chosen by you and your health-care professional. Good choices include pears, brown rice, apples, squash, and carrots (if hypoglycemia is not a problem). The food can be prepared raw, boiled, steamed, or baked. At least one to two quarts of filtered water and/or herb tea should be consumed daily during the mono diet. The mono diet is typically followed for 3-5 days. Break the mono diet by slowly re-introducing foods which are allowed on the Arthritis Diet.

For **UltraBalance Protein Powder**, contact: Metagenics, 166 Fernwood Avenue, Edison, NJ 08837; tel: 800-638-2848 or 732-417-0972.

Juicing

Many people attempt to fast on juice. While juice fasts have positive benefits, the carbohydrates in the juice decrease the rate of toxin removal. Juicing can, however, prepare the body for fasting and should become a part of your daily diet. Fresh juices are a simple way to meet the eight to ten daily servings of fruits and vegetables recommended by the National Cancer Society, National Cancer Institute, and the American Heart Association. Juices help repair damaged body tissues, due to their high concentration of vitamins, minerals, natural sugars, intact enzymes, and phytonutrients. They are easily digested and their nutrients are in a form that can be quickly utilized by the body.

■ Juiced watermelon with rind helps cleanse the kidneys and decrease joint pain.

■ Cherries are especially helpful for gout, due to their anti-inflammatory properties.

■ Okra and cabbage contain the amino acid glutamine, which helps repair the integrity of the intestinal lining. The intestinal lining can disintegrate and allow inflammation-provoking substances to escape into the bloodstream and body tissues.

■ Pineapple and papaya (organic and non-irradiated) contain natural plant enzymes that, when taken on an empty stomach, digest the protein layers of circulating immune complexes (antibody and antigen compounds), which also play a role in causing inflammation.

Add a little ginger to your pineapple juice for extra enzyme power and to soothe gastrointestinal irritations.

"Green" Foods

The green foods (spirulina, chlorella, blue-green algae, wheat grass, and barley grass) are popular juiced drinks available at most health food stores or they can be prepared at home. Green foods are rich in vitamins, minerals, and chlorophyll, the green pigment found in most plants. Chlorophyll has long been used as a healing agent and is well-known for its anti-aging properties. It helps heal wounds of the skin and internal membranes, stimulates the growth of new cells, and hinders the growth of bacteria. Important to detoxifying, chlorophyll also promotes regularity.

■ Blue-Green Algae (*Aphanizomenon flosaquae*)—Blue-green algae is a single-cell freshwater micro-algae plant cultivated in the upper Klamath Lake in Oregon and thrives on the high concentration of minerals in the glacier-fed lake. It is used for increasing physical and mental strength and stamina. Blue-green algae is a source of eight essential amino acids and is high in trace elements, vitamin A and carotenoid complex, and vitamin B12.

■ Chlorella (*Chlorella pyreniodosa*)— Chlorella, a freshwater single-celled green algae, is more popular than vitamin C in Japan. There are an estimated five million people taking this algae every day. Chlorella is approximately 60% protein, including all the essential amino acids, and contains high levels of carotenoids and chlorophyll, important detoxifying agents. It has very high levels of RNA and DNA, which support tissue repair and healing. An antioxidant, chlorella also helps remove heavy metals (cadmium, mercury, lead, and aluminum) and pesticides (DDT and chlordane) from the body. Chlorella

Tips for Juicing

■ Use only organic, non-irradiated fruits and vegetables.

■ If organic produce is not available in your area, wash off pesticide residues using fruit and vegetable washes.

■ Always peel away the skins of citrus fruits before juicing (except lemons and limes). Leave as much of the white layer between the peel and fruit because it contains vitamin C and bioflavonoids.

■ Remove pits, stones, and hard seeds from fruits such as cherries, plums, and mangoes.

■ Juice the stems and leaves of most produce such as beets, grapes, and apples. Remove the greens of carrots and rhubarb.

■ Fruits with a low water content, such as papaya, mango, avocado, and banana, will not juice well; they can be prepared in a blender as smoothies.[14]

absorbs toxins from the intestines, helps relieve chronic constipation, and promotes the growth of healthy intestinal flora. Japanese studies have reported that chlorella is excellent for healing the intestines and for reversing the damage of NSAIDs (nonsteroidal, anti-inflammatory drugs) on the intestinal lining.[15]

■ Spirulina—Spirulina contains eight times more protein than tofu, five times more calcium (in a more easily absorbed form) than cow's milk, and more of certain amino acids than any other vegetables. Spirulina is important in reversing adrenal and thyroid exhaustion, battling depression and mood swings, and is excellent for weight control because it acts as an appetite suppressor. It also has been shown to have anti-inflammatory properties and is the highest vegetable source of vitamin B12, a necessity for vegetarians.[16] Spirulina also chelates (binds with) heavy metals and helps remove them from the body.

■ Wheat Grass—Wheat grass is well-known for its ability to cleanse and detoxify. The variety of wheat grass grown indoors for purposes of juicing is a good source of chlorophyll and used as a purifying tonic. Dehydrated wheat grass, a common ingredient in green food supplements, is more nutritionally rich than the juicing variety. Wheat grass contains beta carotene, calcium, chlorophyll, fiber, iron, vitamins B6, B12, C, and K, folic acid, and trace minerals. Those allergic to wheat or gluten can enjoy wheat grass without any concern, as wheat grass contains no allergic gluten or gliadin.

■ Barley Grass—Barley grass, also found in most green food formulas, contains many of the same nutrients as wheat grass and helps support the growth of "friendly" intestinal bacteria in the digestive tract. Both dehydrated wheat grass and barley grass contain as much vitamin C as oranges (about 60 mg per 100 grams).[17] Vitamin C is important in the formation of collagen, the structural support of connective tissue. We recommend a mixture of these green foods, along with the cereal grasses, as an excellent nutrient-building food before a water fast or in preparation for a mono diet.

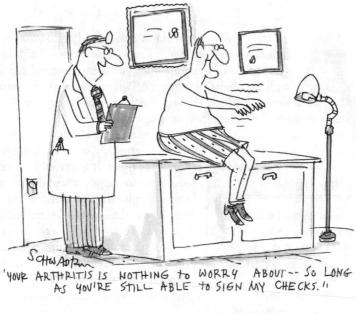

"YOUR ARTHRITIS IS NOTHING to WORRY ABOUT -- So LONG AS YOU'RE STILL ABLE to SIGN MY CHECKS."

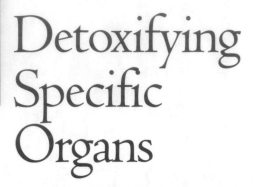

CHAPTER

5 Detoxifying Specific Organs

A S OUR ENVIRONMENT and food are increasingly saturated with pollutants and chemicals, the body's mechanisms for elimination of toxins cannot keep up with the chemical deluge. All organs involved in detoxification, which include the intestines, liver, lymphatic system, kidneys, skin, connective tissue, and respiratory system, can become overloaded. The constant circulation of toxins in the body taxes the immune system, which must continually strive to destroy or eliminate them. It is advisable to take measures to support these detoxification organs and to remove toxins stored in the body. Detoxification therapies designed for specific organs work in conjunction with fasting and the dietary recommendations for general detoxification described in the previous chapter.

In This Chapter

- The Detoxification Defense System
- Toxicity and the Intestines
- Alternative Medicine Therapies for a Toxic Colon
- The Overburdened Liver
- Liver Detoxification Therapies
- Success Story: Detoxification Heals Juvenile Rheumatoid Arthritis
- The Stagnated Lymphatic System
- Therapies for Improving Lymphatic Drainage
- Supporting the Portals: Kidneys, Skin, and Lungs

The Detoxification Defense System

The detoxification system has two lines of defense—specific organs prevent toxins from entering the body and others neutralize and excrete the poisonous compounds that get through this initial line of defense.

When functioning properly, the body's defenses protect healthy tissues and joints from damage by harmful free radicals or circulating toxins. Key components of the detoxification system include:

■ Gastrointestinal barrier, including the small and large intestines

■ Liver

■ Lymphatic system, which transports waste products from the cells to the major organs of detoxification

■ Kidneys, bladder, and other components of the urinary system

■ Skin, including the sweat and sebaceous glands

■ Lungs

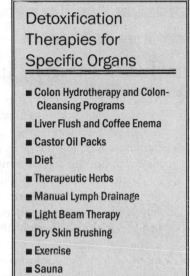

Detoxification Therapies for Specific Organs

■ Colon Hydrotherapy and Colon-Cleansing Programs
■ Liver Flush and Coffee Enema
■ Castor Oil Packs
■ Diet
■ Therapeutic Herbs
■ Manual Lymph Drainage
■ Light Beam Therapy
■ Dry Skin Brushing
■ Exercise
■ Sauna

The gastrointestinal system is typically the first line of defense against toxins and, when compromised, the first place to harbor seeds of disease. Within the 25 feet of the intestinal lining are many hiding places for disease-causing agents, which then break through the intestinal membrane and gain access to the bloodstream. This is one facet of how arthritis begins—once the bowel is toxic, the entire body soon follows. Undigested food materials, bacteria, and other substances usually confined to the intestines escape into the bloodstream, setting off the immune system and inflammation ensues. If the intestines are letting toxins through, then the liver, lymph, kidneys, skin, and other organs involved in detoxification become overwhelmed.

The liver bears most of the burden for eliminating toxins. All antigens (foreign substances) are sent to the liver to be neutralized and expelled from the body. Through enzymes and antioxidants, the liver chemically transforms toxins into harmless substances that can be excreted via the urine or stool. Other toxins are eliminated through the lymphatic system, kidneys, the skin (by sweating), and respiratory system. When imbalances occur in this system, the result can be poor digestion, constipation, bloating and gas, immune dysfunction, reduced liver function, and a host of degenerative diseases, including arthritis. Detoxification can reduce or eliminate the body's "toxic load," restore the proper functioning of the immune and other systems, and help alleviate arthritis.

Detoxification can reduce or eliminate the body's "toxic load," restore the proper functioning of the immune and other systems, and help alleviate arthritis pain and inflammation.

Toxicity and the Intestines

Many illnesses arise from problems in the intestines. Most of the digestion and absorption of nutrients that happens in the body occurs along the 25-foot-long passageway that comprises the small and large intestines. Keeping this passageway clean, free of toxic buildup, and alive with healthy digestive microbes is vital to maintaining health.

Digestion begins in the mouth with proper chewing and digestive enzymes secreted by the salivary glands. From the mouth, food travels to the stomach where hydrochloric acid activates pepsin to break down proteins into absorbable molecular components. The partially digested food then moves to the upper part of the small intestine, where digestion continues with enzymes (produced by the pancreas) and bile. In the next section of the intestine (jejunum), sugar-digesting enzymes are secreted. From the small intestine, the majority of nutrients from food are absorbed into the blood. The large intestine's primary function is to absorb water (about one liter a day) and some minerals. Undigested material is then stored until it can be eliminated.

Around 1900, most people in the U.S. had a brief intestinal transit time—meaning that it took 15-20 hours from the time food entered the mouth until it was excreted as feces. Today, many have a seriously delayed transit time of 50-70 hours. Constipation and sluggish transit time allows for the stool to putrefy, harmful microorganisms to flourish, and toxins to be reabsorbed by tissues and lymph vessels, triggering inflammation throughout the body. In addition, undigested proteins that pass into the small and large intestines without being broken down into their constituent amino acids (due to inadequate levels of hydrochloric acid) produce toxins that further poison the intestines and can escape into the blood or lymph fluids. Inadequate digestion of dietary protein often results in insufficient production of amino acids, hormones, digestive enzymes, and other substances important for proper immune function and overall health.

Mucoid Plaque

Intestinal mucus that is too thick (due to incorrect eating habits and fried or processed foods) makes the stools gummy, causing them to stick to the intestine walls. Mucus also leaves a residue as it passes, which builds up and eventually hardens into plaque, which can be up to one-inch thick in a toxic colon. This "false lining" in the intestine reduces the diameter of the intestinal passageway, leaving only a narrow opening through which waste can travel. As the false lining builds up, it also blocks absorption of essential nutrients into the bloodstream and offers a hiding place for toxins, bacteria, yeast, and parasites that are harmful to human health. These toxins and abnormal life forms can kill off the "friendly" bacteria, such as *Lactobacillus acidophilus*, that inhabit the intestines, leading to an imbalance in the intestinal microflora (see "Friendly and Unfriendly Bacteria," p. 106). Again, the contents of the intestines putrefy and harmful chemicals are generated, which can contribute to numerous health problems.

Serafina Corsello, M.D., director of the Corsello Centers for Nutritional Complementary Medicine in New

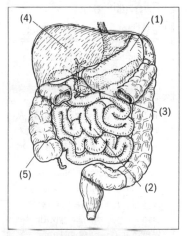

THE DIGESTIVE SYSTEM. Digestion begins in the mouth, then food travels to the stomach (1), where it is further broken down by gastric juices. Next, the partially digested food goes to the small intestine (2) where enzymes from the pancreas (3) and bile produced by the liver (4) act upon the food to extract nutrients for absorption into blood and lymph cells. The unusable food materials are sent to the large intestine (5) for evacuation from the body.

York City and Huntington, New York, states that the large and small intestines are the active front of the immune system, trapping and eliminating pathogens and harmful debris. "The intestines constitute the largest immunological system of the body," Dr. Corsello observes. "The digestive system is one of the first screening systems against the daily load of toxins that, if left unchecked, would constitute a grave threat to our entire immune system." A healthy intestine is immunologically vigilant against undesirable pathogens and toxins. One that is overburdened and compromised fails to perform its immune defensive role and may start contributing to the emergence of an autoimmune illness or other chronic diseases.

Toxins that build up in the colon pass through the intestinal wall and accumulate in the lymphatic system, the network of vessels and nodes that clean and drain the body of toxic substances. When the

Friendly and Unfriendly Bacteria

The estimated 100 trillion bacteria that live in the human intestines do so in a delicate balance. Certain bacteria such as *Lactobacillus acidophilus* and *Bifidobacterium bifidum*, are "friendly" bacteria that support numerous vital physiological processes. They help insure that bowel movements are regular and frequent and they also oppose the overgrowth of yeasts and parasites. Other bacteria, such as *Citrobacter*, *Klebsiella*, and *Clostridium*, are also present, but are considered "unfriendly" because they produce a variety of toxic substances. A healthy proportion of microorganisms in the colon is 85% friendly bacteria to no more than 15% unfriendly bacteria. Unfortunately, in most people, the proportions are the exact opposite. A number of factors can throw off the balance of intestinal flora, including stress, the use of antibiotics and other drugs, and processed foods.

flow of toxins from the colon becomes too heavy, the lymph can become blocked and cause toxins to back up throughout the body. The result can be damage to the liver and other detoxification organs and blood toxicity, eventually compromising the entire immune system.[1]

Factors That Harm the Intestines

These factors can contribute to the formation of mucoid plaque, throw off the balance of the intestinal microflora, and cause a toxic bowel:

■ Acid Diet—Acid-forming foods, such as sugars, processed grains, eggs, and meat, contribute to the formation of intestinal plaque.

■ Processed Foods—Foods made from bleached white flour, such as white bread, pastries, and cakes, contribute to the buildup of intestinal plaque. These foods are almost totally devoid of fiber. In addition, because most of the nutrients have also been bleached out, they tend to deprive the body of enzymes and other wholesome nutrients. Enzymes are specialized living proteins that break down food and change it into a form the body can absorb. Without adequate enzymes, food tends to putrefy in the intestines rather than being digested and absorbed.

■ Stress—Stress can also cause excess acid in the intestine, contributing to the formation of intestinal plaque. Tension also causes the walls of the bowel and sphincter muscles to constrict, hindering the passage of fecal material.

■ Allergies—The intestines may produce mucus in response to a food allergy. Ralph Golan, M.D., a holistic physician from Seattle, Washington, and author of *Optimal Wellness*, says that "any food can be an allergen and cause constipation, cramps, bloating, diarrhea, and other bowel symptoms."[2]

■ Parasites and Yeast—Parasite and yeast infestations in the colon can also cause digestive problems. Parasites commonly enter the body through contaminated food or water supplies (both domestic and from foreign travel). Intestinal parasites can induce a wide variety of reactions, including swelling of joints, asthma, and weight gain. Dr. Corsello is concerned that many physicians refuse to acknowledge that parasite infestation is a major factor in systemic illness. She notes that physicians at her center have observed a strong correlation in their patients between having intestinal parasites and a range of chronic conditions such as arthritis, respiratory problems, heightened allergies, menstrual disorders, and prolonged bowel disorders.

For more information on **food allergies and arthritis**, see Chapter 9: Allergies and Arthritis, pp. 192-207. For more about the **role of bacteria and yeast in intestinal dysbiosis**, see Chapter 6: Eradicating Bacteria and Yeast, pp. 130-151. For more on **parasites and intestinal dysbiosis**, see Chapter 7: Eliminating Parasites, pp. 152-170.

■ Antibiotics—Antibiotics are prescribed by physicians to kill the harmful bacteria causing an infection. Unfortunately, these drugs do not distinguish between the unfriendly and friendly microbes that live in our bodies—they cause a massive die-off of friendly bacteria. Steroids and birth control pills can have a similar effect. Antibiotics are also fed to poultry and beef cattle in alarming amounts; these animal husbandry practices cause large antibiotic residues to remain in meat consumed by most Americans, contributing to the demise of friendly intestinal microbes.

Alternative Medicine Therapies for a Toxic Colon

Cleansing the intestines of this toxic buildup is vital for arthritis sufferers in order to modulate the immune system and stop the chronic inflammatory response that often accompanies an overburdened detoxification system. Repopulating the intestines with friendly bacteria is also important for maintaining healthy digestive functioning.

Colon Hydrotherapy

Colon hydrotherapy (colonics or colonic irrigation) helps to normalize a sluggish intestinal tract, scour the crevices of the intestinal membrane for pathogens, and prevent inflammation (which allows toxins to escape through the intestinal walls). Colon hydrotherapy can decrease parameters of inflammation (such as rheumatoid factor) and reverse many indicators of autoimmune activity (such as antinuclear

How's Your Digestive Function?

An excellent "window" into seeing how digestive inadequacies can contribute to a variety of illnesses is a stool analysis, which consists of a group of nearly two dozen tests performed on a stool sample and can be ordered by your physician. The tests reveal how well you are digesting your food and absorbing nutrients, whether or not your diet contains adequate fiber, if fats are being absorbed, and the status of digestive enzymes. It also tells you whether intestinal bacteria are in balance ("friendly" versus pathogenic) and if yeasts such as Candida are present. All of these factors may be contributing to your symptoms.

For more information on the **Comprehensive Digestive Stool Analysis**, see Chapter 3: Diagnosing Arthritis, pp. 52-77.

antibodies) that contribute to rheumatoid arthritis. Colon hydrotherapy is a safe and minimally uncomfortable procedure that involves the gentle infusion of warm, filtered water into the colon. It is unsurpassed in its ability to detoxify the colon, correct disordered intestinal bacteria (dysbiosis), and treat intestinal permeability or "leaky gut syndrome." It also tones the muscles of the colon and stimulates the wave-like contractions of the intestines to propel food through the digestive tract and prevent the buildup of destructive wastes.

Two to three bowel movements a day, at regular times, soon after the consumption of a meal, are the ideal goal. The average American eliminates less than once per day, which means that most people are actually constipated. With constipation, the stool is hard and dry and hardened fecal stones (fecoliths) get caught in the folds of the colon, contributing to toxic buildup. In traditional cultures, where five to ten times more fiber is eaten than in the Standard American Diet, the stool is typically larger, softer, and more frequent. There is a corresponding lower incidence of colon cancer and other gastrointestinal diseases.

For more about **leaky gut syndrome**, see Chapter 8: Alleviating Leaky Gut Syndrome, pp. 172-190. For more on **rheumatoid factor** and **anti-nuclear antibodies**, see Chapter 3: Diagnosing Arthritis, pp. 52-77.

People with severe heart disease, appendicitis, aneurysm, gastrointestinal hemorrhage, severe hemorrhoids, colon cancer, intestinal wall herniation, pregnancy, severe colitis, and intestinal blockages should not undergo colon hydrotherapy.

The Colonic Procedure—Like an enema, colonic hydrotherapy begins with the insertion of a small, rectal tube (speculum) into the patient by the therapist, nurse, or physician. The colon hydrotherapy machine is a closed system. Water, oxygenated water, food-grade hydrogen peroxide, ozone, botanical anti-microbials, nutritional supplements, or an "implant" of friendly intestinal flora (probiotics) is gently infused into and out of the intestines. The temperature, water pressure, and flow are continuously monitored throughout the treatment. The colonic machine is self-sanitizing, featuring a built-in check valve which prevents waste water from returning and contaminating the water source. All instruments used in the treatment are sterile and disposable, eliminating any possible contamination to the patient.

The water pressure used during the colonic treatment is a safe and gentle five pounds per square inch. The treatment usually lasts for approximately one hour, which includes time for evacuating the bowels after a treatment. A series of 8-12 colonic treatments is often prescribed, depending on the diagnosis. The medications or therapeutic substances are changed often so as to expose the disease-causing microorganisms found in the colon to the widest spectrum of disease fighters, guaranteeing maximum eradication. We recommend using healthy bacteria during colon hydrotherapy (at the end of the treatment), because it is much more effective than taking oral supplements.

Enemas

Enemas can easily be done at home and adding medicinal herbs or the friendly bacteria L. acidophilus makes an enema even more effective. A coffee enema helps to purge both the colon and liver of accumulated toxins, dead cells, and waste products. The enema is prepared by brewing organic caffeinated coffee through a natural brown filter (white filters often contain toxic compounds), letting it cool to body temperature, and delivering it via an enema bag.

Colon-Cleansing Programs

We usually start people on a colon-cleansing program using a combination of psyllium seed powder (½ tsp) and vitamin C powder (1 tsp)

The Origins of Colon Hydrotherapy

Accounts of bowel cleansing date back to ancient Egypt. The *Ebers Papyrus*, an ancient Egyptian health and spiritual manuscript, contains hieroglyphs which depict the use of gourds and rushes as a rudimentary enema bag to infuse liquids into the colon through the anus. In the *Essene Gospel of Peace*, enemas are regularly mentioned as medical and spiritual cleansers, using goat skins and reeds to perform the enema.[3] Eighty years ago, natural health-care pioneer John Harvey Kellogg, M.D., of Battle Creek, Michigan, used colon therapy to avoid surgery in all but 20 of 40,000 patients afflicted with gastrointestinal disease.[4] The popularity of colon therapy reached its zenith in the 1920s and 1930s. At that time, colonic irrigation machines were a common sight in hospitals and physicians' offices. Although interest declined with the advent of pharmaceutical and surgical treatments, colon therapy is once again gaining in popularity and is now commonly used by alternative medicine practitioners.[5]

Colonic Therapy Can Help:

- Autoimmune diseases, including ankylosing spondylitis and rheumatoid diseases
- Psoriatic arthritis and gout
- Fibromyalgia
- Parasitic infections
- *Candida* overgrowth
- Irritable bowel syndrome
- PMS and hormonal problems
- Acne, psoriasis, and eczema
- Headaches, especially migraines
- Chronic colds, allergies, and other immune disorders
- Gallbladder afflictions
- Liver disease

For instructions on preparing a **coffee enema**, see "How to Administer a Coffee Enema," this chapter, p. 115.

in eight ounces of water; drink immediately after mixing ingredients and follow it with an additional eight ounces of water or herb tea; drink once daily. After two days, add these two supplements as support: PlantiBiotic, containing herbs that detoxify the colon, including barberry, wormwood, and cascara (two capsules, twice daily); and GastroGuard, containing nutrients to help rebuild a healthy intestinal lining, including L-glutamine, plaintain, slippery elm, ginkgo, and skullcap (two capsules, twice daily). Continue this protocol daily for one month, then use 1-2 times per week.

Increased interest in colon health has led to a surge in the development of over-the-counter colon-cleansing programs. Most of these programs utilize a cleansing supplement in addition to recommending a basic dietary program. The supplements generally contain a combination of herbs, nutrients, enzymes, and toxin-absorbers designed to help remove the mucoid plaque lining in the colon and enhance digestion and absorption of food. Many of these supplements include ingredients that also cleanse the liver, gallbladder, and lymph.

A.M./P.M. Ultimate Cleanse is a cleansing program designed by Lindsey Duncan, C.N., a nutritionist in Santa Monica, California. The program includes two herbal and fiber formulas called Multi-Herb™ and Multi-Fiber™. The formulas are made from 29 cleansing herbs, amino acids, antioxidants, digestive enzymes, vitamins, and minerals, and five kinds of fiber. Both the Multi-Herb and Multi-Fiber formulas are taken in the morning and evening, in gradually increasing dosages for several weeks. The key to the effectiveness of the formula, Duncan explains, is timing: the morning formula stimulates while the evening formula relaxes. Duncan's formulas target not only the bowel, but the liver, lungs, skin, and lymph. "The goal is to stimulate, feed, and detoxify the complete internal body, not just the bowel," states Duncan. At the end of the program, a person should be having two to three bowel movements every day.

Success Stories: Eliminating Mucoid Plaque Helps Ease Joint Pain

After years of poor diet, constipation, and stagnation, mucoid plaque, a layer of debris, mucus, impacted feces, minerals, and microorganisms, accumulates along the colon wall. It resembles a greenish-black "snake" and is the texture of rubber cement. Although many conventional gastroenterologists dismiss the existence of mucoid plaque, we have observed it on several occasions.

Richard, 48, had chronic psoriasis and psoriatic arthritis and a history of only two bowel movements per week. We recommended colonic hydrotherapy for him. During the fourth treatment, mucoid plaque was dislodged from Richard's colon and expelled. Through colon therapy, nutritional supplements, and adherence to the Arthritis Diet, Richard experienced a reduction in joint pain and psoriasis and eventually a complete remission of all symptoms.

Orlando, 55, developed joint pain and stiffness (particularly unbearable in his spine) a little over 20 years ago. The pain soon inhibited the activities of his daily life and interfered with his job. Conventional doctors put him on prednisone, NSAIDs (nonsteroidal, anti-inflammatory drugs), and gold injections, which brought temporary relief from his joint pain but soon resulted in stomach and gastrointestinal disturbances. Orlando decided to seek the advice of an alternative medical practitioner. We reviewed his case and immediately placed him on a restrictive diet that eliminated his favorite snack, hot dogs, and his evening glass of wine. Removing these two items from his diet resulted in a slight improvement in his symptoms and convinced him of the effectiveness of alternative therapies. We then starting preparing Orlando for a supervised fast. First, he began to juice vegetables every day and slowly cut back on his intake of solid foods, followed by a week of ingesting only water. The entire fasting period lasted 40 days and included a daily colonic. During one colonic treatment, a large section of mucoid plaque was passed. Shortly after this session, Orlando reported a surge of energy and reduction of joint pain. He has since been able to resume a more active life, including athletic hobbies such as biking, swimming, and running, and he even competes in triathlon competitions.

Probiotics

Whenever you undergo any form of intestinal cleansing, all of the bacteria, both friendly and unfriendly, are washed out. It is therefore important to repopulate your intestine with friendly bacteria, particularly *Lactobacillus acidophilus* and *Bifidobacterium bifidum*. Cabbage is one of the best food sources of friendly bacteria; eat it raw daily or juice it. Other foods that can help revitalize the colon and encourage the growth of normal bacteria include rice protein,

For more information on **PlantiBiotic** and **GastroGuard**, contact: Nature's Answer, 320 Oser Avenue, Hauppauge, NY 11788; tel: 800-439-2324 or 516-231-7492; fax: 516-231-8391. For **A.M./P.M. Ultimate Cleanse**™, contact: Nature's Secret, 4 Health Inc., 5485 Conestoga Court, Boulder, CO 80301; tel: 303-546-6306; fax: 303-546-6416.

chicory, onions, garlic, asparagus, and bananas. Friendly bacteria are also found in yogurt and kefir (a fermented milk drink). Another way to repopulate the intestines with friendly bacteria is to take a probiotic supplement. Use non-dairy sources if you have been diagnosed with dairy allergies or if dairy exacerbates your arthritis.

The Overburdened Liver

The liver, located beneath the right lower part of the rib cage, is the largest and one of the most complicated organs in the body, rivaled only by the brain. The liver collects and removes foreign particles and chemicals from the blood and detoxifies these poisons through three systems: (1) the Kupffer cells; (2) Phase I and Phase II systems, involving over 75 enzymes; and (3) the production of bile. Each system feeds into the other, and all three need to be operating at full efficiency for proper detoxification.

Approximately 1,500 milliliters of blood pass through the liver each minute for filtering. The major players in this filtering project are the Kupffer cells, a type of stationary white blood cell that engulfs foreign matter in the blood before it passes through the rest of the liver. When the liver is damaged, toxic, congested, or sluggish, the Kupffer cells become overburdened and the filtration system breaks down, allowing increased levels of antigens, foreign proteins, bowel microorganisms, and dietary waste products to pass through the liver and enter the general circulatory system. Inflammatory agents called cytokines are also released, contributing to the development of arthritis.

The most complex of the liver's detoxification mechanisms are referred to as Phase I and Phase II biotransformation systems. When a toxic chemical like alcohol enters the liver, reactions begin which attempt to break these chemicals down into harmless substances. There are two phases to this complex breakdown process. Phase I is the oxidation phase, in which enzymes "burn" or oxidize chemicals into intermediate substances. Phase II enzymes act to combine these decomposed substances with other molecules (such as sulfur, glutathione, and glycine) to make them more water-soluble and easier for the body to excrete.[6] Bile (excreted by the liver, stored in the gallbladder, and pumped into the small intestine as needed) is a yellowish-brown, orange, or green fluid meant to make intestinal contents less acidic and to emulsify or digest fat; bile prevents putrefaction of intestinal contents. The goal of all the liver's detoxification systems is to convert toxins into a water-soluble form for easy elimination from the body via the stool.

Detecting Defective Detoxification

Defects in the body's ability to activate these detoxification pathways will create an accumulation of toxins in the system or a slowed excretion rate, causing damage to sensitive physiological systems. Overactivation of Phase I causes excessive production of free radicals and toxic by-products. In addition, if Phase II is sluggish, it causes a buildup of damaging molecules in the body. If you want to determine the efficiency of your liver processes, we recommend the Hepatic Detoxification Profile, available through Great Smokies Diagnostic Laboratory.

We regularly test all patients to evaluate their Phase I and Phase II systems. An overwhelming percentage of the arthritis patients we've seen have suffered from the effects of poorly functioning livers and are medically classified as "pathologic detoxifiers." Joseph Pizzorno, N.D., president of Bastyr University of Naturopathic Medicine, in Seattle, Washington, points out that NSAIDs routinely used in the treatment of arthritis are proven inhibitors of the liver's Phase II detoxification enzymes. Other inhibitors include aspirin, acetaminophen, and deficiencies in folic acid, vitamins B12, B complex, and C, and the amino acids glutathione, cysteine, or methionine.

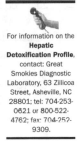

For information on the **Hepatic Detoxification Profile,** contact: Great Smokies Diagnostic Laboratory, 63 Zillicoa Street, Asheville, NC 28801; tel: 704-253-0621 or 800-522-4762; fax: 704-253-9309.

Liver DetoxificationTherapies

Balancing the Phase I and Phase II processes of the liver is extremely important for those with arthritis. Techniques that can help cleanse, tone, and repair damaged liver cells include a liver flush, coffee enema, castor oil packs, and specific herbs, plants, and foods for liver support.

The Liver Flush

"Liver flushes are used to stimulate the elimination of wastes from the body, to open and cool the liver, to increase bile flow, and to improve overall liver function," says Christopher Hobbs, L.Ac., herbalist and author of *Foundation of Health* (Botanical Press, 1994). Here are his instructions for preparing and administering a liver flush:

1. Squeeze enough fresh lemons or limes to produce one cup of juice. Dilute with a small amount of distilled or spring water, if desired, but the more sour, the better it will perform as a liver cleanser.

Orange and grapefruit juice may also be used, provided they are blended with some lemon or lime juice.

2. Add the juice of 1-2 cloves of garlic and a small amount of raw grated ginger juice. Grate the ginger on a cheese or vegetable grater and then press the shreds into a garlic press to get juice, or put a 1-2" piece of ginger root through a juicer.

3. Add one tablespoon of high quality, organic, extra virgin olive oil to the juice. Blend or shake all ingredients.

4. Take the drink in the morning and do not eat any food for one hour afterward.

5. After an hour has elapsed, drink two cups of an herbal blend that Dr. Hobbs calls "Polari Tea." To prepare Polari Tea, combine these dry herbs and simmer for 20 minutes: fennel (one part), flax (one part), burdock (¼ part), fenugreek (one part), and licorice (¼ part). Then, add peppermint (one part) and steep for an additional ten minutes. For convenience, several quarts of Polari Tea may be prepared in advance and refrigerated.

6. Do the flush for ten days, discontinue for three days, then resume for ten days—this is one cycle. Repeat for another cycle. Dr. Hobbs suggests doing the liver flush (two full cycles) twice yearly.

Coffee Enema

The coffee enema, a therapy easily done at home, helps to purge the liver of accumulated toxins, dead cells, and waste products. The enema is prepared by brewing organic caffeinated coffee through a natural brown filter, letting it cool to body temperature, and delivering it via an enema bag (see "How to Administer a Coffee Enema," p. 115). Coffee contains choleretics, substances which increase the flow of bile from the gallbladder.[7] Early research by Max Gerson, M.D., founder of the Gerson Institute, in Bonita, California, and originator of the Gerson Diet Therapy, established that a coffee enema is effective in stimulating the complex system of liver detoxification.[8]

Castor Oil Packs

Castor oil comes from the bean of the castor plant, *Oleum ricini*. The plant itself is quite poisonous, but the oil pressed out of the bean is safe to use, since the toxic constituents remain in the seeds. The Egyptians used castor oil as a laxative for cleansing the bowels and as a scalp rub to make hair grow and shine. Rubbed into sore muscles and joints right before infrared heat treatment, it is said to reduce the pain and swelling of rheumatism and arthritis. Castor oil packs have been used for many conditions, including liver problems, constipation, and other

How to Administer a Coffee Enema

Here is the regimen generally recommended by health researcher Etienne Callebout, M.D., of London, England, for administering the coffee enema:

1) Add three tablespoons of ground organic coffee (not instant or decaffeinated) to two pints of distilled water. Boil for five minutes (uncovered) to burn off oils; then cover, lower heat, and simmer for an additional 15 minutes.

2) Strain and cool to body temperature. Lubricate rectal enema tube with K-Y Jelly or other lubricant. Hang enema bag above you, but not more than two feet from your body; the best level is approximately six inches above the intestines. Lying on your right side, draw both legs close to the abdomen.

3) Insert the tube several inches into rectum. Open the stopcock and allow fluid to run in very slowly to avoid cramping. Breathe deeply and try to relax. Retain the solution for 12-15 minutes. If you have trouble retaining or taking the full amount, lower the bag; if you feel spasms, lower the bag to the floor to relieve the pressure. After about 20 seconds, slowly start raising the bag toward the original level. You can also pinch the tube to control the flow.

4) With symptoms of toxicity, such as headaches, fever, nausea, intestinal spasm, and drowsiness, one may increase the frequency of enemas. Take in one to two pints each time for these conditions.

5) Upon waking the next morning, if you experience headaches and drowsiness, an additional enema is recommended that night. Eat a piece of fruit before the first coffee enema of the day to activate the upper digestive tract. Keep all equipment clean.

ailments involving elimination, as well as non-malignant ovarian fibroid cysts and headaches.[9] The oil helps to draw out toxins, release tension, and improve blood circulation, especially in the lower abdomen (see "Castor Oil Pack Instructions," p. 116).

Dietary Recommendations to Support the Liver

Foods that help the liver include the cabbage family and cruciferous vegetables (Brussels sprouts, cauliflower, and broccoli), which aid the liver in both Phase I and Phase II detoxification. Brussels sprouts are the best of the cruciferous vegetables for the liver, according to John Bastyr, N.D., the namesake of Bastyr University of Naturopathic Medicine, in Seattle, Washington. Other helpful sulfur-containing foods include onions, garlic, leeks, and chives.

Beets contain high levels of betaine, a powerful lipotropic agent (increases the flow of bile). Black radish and artichokes contain cynarin, which has liver-protective properties similar to milk thistle. Olive oil promotes the production of bile in the liver as well as pro-

Castor Oil Pack Instructions

1) Fold a flannel sheet into three sections to fit over your whole abdomen.

2) Cut a piece of plastic one to two inches larger than flannel sheet.

3) Soak flannel sheet in gently heated castor oil. Fold it over and squeeze until some of the liquid oozes out. Unfold.

4) Prepare the surface where you will be lying. Place a large plastic sheet and an old towel over the surface to prevent staining.

5) Lie down on the towel and place the oil-soaked flannel sheet over your abdomen. Place fitted plastic piece over the flannel sheet. Apply a hot water bottle over the area.

6) Wrap towel under and around your torso.

7) Rest for one to two hours.

8) Wash your body with a solution of three tablespoons baking soda to one quart water to rinse off the oil.

9) Repeat as instructed by a physician.

tecting it from microorganisms. Many aromatic cooking spices also aid the liver in its detoxification process. Outstanding among them is rosemary, which assists the production and movement of bile through the liver and gallbladder. Dill, caraway, and fennel aid in Phase II detoxification.

Therapeutic Herbs for the Liver

■ Silymarin (Milk Thistle)— For centuries, European herbalists have used the bioflavonoid silymarin for restoring liver function. Bioflavonoids are plant pigments with beneficial properties: they protect against damage from destructive free radicals in the body and enhance the activity of vitamin C. Silymarin accelerates the process of regenerating damaged liver tissue, thereby freeing the organ to carry out its key functions. It has even been proven effective against certain types of mushroom and petrochemical solvent poisoning. The usual dose is 2-3 capsules (420 mg) daily of milk thistle standardized to 70%-80% silymarin content.

■ *Picrorrhiza kurroa* (Katuka)—Picrorrhiza is a tiny plant that grows in the Himalayas at an altitude of 9,000-15,000 feet. Its active ingredient has been found to be comparable or superior to that of silymarin. Clinical trials on patients with osteoarthritis, rheumatic pains, ankylosing spondylitis, and psoriasis have shown a favorable response.[11] Typical recommended dose: 500 mg, twice daily.

■ Dandelion (*Taraxacum officinale*)—As a liver and digestive tonic as well as blood cleanser and diuretic (urine-increasing agent), dandelion aids in detoxification of the body. As testimony to dandelion's powerful influence on the liver, severe hepatitis has been reversed by dandelion tea along with dietary restrictions in as short a period as a week.[12] Given that chemical or heavy metal toxicity is frequently

How Chinese Medicine Views the Liver

The idea of a congested or sluggish liver is an ancient concept from traditional Chinese medicine (SEE QUICK DEFINITION). The signs of a sluggish or congested liver are often manifested as PMS, fatigue, lethargy, an inability to properly digest foods (particularly fats), multiple allergies, environmental and chemical sensitivities, constipation, and arthritis.

The liver is also the reservoir of anger in the body—anger towards other people or towards the self. Anger affects the liver's ability to govern the flow of qi, blood, and vital nutrients to ligaments, tendons, sinews, joints, bones, and muscles, according to Chinese tradition. One of the main Chinese herbs used in liver ailments as well as arthritis is gardenia. It is known as the "happiness herb," because it has an ability to loosen emotions like anger, stuck due to chronic liver congestion.[10] In TCM, the liver is associated with the wood element and is represented by the color green/yellow. Leafy greens and other substances of that color are considered beneficial for toning and boosting liver function.

Anger and Asparagus—A Chinese doctor once told us that he recommended eating asparagus to all his patients, because asparagus will bring joy and happiness and release anger in the liver. Asparagus contributes to the easy flow of these emotions, he said. This advice is fascinating because most patients with arthritis have a deficiency in a detoxifying enzymatic reaction called sulfoxidation, necessary for digesting sulfur containing compounds. A self-test to see if the sulfoxidation pathway is operating normally is to eat asparagus and notice whether your urine smells after consumption. If it does, your body is having difficulty processing the sulfur in the asparagus due to this enzymatic deficiency.

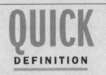

QUICK

DEFINITION

Traditional Chinese medicine (TCM) originated in China over 5,000 years ago and is a comprehensive system of medical practice that heals the body according to the principles of nature and balance. A Chinese medicine physician considers the flow of vital energy (qi) in a patient through close examination of the patient's pulse, tongue, body odor, voice tone and strength, and general demeanor, among other elements. Underlying imbalances and disharmony in the body are described in terminology analogous to the natural world (heat, cold, dryness, or dampness).

involved in arthritis, dandelion can help cleanse the body and support the liver in its own elimination functions. As a digestive tonic, dandelion may also help with the gastrointestinal complaints associated with arthritis. Typical recommended dose: 4-10 g of dried root or three cups of fresh dandelion tea, once daily.

■ Other Phytonutrients—Several other phytonutrients ("phyto" meaning plant) have demonstrated anti-inflammatory activity on the liver through various mechanisms. Catechins (a bioflavonoid) are used by European naturopaths and medical doctors to treat chemical hepatitis, cirrhosis, and other environmental and viral forms of liver disease.[13] Catechins can be taken as a nutritional supplement; typical dose is 250 mg, twice daily. Green tea (2-3 cups a day) is also a good source of catechins.

For **AlteraTonic**, contact: Nature's Answer, 320 Oser Avenue, Hauppauge, NY 11788; tel: 800-439-2324 or 516-231-7492; fax: 516-231-8391; website: www. naturesanswer.com.

Certain botanicals act as Kupffer-cell stimulants, including burdock, goldenseal, baptisia, smilax, Oregon grape root, and echinacea. We have documented improved liver function after using these herbs.[14] One herbal formula we have used to support and tonify the liver and other organs in arthritis patients is AlteraTonic, which contains Siberian ginseng, picrorrhiza, milk thistle, burdock, and dandelion.

Success Story: Detoxification Heals Juvenile Rheumatoid Arthritis

Cam, 7, woke up the day after her birthday party vomiting and running a high fever. Her mother wasn't surprised by her illness; the day before Cam had overdosed on excitement, birthday cake, and ice cream. Cam's symptoms were gone after she took Tylenol® to reduce the fever and got a good night's rest, but her mother noticed that Cam was fatigued and abnormally pale. A few weeks later, her fever returned coupled with joint and muscle pain and a dry, hacking cough. Cam was taken to the family pediatrician who, upon running a complete blood count test, found a high level of white blood cells, suggesting a possible infection. He prescribed antibiotics, and Cam and her mother returned home to wait anxiously for her recovery. But the recovery never came: the fever and migrating joint pain persisted after several months.

Additional blood tests showed that Cam's platelet (a disc-shaped cell produced in bone marrow and released into the blood, where it is essential for clotting) count was dangerously high—Cam's platelet count was 922, normal is 130-400—suggesting either severe anemia, chronic infection, or inflammatory conditions. Her red blood cell count was 9.8 grams per deciliter (normal being 10.3-14.9 g/dl), confirming a moderate case of anemia. An infectious disease specialist initially diagnosed Cam's problems as long-term pneumonia and prescribed a five-day cycle of antibiotics. But Cam's joint pain continued to become more debilitating.

A rheumatologist joined the case, because Cam's physical complaints and anemia matched the symptoms of rheumatoid arthritis

(70% of rheumatoid arthritis patients have anemia). But each test for rheumatoid arthritis came back negative and her doctors, unable to conclusively confirm rheumatoid arthritis, decided that a bacterial or viral infection must be responsible. Cam was placed on prednisone (an anti-inflammatory steroid) and methotrexate (a cancer chemotherapy drug used on rheumatoid arthritis patients to decrease inflammation), methylprednisone (another steroid), and antibiotics.

By this time, she was no longer an active and vibrant seven-year-old. Cam could no longer walk by herself and even had problems standing. She had lost 12 pounds and had developed a rash on her thighs and abdomen; profuse night sweats made it difficult to sleep; and she was always exhausted. The steroid therapy helped ease the pain in her joints for a while but it caused many side effects, including toxicity.

When we first met her, Cam's face was bloated (or moon-shaped) from the disease and the prednisone treatment. Her symptoms—joint and muscle pain, night sweats, and fevers—still suggested rheumatoid arthritis, although her conventional doctors had diagnosed her with infectious arthritis on the basis that her rheumatoid factor (RF—SEE QUICK DEFINITION), at 32, was normal (normal range is zero to 39). But Cam's RF was at the high end of normal, a range where symptoms could begin appearing before her RF rose to abnormal levels. We decided to test for possible parasitic infections, heavy metal toxicity, and delayed food allergies, all contributing factors of rheumatoid arthritis that are commonly overlooked by conventional doctors.

The first darkfield (SEE QUICK DEFINITION) blood analysis showed that Cam's immune system was compromised. She had low numbers of red blood cells and these were abnormally clumped together like a roll of coins. When stuck together, red blood cells are unable to deliver oxygen to the tissues or export toxic waste products out of the body. Another indicator that Cam's body was unable to fight pathogens was the abnormally large and sluggish appearance of her white blood cells, a common side effect of the prescription drugs methotrexate and prednisone. We also found metabolic by-products

EDITOR'S NOTE
This case was supervised by Ellen Kamhi, Ph.D., R.N., under the direction of her clinical colleague Serafina Corsello, M.D., at the Corsello Center for Nutritional Complementary Medicine, 175 E. Main St., Huntington, NY 11743; tel: 516-271-0222.

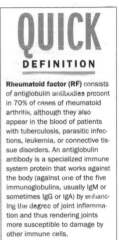

QUICK

DEFINITION

Rheumatoid factor (RF) consists of antiglobulin antibodies present in 70% of cases of rheumatoid arthritis, although they also appear in the blood of patients with tuberculosis, parasitic infections, leukemia, or connective tissue disorders. An antiglobulin antibody is a specialized immune system protein that works against the body (against one of the five immunoglobulins, usually IgM or sometimes IgG or IgA) by enhancing the degree of joint inflammation and thus rendering joints more susceptible to damage by other immune cells.

QUICK

DEFINITION

(due to poor diet or faulty breakdown of waste products) that appeared in the darkfield screen as red and yellow crystals with sharp edges. These crystals can accumulate in joints, muscles, and tissues, causing irritation and pain.

Blood and hair analysis confirmed that Cam had heavy metal toxicity. We found high levels of copper, cadmium, nickel, and aluminum—heavy metals that contribute to liver problems and autoimmune diseases, such as rheumatoid arthritis. Cam also had parasites and the yeast *Candida albicans*, probably due to the antibiotics and her nutritionally poor diet. Taxing an already crippled immune system were food allergies to major components of Cam's diet: wheat, milk, fish, chicken, lamb, cauliflower, celery, squash, and pepper. Cam ate the basic unhealthy American fare, including hot dogs, fast foods, sodas, and lots of processed food.

Our nutritionist put Cam on an allergen-free diet, restricting wheat products and emphasizing low carbohydrates, organic vegetables, soy products, and small amounts of organic meat. Cam would now eat foods rich in organic iron, such as organic beets and leafy greens as well as spirulina or blue-green algae, for her anemia. To ensure that she received enough essential fatty acids, we suggested that her mother give her a salad dressing made from olive oil, flaxseed oil, lemon juice, oregano, and garlic.

Cam was advised not to eat fast foods, sodas, or other processed foods. If she craved a soda, we recommended that she add a little seltzer water to her herbal tea instead. All food preservatives, chemicals, additives, and dyes were to be avoided. We also recommended using a filter for drinking and bathing water, because toxic chemicals can be absorbed through the skin as well as ingested. Cam's system was so sensitive that she could not tolerate the normal levels of toxins most people encounter and accommodate every day.

We also started Cam on a protocol of intravenous vitamin and mineral therapies to support her liver function, reduce inflammation, prevent cellular damage, and stimulate the growth of connective tissue and cartilage. The solution contained sterile water, potassium chloride, vitamin C, magnesium sulfate, heparin, selenium, manganese, zinc, chromium, B complex, B6, and taurine. Cam received intramuscular injections (one per week) of vitamin B12, folic acid, and

Kutapressin® (a liver extract that supports the liver and helps with anemia) for detoxification of her liver.

In addition, Cam took the following supplements:

- Metachel: contains keratin polymer to help chelate (bind and remove) heavy metals and metabolic wastes; 200 mg, twice daily
- Pressidyl: contains shark cartilage to repair damaged cartilage, stimulate the immune system, and relieve pain; 740 mg, twice daily
- Fibroplex: contains malic acid to reduce pain in connective tissues; 500 mg, twice daily
- Micellized vitamin E: 100 IU, three times daily
- Vitamin B12: 1,000 mcg daily
- Folic acid: for nutritional support and to replenish folic acid levels depleted by methotrexate; 400 mcg, once a day sublingually
- Wobenzyme N: contains digestive enzymes; three tablets with meals to help digestion, or two tablets, three times daily, for joint pain
- Adreno-Support: contains vitamins C and B6, and pantothenic acid; for support of adrenal glands under stress from constant steroidal drug intake; three times daily
- *Yunnan Paiyao*: a blend of Chinese and Western herbs; supports the liver by stimulating the production of bile; two tablets, twice daily

For Cam's anemia, an earlier physician had prescribed ferrous sulfate, a type of iron that contributes to free-radical production and is harmful to joints. We replaced it with ferrous fumarate, a non-toxic form of iron, and also gave her yellowdock, an herb with a high iron content.

Several therapies were used to help with her detoxification process. We prescribed a combination of weekly visits to a physiotherapist and nightly baths using Epsom salts and baking soda to relax her aching muscles and joints and pull toxins out through the skin. In addition, every night before bedtime, Cam's mother massaged her with a mixture of these oils: warmed sesame oil for increasing essential fatty acids and rebuilding cartilage, mustard oil for stimulating joints by increasing circulation, and cayenne pepper, a mild analgesic for pain relief.

After four months on the regimen, Cam started to have pain-free days and less inflammation. She has been able to gradually decrease the levels of her conventional medications. Cam has continued on our therapies for over a year, during which time her symptoms have slowly receded. She stopped having night sweats or fevers and her joint pain lessened, although she still experiences occasional stiffness.

For information on **supplements** used to treat Cam, contact: Global Nutrition, 175 E. Main Street, Huntington, NY 11743; tel: 888-461-0949. Environmental Detoxification Consultants, 413 Grassy Hill Road, Woodbury, CT 06798; tel: 203-263-2970.

A recent urine analysis test showed that her body is adequately absorbing essential nutrients, but we are still working to reverse her anemia and raise her red blood cell count, which remains a little below normal. Her mother told us that she is relieved to see her daughter active and running around the playground again.

The Stagnated Lymphatic System

The lymphatic system is the body's master drain, collecting and filtering lymph (a clear to milky fluid containing waste products and cellular debris that accumulates in the tissue spaces between cells) and conveying it from tissues to the bloodstream for elimination from the body. The lymph system comprises a network of ducts and channels. Interspersed throughout the lymph channels are the lymph nodes, clusters of immune tissue that work as immunological inspection stations for detecting foreign and potentially harmful substances in the lymph fluid. Each lymph node contains scavenger cells (macrophages and reticuloendothelial cells) that help destroy and degrade toxins and microbes. Lymph nodes are clustered in strategic junctures of the body, like the head and neck, the armpits, and the groin. The gastrointestinal tract, including the appendix, contains a tremendous quantity of lymph nodes called the Gut Associated Lymphoid Tissue (GALT), a primary filter for the bloodstream.

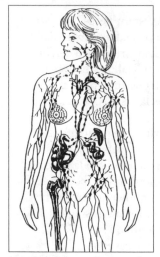

Lymph nodes are clusters of immune tissue that work as filters or "inspection stations" for detecting foreign and potentially harmful substances in the lymph fluid. Lymph nodes are part of the lymphatic system, which is the body's master drain.

The lymph system does not have its own pump (like the heart for the circulatory system). Instead, it is dependent on the movement of skeletal muscles, through normal day-to-day activities, exercise, and breathing, as well as massage and other lymphatic drainage techniques. As the muscles contract and relax, they push the lymph fluid along and backflow is prevented by valves throughout the lymphatic system. The lymph is full of nutrients on their way to all the cells and waste products that must be removed. Any interference with this flow can create serious problems for the body.

Stagnant lymphatic fluid changes in consistency. It goes from a clear, thin fluid to a thick and cloudy consistency in the early stages of toxemia. If the lymph remains stationary, it will progress to a glutinous consistency of thick cream and eventually cottage cheese. Viscous lymphatic fluid becomes an oxygen-deprived sludge that impedes the flow of nutrients to the cells and barricades toxic substances from exiting the extracellular spaces. Lack of nutrients to tissues combined with the stagnation of waste products leads to degenerative diseases, including cancer and arthritis.

Lymphatic stagnation can be caused by allergic and mucus-forming foods, chronic constipation, musculoskeletal imbalances, lack of exercise, improper breathing, prescription drugs, and impairment of local or systemic circulation due to complications of diabetes or arteriosclerosis.

Therapies for Improving Lymphatic Drainage

Preventing the stagnation of the lymphatic system is of paramount importance in treating most diseases, including arthritis. Through detoxification, the lymphatic fluid can circulate freely and easily throughout the body. Techniques that encourage lymphatic drainage include manual lymph drain massage, light beam therapy, dry skin brushing, exercise, and herbs.

Manual Lymph Drainage

Manual lymph drainage is a specially designed massage technique that uses gentle stationary circular motions on the lymph nodes, palpating with the tips or the entire length of the fingers. These motions act like an external pump that pulls lymphatic fluid through the channels and enhances the release of toxins. Lymph drain massage should not be confused with conventional massage techniques, as it relies on gentle and directed manipulations designed to induce lymph flow. The lymph should only be massaged lightly, as too much pressure can cause thickening. Lymph drain massage is a commonly prescribed technique in Europe, especially in Germany, Austria, France, and the Scandinavian countries. The technique has recently gained increased attention in North America, with about 160 certified therapists now practicing.

For referrals to certified lymph massage therapists, contact North American Vodder Association of Lymphatic Therapy, 11526 Coral Hills Drive, Dallas, TX 75229; tel: 214-240-5959; fax: 214-243-3227. National Lymphedema Network, 2211 Post Street, Suite 404, San Francisco CA 94115; tel: 800-541-3259. For information about lymphatic detoxification and the Lymph Pho/Laser™, contact: Marika von Viczay, Ph.D., N.M.D., 16 Arlington Street, Asheville, NC 28802; tel: 704-253-8371; fax 704-258-1350. For the Light Beam Generator™, contact: ELF Teslar, Star Route 1, Box 21, Francisville, IL 62460; tel: 618-948-2393; fax: 618-948-2650

Light Beam Therapy

High-tech lymphatic drainage uses various types of light beam generators, such as the Lymph-Pho/Laser™ and the Light Beam Generator™, to break up lymph blockage. The light beam generator looks like a flashlight with a long, extensible hose. Practitioners use this hand-held device to focus energy on blocked lymph areas. The energy from the generator breaks the electrical bonds that hold clusters of lymph protein molecules together, thus unclogging stagnated lymph fluid. This therapy is often used to enhance the benefits of lymph massage.

Dry Skin Brushing

Dry skin brushing improves flow in the lymphatic system by stimulating the lymph nodes under the skin. This technique is based on acupuncture, which states that there are an estimated three million nerve points spread over the surface of the skin, 700 of which are nodal, meaning they can serve as treatment nodes in acupuncture. By applying friction to the skin with a soft, natural fiber brush (called a "dry skin brush" at most health food stores), a loofah, or a towel (tightly rolled), one can stimulate all of these nerve points, which correspond to specific organs, glands, and muscles.

The physical motion of dry skin brushing moves lymph fluid through the lymphatic channels to encourage drainage and prevent stagnation. Blood and lymphatic circulation and metabolism are stimulated in all organs and tissues as well. Brushed skin is better able to eliminate toxins from the body, as oils (sebum) and dead skin are removed and pores are unclogged. Toxins are transferred into the main lymphatic drainage ducts, which go directly to the liver for elimination. *Qi* or life energy can move freely through the meridians, thus relieving the pain caused by obstruction. White blood cells (lymphocytes) also migrate into the skin after brushing and enhance the function of the immune system.

How to Perform Dry Skin Brushing—To proceed, simply begin gently brushing from the ends of the arms with long strokes that sweep towards the trunk of the body. Do all sides of the arms. Then brush the head and neck with downward strokes towards the clavicle (collar bone). Brush the feet and legs upward towards the groin area; again, be sure to brush all areas of the legs. As you brush the trunk, use upward-sweeping motions towards the heart. The ideal time to perform the dry skin brushing is prior to showering; then jump into the shower to remove the dead skin cells. Be sure to clean the brush thoroughly with soap and water and then hydrogen peroxide after each use.

Exercise

Any exercise helps to pump the lymph, because of the contracting and relaxing motions of the muscles. "During exercise the rate of lymph flow can increase to as high as 14 times normal because of the increased activity," according to Arthur C. Guyton, M.D., chairman of the Department of Physiology and Biophysics at the University of Mississippi School of Medicine, and author of *Basic Human Physiology*.[15] Light bouncing on a mini-trampoline, also called a "rebounder," is especially effective in helping to restore lymph flow. The mini-trampoline used for rebounding has a flexible jumping surface, measuring 28-26 inches in diameter and set 6-9 inches off the ground. Bouncing on the mini-trampoline allows the rapid changes in gravity to act as a powerful lymphatic pump, causing expansion of lymph ducts and channels for increased circulation. When you land on the rebounder, you land with twice the force of gravity, which makes rebounding more effective than running in stimulating the lymph.[16] Rebounding exercise can be tailored to an individual's fitness level. To see improved lymphatic drainage, it takes only 5-10 minutes of rebounding exercise per day.

Herbs That Stimulate Lymphatic Drainage

■ Poke Root (*Phytolacca americana*)—We have found poke root to be one the most potent immune tonics and stimulators. It is used to stimulate white blood cells (B and T lymphocytes) to assist the immune system in fighting off viruses, such as Epstein-Barr, and is a powerful remedy in laryngitis, swollen tonsils, and sore throat. Poke root

For information on **rebounders** and books and videos about rebounding exercise, check your local fitness and sporting goods store, or contact: Best of Health, Unit #1758 W.E. Mail 8770-170st, Edmonton, Alberta T5T-4J2, Canada; tel: 800-561-1513 or 403-407-7898; fax: 403-444-1048.

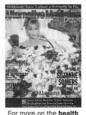

Lymph movement can also be aided by physical therapies, including contrast hydrotherapy, yoga, *qi gong*, and massage. For more information about **physical therapies**, see Chapter 14; Exercises and Physical Therapies, pp. 314-339.

For more on the **health benefits of rebounding**, see "Rebounders: Bounce Your Way to Better Health," *Alternative Medicine Digest* 20 (October/November 1997), pp. 42-46; to order, call 800-333-HEAL.

is also used when the lymphatic glands throughout the body are swollen; it is one of the most potent herbs for lymphatic drainage.

■ Cleavers (*Galium aparine*)—Cleavers, also known as goose grass or bedstraw, is a safer alternative to poke root. Cleavers reduces swelling and edema and is also a kidney tonic. It benefits arthritis by removing "damp congestion," the traditional Chinese medicine designation for the pain associated with arthritis, from the body and by cleansing the lymph system. Fresh, preserved juice can be regularly added to vegetable juices or you can make a spring tonic by combining cleavers with dandelion greens and chickweed, or mixed with carrot/apple/ginger juice. Typical suggested dose: 300 mg, twice daily.

Supporting the Portals: Kidneys, Skin, and Lungs

An effective detoxification protocol must include therapies that enhance the body's ability to expel waste products through all the detoxification pathways. These exit routes or portals—the kidneys, skin, and lungs—must be supported to ensure that toxins are efficiently removed. If there is an imbalance in these organs, toxins can be reabsorbed, compromising detoxification and preventing the healing process.

Kidneys

The kidneys assist the body in removing nitrogenous wastes originating from proteins, xenobiotics (environmental estrogens), drug residues, and a host of other water-soluble toxins. They also regulate sodium and potassium levels as well as blood pressure. During detoxification of specific organs or a general cleansing, it is important to increase the amount of urine being excreted from the body and to keep the urine very diluted. Concentrated urine, especially during detoxification, contains high levels of toxins, which can cause unintended kidney damage. Periodic laboratory measurements of kidney and liver function during a detoxification program are mandatory.

Botanicals which assist the kidneys in excreting waste are referred to as diuretics. Diuretics induce the flow of urine via many physiological mechanisms. Some diuretics increase blood flow to the kidney, while others work by inhibiting the reabsorption of water, which enhances urination. If a person consumes a diet high in animal products for a long time, they are more likely to have high levels of uric acid in the blood; botanical diuretics are also helpful in reducing uric acid levels (important for gout).

■ Dandelion (*Taraxacum officinale*)— Dandelion leaves are one of the best diuretic herbs, and dandelion also has other beneficial functions, such as supporting the liver, for those with arthritis. Typical recommended dose: 4-10 g dried leaves daily.

■ Parsley (*Petroselium sativa*)—Parsley is used to support kidney function because of its diuretic action. It's much more than just a plate garnish—include fresh parsley juice in vegetable juices and eat it regularly as a vegetable. Suggested dosage: one large bunch of fresh parsley daily.

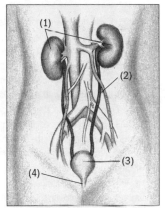

THE URINARY SYSTEM. The kidneys (1) filter water-soluble toxins and other wastes from the blood. These substances make up urine, which is sent through the ureter (2) to the bladder (3) for temporary storage until it can be expelled from the body through the urethra (4).

■ Horsetail (*Equisetum arvense*)— Horsetail, also called Scouring Rush because it was used by native peoples to scour dishes, is an excellent diuretic that has specific benefits to the arthritis patient. It contains the mineral silica, which is a critical nutrient for bone, muscle, and cartilage formation, and has a long history of use in rheumatism.[17] Typical dosage: 250 mg daily.

Skin

Often referred to as "the third kidney," the skin is the largest organ of the body and one of the first lines of defense against external pathogens. The pores and glands of the skin are important organs of elimination as well, through which toxic chemicals can be excreted via either sweat or sebum (oil secreted by the skin).[18] William Rea, M.D., director of the Environmental Health Center in Dallas, Texas, has discovered that certain chemicals—formaldehyde, phenol, various insecticides, chlorine, and petroleum products—can induce rheumatoid diseases. In addition to entering the body through inhalation, these chemicals can be absorbed through the skin, from drinking tap water or through bathing.

EDITOR'S NOTE
The authors, Eugene Zampieron, N.D., A.H.G., and Ellen Kamhi, Ph.D., R.N., conduct workshops nationally on the identification of wild edible and medicinal plants, in which they gather indigenous flora, cook it into a wild stir-fry, and make tinctures, salves, and teas. For more information on workshops, call 800-829-0918.

Sauna Brew

This herb tea is recommended for people using sauna therapy. The tea expedites sweating, especially if consumed as a hot tea before and during the sauna treatment, thereby enhancing the removal of toxins from the body. Patients have commented that this blend also tastes exceptionally good. Combine equal parts of the following herbs (which can be purchased in bulk at health food stores):

- Cinnamon (*Cinnamonium zeylanicum*)
- Ginger (*Zingiber officinale*)
- Boneset (*Eupatorium perfoliatum*)
- Yarrow (*Achillea millefolium*)
- Peppermint (*Mentha piperata*)
- Elder (*Sambucus nigra*)

Use one tablespoon of the herb mixture per cup of tea. Pour one cup of recently boiled water over the herbs, cover, and allow to steep for 20 minutes.

For information on medically supervised **sauna detoxification treatments**, contact: William Rea, M.D., Environmental Health Center, 8345 Walnut Hill Lane, Suite 220, Dallas, TX 75231; tel: 214-368-4132; fax: 214-691-8432.

Dry Skin Brushing—To enhance the skin's ability to detoxify, use a loofah sponge or dry skin brush. Brush the skin with long strokes towards the heart, before bathing or showering. This helps to debride the top layer of dead skin cells and stimulates lymphatic drainage.

Sauna (Heat Stress Detoxification)— Using a sauna can effectively clear the body of fat-soluble toxins. The heat of the sauna helps arthritis by making the muscles, joints, and sinews more pliable and by increasing blood flow to the joints. Studies of fat biopsies before and after a heat stress detoxification protocol revealed an average of 21.3% reduction in the body levels of 16 toxic chemicals, including PCBs and PBBs, with a 64%-75% reduction in harmful toxins.[19] After discontinuing the heat and detoxification therapy, the study found that toxins in patients continued to decrease for up to four months after treatment. Dr. Rea has published documentation showing that his detoxification program, which includes fasting, juicing, sauna therapy, exercise, and lymphatic drainage, produced a reduction of various pesticide residues ranging up to 66%.[20]

Lungs

During the energy crisis in the 1970s, building construction practices changed: homes, offices, schools, and all buildings were insulated and sealed tightly. This method saves a great deal of energy, but tends to trap indoor air pollution, including pollens, oils, dry cleaning fluid (a known liver toxin), and other allergens. Chemicals, such as benzene (a carcinogen), are released from paint, new carpets, drapes, and upholstery. Formaldehyde vapors rise up from plywood, new cabinets, furniture, carpets, drapes, wallpaper, and paneling. All enter the body through the lungs.

Herbs for Lung Detoxification—Herbs are frequently used to target specific aspects of lung contamination and detoxification:

- Fenugreek and horehound help decrease production and thickness of mucus secretions; a typical dose is 500 mg daily.
- Wild cherry bark is an expectorant that helps remove mucus and congestion; typical recommended dose is 250 mg daily.
- To strengthen lung tissue, use the herbs mullein (500 mg), elecampane (500 mg), and grindelia (250 mg).
- Eucalyptus and thyme oil (2-3 drops each) are antiseptics that kill microbial organisms; a combination of these herbs can be taken as a tincture (½ tsp, three times per day).

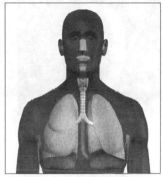

The lungs and respiratory system are important avenues of detoxification.

Inhalation Therapy—Steam inhalation can be very helpful for detoxifying the lungs. To a pot of boiling water, add two to three drops of eucalyptus and thyme oils. Remove the pot from the stove and place your head above the steam. Create a "tent" by covering your head with a towel and inhale the steam vapors. Be sure to keep your head far enough above the steam so as not to get burned.

For more information about **yoga breathing techniques**, see Chapter 14: Exercises and Physical Therapies, pp. 314-339.

Exercise—Exercise helps the lungs by increasing the perfusion of blood, which causes an enhanced intake of oxygen and *qi* (vital life force energy) and increased expiration of waste products. Aerobic exercises, such as running, cycling, and walking, can help clear the lungs. However, aerobic activity needs to be done in fresh, clean air— running in a polluted environment only increases the overall body burden of toxins and should be avoided. Yoga breathing techniques are excellent for cleansing the lungs and increasing oxygen levels in the body. They are especially useful for arthritis patients, who may be in too much pain to do aerobic exercises.

6 Eradicating Bacteria and Yeast

THERE ARE OVER 400 SPECIES of bacteria living in the human body and the majority of these bacteria reside in the gastrointestinal tract. Under conditions of intestinal health, "friendly" bacteria (such as *Lactobacillus acidophilus* and *Bifidobacterium bifidum*) predominate and contribute to digestion and the overall health of the body. But, increasingly, the shift observed today is towards a predominance of pathogenic bacteria, a condition of intestinal imbalance called dysbiosis. The unfriendly or pathogenic bacteria that dominate the intestines impair digestion, the absorption of nutrients, and the normal elimination cycle.

In This Chapter

- What Causes Intestinal Imbalance?
- The Role of Intestinal Toxins in Arthritis
- Bacteria and Arthritis
- Success Story: Treating *Candida* Relieves Juvenile Arthritis
- Illuminating the *Candida* Connection
- Diagnosing a Yeast Overgrowth
- Ridding the Arthritic Body of *Candida*

They also provoke allergic reactions to food and contribute to the erosion of the intestinal membrane and the infiltration of inappropriate substances into the bloodstream—a condition referred to as "leaky gut syndrome."

Dysbiosis is considered a primary cause or major cofactor in the development of many health problems, such as rheumatoid arthritis, acne, chronic fatigue, depression, digestive disorders, bloating, food allergies, PMS, and cancer. Of the pathogenic bacteria most significantly implicated in arthritis, there are three of special interest—the bacteria *Klebsiella* and *Proteus* and the yeast-like fungus *Candida*. Until they are eliminated and intestinal balance is restored, it is unlikely that individuals with arthritis will have their problem completely reversed.

What Causes Intestinal Imbalance?

The modern North American way of eating is largely responsible for dysbiosis. The foods we eat are not pure and, to an extent, full of poi-

---

Alternative Medicine Therapies for Bacteria and Yeast

- Dietary Recommendations
- Ayurvedic Anti-Fungal Therapies
- Herbal Remedies
- Nutritional Supplements
- Probiotics

---

sons. The typical diet is replete with meat products, which contain large amounts of chemical residues from the pesticides and herbicides used in livestock feed, and hormones and antibiotics used to make the animals grow larger and more rapidly. Ingestion of antibiotics, either through food products or prescribed medication, severely alters the intestinal flora by killing off bacteria, including beneficial microorganisms. As the bacterial communities repopulate after prolonged use of antibiotics, the colonic environment favors the growth of disease-causing organisms in lieu of the healthier bacteria.

We also tend to eat too many of the nutritionally wrong foods. Consider the huge amount of sugar and refined carbohydrates found in what's called the Standard American Diet (SAD). It is a sad diet indeed, for it has led to a nation with a staggering number of obese individuals and has caused chronic aberrations in the digestive flora. The SAD decreases the amount of intestinal secretions that aid in the proper breakdown of foods and this favors the overgrowth of pathogenic microorganisms.

In addition, we're not completely digesting the foods we eat. To properly handle foods we've eaten, the body depends on the stomach's digestive juices and enzymes (SEE QUICK DEFINITION) secreted by the pancreas. But many people now have a deficiency of both hydrochloric acid (the stomach's main digestive acid) and the four main forms of pancreatic enzymes, and this leads to incomplete digestion. When foods are not digested properly, especially amino acids (from

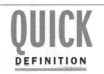

QUICK
DEFINITION

Enzymes are specialized living proteins fundamental to all living processes in the body, necessary for every chemical reaction and the normal activity of our organs, tissues, fluids, and cells. Enzymes are essential for the production of energy required to run cellular functions. There are hundreds of thousands of these "Nature's workers." Enzymes enable the body to digest and assimilate food: protease digests proteins, amylase digests carbohydrates, lipase digests fats, cellulase digests fiber, and disaccharidase digests sugars. Enzymes also assist in clearing the body of toxins and cellular debris.

Dysbiosis is a major cofactor in the development of many health problems, such as rheumatoid arthritis, acne, chronic fatigue, depression, digestive disorders, food allergies, PMS, and cancer. Until eliminated, it is unlikely that individuals with arthritis will have their problem completely reversed.

For more about **the role of enzymes in health and disease**, see *The Enzyme Cure* (Future Medicine Publishing, 1998; ISBN 1-887299-22-X); to order, call 800-333-HEAL.

For an **in-depth discussion of leaky gut**, see Chapter 8: Alleviating Leaky Gut Syndrome, pp. 172-190.

proteins), they putrefy in the intestines and release toxins (endogenous toxins, or endotoxins, meaning toxins produced within the body) into the system. For example, the amino acids arginine and ornithine are ingested in the course of a normal diet, but if your system is unable to process them completely, they undergo unfavorable chemical changes. Ornithine is converted into a toxic substance called putrescine, which then degrades into polyamines, such as spermadine, spermine, and cadaverine. These endotoxins tend to be elevated in individuals with psoriatic arthritis and other forms of arthritis.

Leaky Gut

In an unhealthy state of dysbiosis, the cellular "glue" that keeps the mucosal membrane of the intestines intact is slowly attacked and eventually develops gaping holes—initiating leaky gut syndrome. The substances that were once sealed off from the body can now easily pass through and trigger inflammatory cascades, allergic reactions, and more serious illnesses such as arthritis. As the intestinal "garbage" escapes into the bloodstream, the immune system attacks what it perceives as antigens (foreign bodies) and inflammation results. This inflammation produces the symptoms of most gastrointestinal disorders (bloating, flatulence, heartburn, diarrhea, constipation) when it occurs locally or the symptoms of arthritis when inflammation occurs in joints or skin. Endotoxins are often elevated in the blood of people with arthritis as well as those with migraine headaches, acne, and eczema.[1]

The overall body burden of circulating immune complexes (SEE QUICK DEFINITION) increases as a result of leaky gut. According to Joseph Pizzorno, N.D., some of the toxic by-products produced by pathogenic microorganisms are carcinogens (cancer-causing agents). They mimic neurotransmitters that then damage brain and nervous system tissues and interfere with neurological functions. Intestinal endotoxins also block the energy pathways of the body, particularly the Krebs cycle (SEE QUICK DEFINITION), which occurs in the mitochondria (energy-producing centers) of all the body's cells.[2]

The Role of Intestinal Toxins in Arthritis

Intestinally produced toxins can contribute to the arthritis process by stimulating non-cellular inflammatory cascades in the body. Specifically, inflammation is triggered by endotoxins, various bacteria such as *Streptococcus*, *Candida spp.* and other members of the yeast family, compounds produced by the yeast as part of their metabolic processes, and various food allergens (particularly yeast, either brewer's or baker's). To understand what this means, consider that inflammation in itself is a good thing—a homeostatic (balance-maintaining) mechanism by which the body deals with foreign material that doesn't belong within its tissues. The inflammatory response or process includes the biochemical pathways initiated by the immune system and the migration of additional white blood cells (immune defense cells) into a particular problem area.

Intestinal toxins can trigger inflammation (remember, this is one of the hallmarks of arthritis) by stimulating a non-cellular part of the immune system known as the complement pathway. This is a technical term referring to a series of 28 proteins that are activated in a chain reaction when the immune system senses a foreign protein (antigen) present. The complement system's legitimate job is to amplify inflammation, because the body's goal is to clean itself out, to flush out of the tissues the circulating immune complexes. The complement system summons additional white blood cells to the contaminated tissues to start cleansing them of this inappropriately deposited foreign matter. When the inflammatory response gets out of control, however, then the condition shifts into a

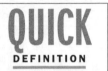

QUICK
DEFINITION

Circulating immune complexes (CICs) form in the body when poor digestion results in undigested food proteins "leaking" through the intestinal wall and into the bloodstream. The immune system treats these foreign substances or antigens as invaders, causing antibodies to form and couple with them. This antigen and antibody combination is known as a CIC. In a healthy person, CICs are neutralized and filtered out by the liver, but in someone with a compromised immune system, they tend to accumulate in the blood where they burden the detoxification pathways or initiate an allergic reaction. If too many CICs accumulate, the kidneys and liver cannot excrete enough of them via the urine or stool. The CICs are then stored in soft tissues, causing inflammation and bringing stress to the immune system. The overload can lead to a variety of chronic health conditions.

The **Krebs cycle** (also known as the citric acid cycle) is a metabolic process that occurs in each cell of the body in a small organelle called the mitochondria. It is an essential step in cellular respiration (the exchange of oxygen and carbon dioxide between the cell and the environment) and can be compared to the refinement of crude oil into high-grade, octane-rich petroleum. Foods consumed are transformed by digestion into smaller molecules of glucose, fatty acids, and amino acids; these are further converted into carbon compounds called pyruvates and acetates. In the Krebs cycle, acetates and pyruvates are converted into carbon dioxide and four pairs of electrons. It is the energy found in these electrons that is eventually stored in the molecule called adenosine triphosphate (ATP). ATP is analogous to refined gasoline and is the human fuel that provides energy to every cell.

disease process and localized healthy tissues start getting damaged by the excessive white blood cell activity. White blood cells release powerful peroxides (like hydrogen peroxide) that oxidize invaders as well as healthy tissues. When this continues long enough, arthritis begins.

The liver is also involved in this short-lived, natural inflammatory response. Under normal conditions, the liver traps about 99% of the bacteria that has escaped from the intestines.[3] Intestinal endotoxins activate the liver's Kupffer cells, immune cells residing in the liver, which cause a release of interleukin 2. Interleukin 2 is a lymphokine, a chemical that calls in other white blood cells to the area to clean up the "gut garbage," a process that increases inflammation.[4] If the liver is overburdened, weakened, or compromised by poor diet, excessive toxins, or other factors, it becomes less efficient at processing the circulating immune complexes. These complexes then escape the liver's filtering system and enter the body's connective tissues, producing inflammation and eventually tissue damage. Another side effect of increased toxins and subsequent white blood cell infiltration is an elevation in the number of free radicals. These free radicals generated by the white blood cells can quickly deplete the body's supplies of antioxidants and initiate inflammation and damage throughout the body.

Bacteria and Arthritis

In the 1970s, a British immunologist named Alan Ebringer, M.D., a member of the Department of Rheumatology at both Middlesex Hospital and Kings College in London, suggested a correlation

Microorganisms Implicated in the Development of Arthritis

Severe Pathogens

Streptococcus species (spp.)	*Campylobacter spp.*
Yersinia enterocolitica	*Yersinia pseudotuberculosis*
Shigella spp.	*Salmonella spp.*

Dysbiotic Organisms (organisms of low intrinsic virulence that can induce disease in host if conditions warrant)

Hemolytic E. Coli	*Mucoid E. Coli*
Citrobacter freundii	*Bacillus spp.*
Bacteroides fragilus	*Morganella spp.*
Enterobacter spp.	*Pseudomonas spp.*
Klebsiella spp.	*Proteus spp.*
Aeromonas spp.	

Fungi/Yeast Associated With Arthritis

Candida albicans	*Candida tropicalis*
Candida spp.	*Rhodotorula*
Geotrichum	*Trichospora spp.*
Fungal conidia	

between ankylosing spondylitis (a type of arthritis that affects the back and spine), a specific bacteria, and a specific human gene. People suffering from ankylosing spondylitis often carry a genetic marker called HLA-B27, Dr. Ebringer said.[5] In fact, he found that 96% of ankylosing spondylitis patients have the gene. When the HLA-B27 gene is expressed or activated, it forms a particular pattern on the surface of the cell. These patterns are how the immune system recognizes a friend or a foe in the body and keeps it from attacking "friendly" tissues.

The *Klebsiella* bacteria has cell surface markers very similar to the pattern on human cells with the gene HLA-B27, a phenomenon called "molecular mimicry." The similarity acts as an effective camouflage technique for the bacteria, allowing them to hide from the host's immune system. However, once the immune system does recognize the bacteria and begins to attack it, it then also attacks its own body tissues with similar cell surface markers.[6] The body's reaction to its own tissues as something foreign is called an autoimmune disease, a potentially serious health problem.

Dr. Ebringer found that many ankylosing spondylitis patients have intestinal overgrowth of *Klebsiella* and high blood levels of *Klebsiella* antibodies, and that *Klebsiella* antigens (proteins recognized by the immune system as foreign substances) cross-react with HLA-B27, initiating inflammation and leading to bacterial reactive arthritis.[7] This condition arises when the immune system begins to attack the *Klebsiella* bacteria and simultaneously begins attacking the body's own tissues. In essence, Dr. Ebringer proposed that *Klebsiella* microbes present in the bowel act as triggers for the development of ankylosing spondylitis. Dr. Ebringer also found that men had more *Klebsiella* in their bowels than women, and this, he thought, may explain why ankylosing spondylitis is almost three times as prevalent in men as it is in women. His research further indicated that *Klebsiella* can inhabit areas of the body other than the digestive system, triggering a process of tissue self-destruction. Other bacteria, such as *Salmonella*, *Yersinia*, and *Shigella*, can also trigger inflammatory reactive arthritis.

Ankylosing spondylitis patients suffer increased stiffness and pain in the back, spine, and buttocks, particularly of the low back in the morning. Chronic inflammation in this region of the body leads to the development of bone bridges or osteophytes; eventually these can take an otherwise mobile joint and "ankylose" or fuse it. Dr. Ebringer contended that ankylosing spondylitis is actually the end stage disease of repeated flare-ups or episodes of *Klebsiella*-reactive arthritis. Thus, *Klebsiella*, thought to be a semi-pathogenic resident of the colon, now seems to be linked with arthritis.

Evidence also exists that rheumatoid arthritis may be linked with the *Proteus* bacterium, specifically *Proteus vulgaris* and *Proteus mirabilis*. These bacteria have similar markers to cell surfaces that carry the HLA-DR4 gene. High levels of antibodies to *Proteus* have been found in rheumatoid arthritis patients.[8] It's possible, Dr. Ebringer speculated, that the reason two thirds of sufferers of rheumatoid arthritis are women is because *Proteus* also causes urinary tract infections, to which women are far more susceptible than men (because of the anatomical proximity of the anus to the vaginal opening).

Our clinical research, based on the results of numerous stool analyses from patients, is that many other microorganisms are associated with arthritis, specifically with rheumatoid arthritis. For instance, in people with juvenile arthritis, species of *Streptococcus*, some of which are considered to be non-problematic, tend to be among the most dominant flora of the colon. These patients often have high levels of antibodies to *Streptococcus* bacteria, which, incidentally, may also derive from infected root canals and underlying gum disease. Many times when these patients have dental work, they have a strong exacerbation of their symptoms, such as an increase in stiffness and joint swelling and elevation of inflammation, developments that suggest a link between these bacterial species and rheumatoid arthritis.

Diagnosing Pathogenic Bacteria Overgrowth

The stool analysis is a way of seeing how digestive inadequacies may be contributing to your illness. It consists of a group of nearly two dozen tests performed on a stool sample and can be ordered by your physician. The tests reveal how well you are digesting your food and absorbing nutrients, the proportions of friendly versus unfriendly bacteria in your intestine, if bacteria and yeasts such as *Candida* are present, and whether or not your diet contains adequate fiber. All of these factors may be contributing to your arthritis.

For information about the **Comprehensive Digestive Stool Analysis**, contact: Great Smokies Diagnostic Laboratory, 63 Zillicoa Street, Asheville, NC 28801; tel: 800-522-4762 or 704-253-0021. Lab staff will also make referrals to physicians

The Anti-*Klebsiella* Starch-Free Diet

Dr. Ebringer discovered that *Klebsiella* (like *Candida*) thrives on a diet rich in refined carbohydrates and starch. If you cut out starchy carbohydrates, such as rice, potatoes, and flour products, as well as refined sugars and fruit juices, then you reduce the number of *Klebsiella* in the intestines. Subsequently, fewer antibodies to this bacteria are produced, which otherwise would cause inflammation as the body began to attack itself (the inflammatory cascade). Dr. Ebringer contends that this low-starch diet leads to a reduction in the total amount of IgA (a specific antibody usually associated with the gastrointestinal tract) in the blood, thereby decreasing inflammation and symptoms of ankylosing spondylitis.

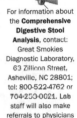

For more detailed information on the **Comprehensive Digestive Stool Analysis**, see Chapter 3: Diagnosing Arthritis, pp. 52-77. For **detailed dietary recommendations for arthritis**, see Chapter 12: The Arthritis Diet, pp. 250-278. For **colon-cleansing programs**, see Chapter 5: Detoxifying Specific Organs, pp. 102-129.

Dr. Ebringer's diet is devoid of bread, flour, potatoes, rice, pasta, and other starchy products.[9] The diet does allow for protein sources, eggs, fruits, and vegetables, particularly the non-starchy vegetables (dark leafy greens, such as kale, Swiss chard, and broccoli), to be eaten without restriction. Our modifications of this diet include adding digestive enzymes (to properly break down the starches, proteins, and other substances) and antimicrobial therapy (such as herbs that fight microbes and colon-cleansing programs) to kill the *Klebsiella* bacteria. Using these dietary recommendations, along with the Arthritis Diet, will help the body fight off any kind of invading microorganism, curing ankylosing spondylitis.

Success Story: Treating *Candida* Relieves Juvenile Arthritis

Essie, 16, presented with a case of juvenile rheumatoid arthritis (RA). Her family history, including a cousin who had also suffered from juvenile arthritis and an aunt with lupus (an autoimmune condition characterized by skin lesions), indicated a genetic predisposition for her condition. The onset of RA occurred suddenly, initially with symptoms of fatigue, musculoskeletal pains, nausea, and loss of appetite. Essie's pediatrician had put her on a course of antibiotics, which had provided her with no relief whatsoever. She was then treated with a series of drugs—including nonsteroidal, anti-inflammatory drugs (NSAIDs), prednisone, Imuran®, and gold injections, among others—none of which led to any relief. In fact, the medications caused a number of severe side effects, including nausea, chronic headaches, liver inflammation, anemia, and fatigue.

When we first examined Essie, she had large synovial pouches (areas of swelling containing joint fluid) at the wrists, elbows, knee joints, and ankles. Earlier blood tests had revealed an elevated sedimentary rate and elevated rheumatoid factor, both diagnostic indicators for arthritis.

We ran a food allergy (IgG ELISA) test, which showed that Essie was sensitive to barley, wheat and buckwheat, broccoli, grapefruit, oranges, beef, and lamb. Wheat, broccoli, and orange juice were foods she consumed in large quantities. A hair analysis to test for heavy metals revealed high levels of copper, mercury, and aluminum. The test also revealed that Essie was deficient in two trace minerals, molybdenum and germanium.

Another blood test revealed high levels of the immunoglobulin (SEE QUICK DEFINITION) IgM, indicating an infection of the yeast-like fungus *Candida albicans*. Her IgM antibody level was 51.5; a normal level would be less than 12.5. A urinalysis showed an elevated level of leukocytes (white blood cells), protein in the urine as well as blood, a high specific gravity (indicating excess sediments in the urine and kidney stress), and a trace amount of ketones (indicating excess protein in the urine). These test results made us suspect bladder inflammation or a urinary tract infection.

Using a darkfield microscope (SEE QUICK DEF-INITION), we examined Essie's blood. Her red blood cells were slightly low in number (anemia) and were abnormally clumped together. We also saw long tubules in the blood, which usually indicates the presence of parasites or other infectious microorganisms. Red and yellow crystals in the blood corresponded to her joint pain. Finally, her blood contained high levels of yeast forms, confirming the presence of *Candida*.

The last test we ran was a stool analysis, which showed that Essie was producing insufficient amounts of digestive enzymes and hydrochloric acid (the primary stomach acid). We also found occult (hidden) blood, an indication of bleeding in the intestinal tract, perhaps caused by her drug therapy. She had a zero reading on the friendly bacteria *Lactobacillus acidophilus*, which indicated an imbalance in her intestinal flora, and a positive finding for parasite infection.

Clearly, we needed to address not just Essie's arthritis symptoms but her underlying health problems as well. Our goal was to reduce the number of drugs she was taking, which were adversely affecting her. We needed to treat the *Candida* and parasite infections, rebuild her digestive system, decrease the pain and swelling in her joints, and decrease her fatigue and other symptoms.

To begin, we gave Essie an intravenous infusion of vitamins, minerals, antioxidants, and amino acids to build up her depleted nutrient reserves and to support her liver function. We started her on several homeopathic remedies (SEE QUICK DEFINITION) from Professional Health Products in Pittsburgh, Pennsylvania: Opsin I (ten drops with meals) for her food allergies and several formulas, Joint Pain Formula for Large Joints, Pain Formula, Rheuma Pain Drops, and Anti-Rheumatic Drops (ten drops of each formula, three times daily, between meals), for pain.

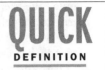

DEFINITION

An **immunoglobulin** is one of a class of five specially designed antibody proteins produced in the spleen, bone marrow, or lymph tissue and involved in the immune system's defense response to foreign substances. The main types of immunoglobulins, grouped according to their concentration in the blood, are: IgG (80%), IgA (10%-15%), IgM (5%-10%), IgD (less than 0.1%), and IgE (less than 0.01%).

Darkfield microscopy is a way of studying living whole blood cells under a specially adapted microscope that projects the dynamic image, magnified 1,400 times, onto a video screen. The skilled physician can detect early signs of illness in the form of microorganisms in the blood known to produce disease. Relevant technical features in the blood include color, variously shaped components (such as spicules, long tubules, and roulous), and the size of certain immune cells. The amount of time the blood cell stays viable and alive indicates the overall health of the individual. Specifically, darkfield microscopy reveals distortions of red blood cells (which indicate nutritional status), possible undesirable bacterial or fungal life forms, and blood ecology patterns indicative of health or illness.

Homeopathy was founded in the early 1800s by German physician Samuel Hahnemann. Today, an estimated 500 million people worldwide receive homeopathic treatment; in Britain, homeopathy enjoys royal patronage. Homeopathy is now practiced according to two differing concepts. In classical homeopathy, only one single-component remedy is prescribed at a time, in a potency specifically adjusted to the patient; the physician waits to see the results before prescribing anything further. In complex homeopathy, typified by *Hepar compositum*, a prescription involves multiple substances given at the same time, usually in low potencies.

To treat her *Candida*, we gave Essie a probiotic supplement containing the friendly bacteria *L. acidophilus* and *B. bifidum*. Friendly bacteria are beneficial microbes inhabiting the human gastrointestinal tract where they are essential for proper nutrient assimilation. Friendly bacteria are natural antagonists for *Candida* and supplementing with them helps normalize intestinal flora.

We gave her Adreno-Max and Chronic Fatigue Support Formula, two supplements developed by Serafina Corsello, M.D., of New York City. Adreno-Max supports the adrenal glands and contains vitamin C, pantothenic acid, and raw adrenal concentrate. The other formula is excellent for fighting fatigue and supporting the immune system. Ingredients include multiple vitamins and minerals, echinacea, shiitake mushroom, burdock root, licorice, and digestive enzymes, among others. For joint support, we gave her another Corsello formula called Bone Plus, containing calcium, magnesium, and vitamins D and K1.

We recommended a number of dietary changes for Essie. Clearly, she needed to avoid the foods that she had tested positive to on the allergy test. We also advised her to avoid nightshade vegetables (tomatoes, green peppers, white potatoes) as these seem to aggravate arthritis symptoms. Her diet was to consist of free-range, organic turkey, chicken, and fish, once per week for each; otherwise, she was to follow a vegetarian diet high in dark-green leafy vegetables and lots of steamed vegetables of different colors. We encouraged her to eat several small meals throughout the day and to chew each bite thoroughly to ease the stress on her digestive system.

It is also important for arthritis patients to get the right oils or essential fatty acids (EFAs—SEE QUICK DEFINITION) in their diet because of their effect on inflammation. Essie was to use a salad dressing, made with organic flaxseed and olive oils, lemon juice, and herbs, on her salads and vegetables. Flaxseed and olive oils are excellent sources of omega-3 EFAs. She also started supplementing with Omega Balance (one capsule, twice daily), a balanced blend of EFAs.

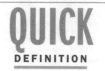

QUICK DEFINITION

Essential fatty acids (EFAs) are unsaturated fats required in the diet. Omega-3 and omega-6 oils are the two principal types. The primary omega-3 oil is alpha-linolenic acid (ALA), found in flaxseed and canola oils, as well as pumpkins, walnuts, and soybeans. Fish oils, such as salmon, cod, and mackerel, contain the other important omega-3 oils, DHA (docosahexaenoic acid) and EPA (eicosapentaenoic acid). Linoleic acid is the main omega-6 oil and is found in most vegetable oils, including safflower, corn, peanut, and sesame. The most therapeutic form of omega-6 oil is gamma-linolenic acid (GLA), found in evening primrose, black currant, and borage oils. Once in the body, omega-3 and omega-6 are converted to these oils into prostaglandins, hormone-like substances that regulate many metabolic functions, particularly inflammatory processes.

Reflexology is based on the idea that there are reflex areas in the hands and feet that correspond to every part of the body, including the organs and glands. By applying gentle but precise pressure to these reflex points, reflexologists can release blockages that inhibit energy flow and cause pain and disease. Practitioners often focus on breaking up lactic acid and calcium crystals accumulated around any of the 7,200 nerve endings in each foot. Eunice Ingham, a physiotherapist, pioneered the discipline in this country in the late 1930s. He mapped out reflexes on the feet and developed techniques for inducing healing effects in those areas.

We also recommended physical therapy for Essie. She paid weekly visits to a chiropractor and massage therapist and we taught her mother to give her reflexology (SEE QUICK DEFINITION) and massage treatments. We also instituted energy balancing using reiki and similar techniques. After several months on this treatment protocol, Essie's attitude and energy levels were greatly improved. She had adjusted to the rotation diet and her bowel movements were much more regular as well, indicating that her gastrointestinal tract was improving. We started her on anti-parasitic herbs at this stage. After another month, Essie was able to go completely off the medications she had been taking for her arthritis. After a year-and-a-half on the program, Essie was pain-free except for occasional bouts of inflammation due to stress or lapses in her diet, her *Candida* infection was under control, and she felt considerably better.

For more information on **homeopathic remedies**, contact: Professional Health Products, P.O. Box 5897, Pittsburgh, PA 15209; tel: 800-245-1313; fax: 412-821-0520. For **Adreno-Max, Bone Plus, Chronic Fatigue Support Formula**, and **Omega Balance**, contact: Global Nutrition, 175 E. Main Street, Huntington, NY 11743; tel: 888-461-0949 or 516-271-0222; fax: 516-271-5992.

Illuminating the *Candida* Connection

While there are many species of microorganisms that can overgrow in the body and cause an increase in intestinal permeability, of prime concern here is *Candida albicans*. This is a yeast-like fungus found widely in nature, in the soil, on vegetables and fruits, and in the human body. It is frequently present in small quantities in the intestines and in the vagina. *Candida* overgrowth, a condition called candidiasis, can become pathogenic and cause allergic reactions throughout the body. These reactions can lead to a wide range of symptoms, including depression, fatigue, weight gain, anxiety, rashes, headaches, and muscle cramping.

Predisposing factors for candidiasis include the use of steroid hormone medications such as cortisone or corticosteroids, which are often prescribed for skin problems; prolonged or repeated use of antibiotics; oral contraceptive use; estrogen therapy; and a diet high in sugar, both natural and refined. Certain illnesses, such as AIDS, cancer, and diabetes, which are accompanied by extreme immune suppression, can also increase susceptibility to *Candida* overgrowth.

This organism changes form as it develops, and sends hyphae (microscopic "root-like" filaments) through the intestinal wall, similar to the way English ivy grows up a wall and adheres to the bricks. This analogy is helpful in understanding how *Candida* produces illness. The ivy's rootlets infiltrate the mortar between the bricks and severely

Candida—A Stealth Pathogen

The concept that *Candida albicans* (or other strains of *Candida*) can pass through the intestines into general blood circulation was first established many years ago, yet in conventional medical circles, the importance of *Candida* involvement in health is still largely undervalued. In 1969, W. Krause, Ph.D., demonstrated that intact *Candida albicans* organisms are capable of escaping the intestinal tract and reaching the blood and urine in humans.

After he was carefully screened for any prior illness or exposure to *Candida*, Dr. Krause ingested a large dose of *Candida albicans* orally. In a surprisingly short time, just a few hours later, he developed numerous symptoms, including headaches and fever. The scientists working with Dr. Krause were able to culture *Candida* organisms from his blood and urine; the colonies were found to be identical to the strain administered.[11] Dr. Krause's bold experiment proved that it is possible for *Candida* to cross the gastrointestinal tract in a viable form and cause systemic illness in healthy patients.

The researchers also concluded that antibiotic use may be a common precursor in cases of systemic candidiasis and increased intestinal permeability. Despite Dr. Krause's experiment, there is still controversy over the idea that *Candida* can systemically translocate to distant sites in the body as a kind of "stealth pathogen" and cause illness.

damages it, eventually to the extent of disintegration. Similarly, *Candida*'s root-like filaments become attached to the intestinal wall and loosen the intracellular "cement" (the connective tissue between cells), create holes through the cell membranes, and release toxic waste products that circulate throughout the system, causing an increase in toxemia in the body. This results in joint and connective tissue damage through stimulation of the complement system (immune response).

Yeasts like *Candida* contain decarboxylases, enzymes that convert (and putrefy) amino acids (protein building-blocks) into vasoactive amines (such as putrescine from arginine and ornithine, and indican from tryptophane), which cause alterations in the permeability of blood vessels and other tissues and affect how easily materials penetrate the walls of cells. Vasoactive amines can cause leaky gut syndrome and dissolve the intestinal membrane that holds the cells of the gastrointestinal system together.

Candida albicans can also produce over 400 mycotoxins, any of which can cause systemic illness. A mycotoxin is a fungal poison; more specifically, it is a toxic chemical released into the blood as a by-product of the yeast's metabolism or from cell fragments from dead yeast cells. Some of these mycotoxins, like acetylaldehyde and alcohol, can produce the feelings of being "hung over" that many patients affected with *Candida* tend to experience. One mycotoxin in particular, gliotoxin, has been shown to suppress the immune system, particularly the ability of the white blood cells to engulf foreign material. It suppresses the thymus gland, the lymph nodes, the spleen, and the bone marrow in the production of white blood cells. Gliotoxin also interferes with normal glutathione metabolism within the cell; the depletion of glutathione not only robs the person of this important antioxidant needed for liver detoxification, but it contributes to other systemic illnesses associated with low levels of glutathione, such as allergies and symptoms of chemical hypersensitivity.[10]

Arthritis and *Candida*

The presence of elevated levels of *Candida* in the body is highly relevant for arthritis patients. Muscle aches, pain and swelling in the joints, loss of energy, and chronic muscular tightness—in other words, the key symptoms of arthritis—are all symptoms of *Candida albicans* overgrowth. Yeast also acts as a direct instigator of the complement pathways, leading to inflammation and joint dysfunction.

Although activation of the complement system can help the body rid itself of invading foreign organisms, over-activation by a *Candida* infection can cause significant damage to healthy body tissues. *Candida* stimulates the immune system to summon aggressive white blood cells. Once stimulated, these white blood cells destroy all cells in the area, including *Candida* and other pathogens as well as the body's own cell membranes and tissues. In patients with arthritis, significant damage occurs in the joints through this mechanism, because the tissues attacked include the lining of the joints and the cartilage.[12] In addition to *Candida* and fungal forms present in the intestines, many other infective agents can initiate joint inflammation, even though they originate in other areas of the body. Some examples include chronic bacterial inflammation of the sinus cavities, infections of the

An elevated level of *Candida* in the body is highly relevant for arthritis patients. Muscle aches, pain and swelling in the joints, loss of energy, and chronic muscular tightness—in other words, the key symptoms of arthritis—are all symptoms of *Candida albicans* overgrowth.

gums and teeth (including abscesses, cavities, and root canals), and inflammation of the adenoids or tonsils. All provide constant sources of bacteria that can initiate or worsen any arthritis already present.

Scientific studies have observed the role of yeast in psoriasis. E.W. Rosenburg, M.D., professor and researcher at the University of Tennessee Center for Health Sciences in Memphis, reported that his patients with psoriasis responded favorably to oral nystatin, a conventional drug typically used for yeasts in the gastrointestinal tract.[13]

Diagnosing a Yeast Overgrowth

The diagnosis of a *Candida albicans* overgrowth in those with arthritis can be made using any or all of these means:

Symptom Questionnaire—William Crook, M.D., author of *The Yeast Connection*, popularized the idea that *Candida* can create numerous health problems. During the course of his research, Dr. Crook developed a reliable questionnaire for assessing potential *Candida* involvement in a patient's health picture. Among the questions are the following (positive answers may indicate a yeast infection):

- Have you taken repeated courses of antibiotics or steroids (e.g., cortisone)?
- Have you used birth-control pills?
- Have you had repeated fungal infections ("jock itch," athlete's foot, ringworm)?
- Do you regularly have any of these symptoms—bloating, headaches, depression, fatigue, memory problems, impotence or lack of interest in sex, muscle aches with no apparent cause, brain fogginess?
- Do you experience symptoms of PMS (pre-menstrual syndrome)?
- Do you have cravings for sweets, products containing white flour, or alcoholic beverages?
- Do you repeatedly experience any of these health difficulties—inappropriate drowsiness, mood swings, rashes, bad breath, dry mouth, post-nasal drip or nasal congestion, heartburn, urinary frequency or urgency?[14]

A study conducted at Bastyr University showed the degree of *Candida albicans* growth in stool cultures correlated well with the symptomatic scores (for the same patients) on Dr. Crook's *Candida* questionnaire.[15] In another study, published in 1997, out of 854 patients considered, the predominant fungal species isolated were *Candida albicans* (64.5%), followed by *Candida tropicalis* (23.3%) and *Candida krusei* (6.9%).[16] Other fungal species, such as *Trichosporon*,

Geotrichum, Rhodotorula, and *Conida,* are lesser-known fungi that can also contribute to the "yeast connection" and, ultimately, to arthritis.

Candida Antibody Titer Blood Test—This tests for the body's reaction to the presence of *Candida* as indicated by the levels of antibodies IgA, IgM, and IgG, rather than measuring the level of *Candida* directly. The test is useful, but not totally reliable. If positive, it can indicate past or present *Candida* infection somewhere in the body, but it may not indicate intestinal overgrowth. If negative, it may mean that although *Candida* is present, the body's immune mechanisms did not react appropriately to create the antibodies against *Candida.* This occurs in individuals with a compromised immune system.

Comprehensive Digestive Stool Analysis—This is a complete survey of the contents of the patient's stool sample. It can indicate digestive strengths or weaknesses and pinpoint causes of dysbiosis, including yeast overgrowth and parasitic infestation.

Darkfield Microscopy—Darkfield microscopy is a way of studying living whole blood cells under a specially adapted microscope that projects the dynamic image, magnified 1,400 times, onto a video screen. Although there is controversy about whether or not yeast can be seen in the blood, we have used the darkfield microscope to view fungal forms in living blood samples. We have also used yellow phosphorescent cellulose binding dye to identify different kinds of yeast forms.

Ridding the Arthritic Body of *Candida*

Successful treatment of candidiasis requires the reduction of factors that predispose a person to *Candida* overgrowth and the strengthening of immune function. Diet, nutritional supplements, herbal and Ayurvedic remedies, acupuncture, and enzyme therapy are some of the choices that can be used to help accomplish these ends.

Recovery from chronic candidiasis seldom takes less than three months and it may take much longer. However, many patients experience relief from some symptoms after only one week. For example, Adriane, 45, had joint swelling, fatigue, bloating after eating, and an inability to think clearly. She came to see us for help in discontinuing some of the NSAIDs and other drugs she was taking for her arthritis. After a full examination, we found that she had a high level of *Candida albicans* (four out of a possible score of five). Adriane agreed to start an anti-yeast diet individually tailored to her specific food allergies. Three days after starting this diet, Adriane noticed that, although she still had some joint pain, her stomach was much less bloated after eating and she was able to think more clearly. It took Adriane two years to completely resolve her arthritis, but she got the *Candida* under control in one month.

Dietary Recommendations

Reduce Dietary Sugars—Yeast thrives on any sugar, so to overcome candidiasis, sugar must be avoided in all its various forms. These include sucrose, dextrose, fructose, fruit juices, honey, maple syrup, molasses, milk products (which contain lactose), most fruits (except berries), and potatoes (their starch converts into sugar). Those with candidiasis should also avoid all alcohol since it is composed of fermented and refined sugar.

Arthritis patients are advised to avoid yogurt because of its high lactose (milk sugar) content and allergenicity, despite its high concentration of *Lactobacilli*, which suppress harmful bacteria and keep other organisms under control. Freeze-dried, nondairy-derived *acidophilus* supplements in capsule form are more effective in reducing bacteria than unsweetened raw yogurt.

Minimize Non-Organic Animal Protein Intake—Meat, dairy, and poultry consumption can foster *Candida* growth due to the large amount of antibiotics used in animal feed. Traces of antibiotics given to dairy cows can later show up in milk.[17] For example, the antibiotic tetracylcine is regularly used as a growth enhancer in poultry; traces of this antibiotic remain in the poultry tissue, then are passed on to humans who consume it. Antibiotics kill off all microflora living in the colon and give opportunistic organisms, such as *Candida*, a chance to repopulate areas once dominated by beneficial bacteria. Organic (hormone and antibiotic-free) meat and poultry should be consumed whenever possible. For people with candidiasis, seafood (free of mercury toxins) and vegetable protein are preferable, since they are not only antibiotic-free, but lower in fat.

Reduce Yeasted Foods Intake—Many people with candidiasis have allergies and sensitivities to various foods. Although *Candida albicans* is not the same as the yeast used in foods (such as bread), a cross-reactivity between yeasts and fungi frequently occurs. All foods containing or promoting yeast growth should be avoided, such as baked goods, alcohol, vinegar, and all vinegar-containing condiments. Rice cakes and rye crackers are good bread substitutes. Make your own vinegar-free salad dressing with olive oil, flaxseed oil, herbs, spices, and lemon juice; lime or vitamin C crystals can also be used to replace vinegar, as each can impart a suitably tangy taste. Probiotics such as *Lactobacillus acidophilus* and *Bifidobacteria* strains are important supplements in any anti-*Candida* program.

Avoid Molds—Molds are another aspect of *Candida* sensitivity. These include food molds (found in cheeses, grapes, mushrooms, and fermented foods) and environmental molds (found in wet climates, in damp basements, in plants, and outdoors). Mold and yeast can also exchange forms. Therefore, the ingestible molds of cheeses and fermented foods should be avoided. Avoiding food yeast and mold does not affect the *Candida* yeast itself, but is an attempt to ease stress on the immune system caused by substances which can trigger allergies.[18] Still, food yeast and mold avoidance should be considered on an individual basis.

Ayurvedic Anti-Fungal Therapies

Ayurvedic medicine (SEE QUICK DEFINITION) considers candidiasis to be a condition caused by ama, the improper digestion of foods, according to Virender Sodhi, M.D. (Ayurveda), N.D., of Bellevue, Washington. As do other alternative physicians, Dr. Sodhi attributes this malfunction, and thus candidiasis, to the widespread use of antibiotics, birth control pills, and hormones, environmental stress, and society's addiction to sugar in the diet. "Ayurvedic medicine believes that these stresses on the system cause carbohydrates to be digested improperly," he says. "Furthermore, the immune system in the gut becomes worn down." Dr. Sodhi's candidiasis protocol involves strengthening the immune system and improving digestion through stimulation of secretory IgA, the immunoglobulin, or antibody, found in the mucoid lining of the intestines and lungs; it may help prevent invasion of those surfaces by disease-producing bacteria and viruses.

To address the *Candida* overgrowth and thus bolster immunity, Dr. Sodhi uses grapefruit seed oil and tannic acid, which act as antifungals and

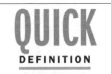

DEFINITION

Ayurveda is the traditional medicine of India, based on many centuries of empirical use. Its name means "end of the Vedas" (which were India's sacred scripts), implying that a holistic medicine may be founded on spiritual principles. Ayurveda describes three metabolic, constitutional, and body types (doshas), in association with the basic elements of Nature in combination. These are *vata* (air and ether, rooted in intestines), *pitta* (fire and water/stomach), and *kapha* (water and earth/lungs). Ayurvedic physicians use these categories (which also have psychological aspects) as the basis for prescribing individualized formulas of herbs, diet, massage, breathing, meditation, exercise and yoga postures, and detoxification techniques.

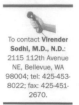

To contact **Virender Sodhi, M.D., N.D.**: 2115 112th Avenue NE, Bellevue, WA 98004; tel: 425-453-8022; fax: 425-451-2670.

antibiotics, and *acidophilus*, which helps restore the balance of friendly bacteria in the intestines. Long pepper, ginger, cayenne, and the Ayurvedic herbs trikatu and neem taken 30 minutes before meals increase immunoglobulin and digestive functions. He further recommends that his patients cleanse toxins from their systems using the *pancha karma* program, which involves herbs and dietary modification. With Dr. Sodhi's approach, candidiasis can usually be eliminated in four to six months.

Herbal Remedies

Herbs are often used to kill harmful yeasts and to shore up immune function. Herbs containing berberine (an alkaloid) have proven to be particularly useful for *Candida*. These include goldenseal, Oregon grape root, and barberry. Berberine acts as a natural antibiotic against *Candida* overgrowth, normalizes intestinal flora, helps digestive problems, and stimulates the immune system.[19] Other herbs helpful for candidiasis include artemisia, quassia bark, red clover, and pau d' arco. The commercial formula PlantiBiotic (which contains barberry, berberine, citrus seed extract, thyme oil, oregano oil, tea tree oil, garlic, and other herbs) is also helpful in treating *Candida* infections. We typically recommend a dose of two tablets, three times a day with food.

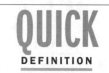

DEFINITION

Soil-based organisms (SBOs) are beneficial microbes, or probiotics, found in soil. Before chemical farming, the earth was rich in these organisms which naturally destroyed molds, yeast, fungi, and viruses in the soil . Transmitted to humans in the food supply, SBOs performed the same function in the human body, working with the "friendly" bacteria inhabiting the gastrointestinal tract to maintain balance in the intestinal flora and thus ensure a healthy digestive system. Since soil has become depleted of SBOs, the ratio of good to bad bacteria in the intestines has become skewed and a host of health problems, including allergies, candidiasis, and Crohn's disease among other gastrointestinal conditions, are the result.

Nutritional Supplements

Enzyme therapist Lita Lee, Ph.D., author of *The Enzyme Cure*, has three recommendations for treating candidiasis. First, Citricidal (grapefruit seed and pulp extract) which is a nontoxic antibacterial, anti-parasitic, anti-fungal, and antiviral; it kills 11 fungi, including *Candida albicans*. Typical dosage: 1-2 tablets (each tablet contains four drops), three times daily.

Second, Dr. Lee recommends soil-based organisms (SEE QUICK DEFINITION). This is an intestinal formula of beneficial bacteria, which kill pathological microbes and help prevent proliferation of toxins in the intestines. Typical dosage: one capsule daily, increasing by one capsule per week up to six capsules daily, in divided doses.

Third, Dr. Lee advises taking a multiple–digestive enzyme formula, determined by urinalysis, to address the foods the person has difficulty digesting or eats in excess. She also recommends a product called Thera-zyme SmI, which contains a form of cellulase (the enzyme that digests plant fiber) that breaks down pathogenic yeast into nontoxic particles, which are then eliminated through the urine and stool. The formula also contains *L. acidophilus* and *B. bifidum*, which reestablish friendly bowel flora, thus lessening the likelihood of yeast overgrowth in the future.

Probiotics—High-doses of probiotics or friendly bacteria such as *Bifidobacterium bifidum* and *Lactobacillus acidophilus, bulgaricus, plantarum,* and *salvarius,* are available as nutritional supplements. Treatment may last from eight to 12 weeks. Leon Chaitow, N.D., a British naturopath, reports an 80% success rate using this method in cases of seriously ill people afflicted with yeast overgrowth and parasites. Recolonizing the intestines with friendly bacteria can also help prevent illness by depriving the pathogenic (disease-causing) bacteria of the opportunity to overgrow and flourish.

Caprylic Acid (Capricin)—This is a fatty substance found in coconut oil that is an effective anti-fungal agent. Caprylic acid is readily absorbed into the body and should be taken in coated tablets or in a sustained-release form that ensures release in the small intestine rather than the stomach. In one study, 16 patients were given 1,800 mg daily of caprylic acid for 16 days, three patients were given 2,700 mg daily, and six received 3,600 mg per day. The results were a 30%-90% reduction in *Candida* levels among those with the 1,800-mg dosage; a 70%-100% reduction in the three patients taking 2,700 mg; and complete elimination in two weeks in all of those taking 3,600 mg.[21]

However, we have seen (through darkfield blood analysis) an increase in the fragility of red blood cells in patients who stay on caprylic acid for more than two months; perhaps the same factors that attack *Candida* also begin to attack blood cell membranes. We use caprylic acid only for

Why Friendly Bacteria are Essential to Your Health

A study of 154 newborns found that *L. acidophilus* given shortly after birth encouraged the growth of normal intestinal flora and reduced the number of opportunistic infections (particularly by the *Klebsiella* and *Staphylococcus aureus* bacteria) and inflammatory diseases in those infants. Another study demonstrated that *L. acidophilus* prevents the attachment of harmful bacteria to human intestinal cells, thus providing a barrier against these bacteria in the digestive system. The pathogenic bacteria affected included *E. coli*, *Salmonella typhimurium*, and *Yersinia pseudotuberculosis*. *L. acidophilus* is also effective against *Campylobacter pylori*, a common bacteria that causes acid-peptic disease. Researchers concluded that *L. acidophilus* is "a highly active antagonist for the treatment and prophylaxis of intestinal dysbacteriosis"; that is, it helps maintain the levels of healthy bacteria and fights off the unhealthy ones.

One of the common side effects of treatment with antibiotics (especially the broad-spectrum type) and with radiation therapy is that levels of both friendly and pathogenic bacteria are killed off, opening the door to yeast infestation and gastrointestinal distress, particularly diarrhea. Steroids, such as cortisone, and birth control pills can contribute to probiotic damage as well. Supplementing with *Lactobacilli* and other probiotics can restore the normal intestinal microflora damaged by antibiotics, according to several studies. In one double-blind study, 98 patients taking the antibiotic ampicillin were divided into two groups, one receiving a *Lactobacilli* supplement (four times daily for five days) while the other group received a placebo. There were no cases of ampicillin-induced diarrhea in the group receiving *Lactobacilli*, while 14% of the placebo group had diarrhea as a result of the antibiotics. Another study involved 27 patients with ear, sinus, or throat infections who were given the antibiotic amoxicillin/clavulanate; some of the patients were also given *L. acidophilus* at the same time as the antibiotic. According to the researchers, there was "a significant decrease in patient complaints of gastrointestinal side effects and yeast superinfection" in the group given *L. acidophilus* supplements.[20]

short-term intervention and rely on dietary and lifestyle changes for a long-term cure. Typical dosage: 1,800 mg to 3,500 mg per day. We often use a product called Mycopryl 680; the dosage is two capsules (680 mg each) with each meal, for up to eight weeks.

Garlic—It was Louis Pasteur, the 19th-century formulator of modern germ theory, who first recognized the antibiotic properties of garlic. Although now eclipsed by penicillin and other antibiotics, garlic often is more effective and more versatile in treating fungal, bacterial, and viral infections.[22] In treating the overgrowth of *Candida albicans*, researchers in the United States and Europe found that an injection of fresh raw garlic extract into *Candida*-infected cells inhibited growth of the fungus by 70%. Garlic far exceeded the success of other antibiotics and anti-fungals tested in that study. Allicin, the active anti-fungal component in garlic, attacks the surface of the *Candida* cells, alters its fat content, and oxidizes a group of its essential enzymes.[23] Allicin is potent—only a small concentration is needed to kill *Candida*—and garlic has the added benefit of stimulating the immune system rather than depressing it. Recommended dosage: two fresh cloves daily.

Oregano Oil—Oil of oregano, distilled from a species of oregano that grows prolifically on Mediterranean hillsides, is used to treat topical and internal candidiasis. Its powerful antimicrobial properties come from a combination of carvacrol, a naturally occurring antiseptic, and thymol, a compound similar to that found in thyme. Carvacrol is a phenol that rivals in strength the synthetic phenol known as carbolic acid, once used to sterilize medical instruments. For internal *Candida* infections, a relatively small amount of oil of oregano is needed to kill the overgrown fungi. But while this amber-colored liquid may look mild, it has a strong and almost spicy flavor, so we recommend mixing it with vegetable juice. Oil of oregano is also a safe alternative to commercially produced anti-inflammatory drugs, such as aspirin, Motrin, and Indocin, which are the leading cause of sudden death in arthritics.[24] Typical dosage: a few drops sublingually, two or three times a day, for two weeks.

Tea Tree Oil— An Effective Germ-Fighter

The essential oil from the leaves of the tea tree (*Melaleuca alternifolia*) is impressively effective as a natural, nontoxic medicinal agent against infections, fungi, and other microbes on the skin. It is effective against numerous conditions, including candidiasis, acne, insect bites and sunburn, athlete's foot, cuts, muscle aches, and shingles. Depending on the condition, tea tree oil can be used at full strength or diluted in water or with another oil. In a 1995 study published in the *Journal of Applied Bacteriology*, scientists at the University of Western Australia in Nedlands tested eight components of tea tree oil against infectious microorganisms, including *Candida, E. coli, Pseudomonas aeriginosa*, and *Staphylococcus aureus*. The researchers concluded that no single element in tea tree oil accomplishes its remarkable germ-fighting ability; rather the interaction of at least eight distinct chemicals in the oil seemed to produce the effects.[25] Typical recommended dosage: ¼ teaspoon in one quart of lukewarm water as a douche; a few drops applied directly to the skin for skin irritation.[26]

Tea tree oil is meant for topical, not oral, use.

151

CHAPTER

7

Eliminating Parasites

UNDETECTED, UNTREATED infestation of the intestines, and sometimes of other organs, by parasites (protozoa and worms) is a major factor underlying the creation and persistence of many health problems, from arthritis and cancer to allergies, unexplained fatigue, and chronic intestinal dysbiosis. In this chapter, we explain how a parasite infestation may be a causative factor in arthritis, leading to inflammation and deterioration of the joints. We also outline how alternative medicine—through colon cleansing, herbs, and dietary recommendations—can help you eliminate parasites and alleviate your arthritic problems.

What is a Parasite?

A parasite is an organism that lives off the life and nutrients of another organism, to the host's detriment. Specifically, parasites are

the protozoa (single-cell organisms), arthropods (insects), and worms that infect the body and cause serious damage to tissues and organs. Parasites tend to reside in the intestines, but they can also migrate to the blood, lymph, heart, liver, gallbladder, pancreas, spleen, eyes, and brain, as well as inside the joints.

It is estimated that more than 300 kinds of parasites can live in the human body, where they often reside as what microbiologists call the "great masqueraders." They generate numerous symptoms that are usually, mistakenly, associat-

In This Chapter

- What is a Parasite?
- The Link Between Parasites and Arthritis
- Success Story: Reversing Arthritis by Eliminating Parasites
- Diagnosing Parasite Infestations
- Natural Parasite Elimination Techniques

ed with other illnesses by conventional medicine, while a parasitic infestation is overlooked. For example, if you have parasites, you may have headaches, back pain, energy loss, "spaciness," vomiting, weight loss, colitis, gas, uncontrolled appetite, acne, and many other symptoms. You could easily wander through a labyrinth of unsuccessful treatments for each of the symptoms as the attending physicians never suspect—and therefore never treat—a parasite involvement.

In the United States, the most common parasites, apart from head lice, are microscopic protozoans. These include *Giardia lamblia*, a virulent form found in the contaminated waters of lakes, streams, and oceans, and a common cause of traveler's diarrhea;[1] *Entamoeba histolytica*, which can cause dysentery and injure the liver and lungs; *Blastocystis hominus*, which is increasingly linked to acute and chronic illnesses; *Dientamoeba fragilis*, associated with diarrhea, abdominal pain, anal itching, and loose stools; and *Cryptosporidia*, which is particularly dangerous to those with compromised immune function. Arthropod parasites, which include mites, fleas, and ticks, can carry smaller parasites that are also infectious to humans. Of particular interest to arthritis patients is *Borrelia burgdorferi*, a parasite that causes Lyme disease, a condition with many arthritis-like symptoms. Larger parasites include pinworms, tapeworms, roundworms, hookworms, filaria (thread-like worms that inhabit the blood and tissues) and flukes (which invade the liver).

In case you think it's necessary to travel abroad in undeveloped countries to pick up internal parasites, you are quite mistaken. Many authorities in the field of parasitology now confirm that humans are the vessels of many unreported parasites. In a recent study done at Johns Hopkins Hospital in Baltimore, Maryland, 18% of a random selection of blood samples showed a past or present infection of the parasite *Giardia lamblia*. Parasites can easily evade detection by sophisticated testing; they have life-cycle phases in which they leave the gastrointestinal system (the site of most parasite testing) and enter the liver, lungs, eyes, kidneys, lymphatic system, or the joints and articular cells.

The Link Between Parasites and Arthritis

Parasites can cause arthritis-like joint pain in two ways: 1) by directly invading a joint; and 2) through the production of toxic waste products that increase the body burden of circulating immune complexes (SEE QUICK DEFINITION), which initiate an exaggerated immune

Undetected, untreated infestation of the intestines, and sometimes of other organs, by parasites is a major factor underlying the creation and persistence of many health problems, from arthritis and cancer to allergies, unexplained fatigue, and chronic intestinal dysbiosis.

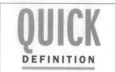

DEFINITION

Circulating immune complexes (CICs) form in the body when poor digestion results in undigested food proteins "leaking" through the intestinal wall and into the bloodstream. The immune system treats these foreign substances or antigens as invaders, causing antibodies to form and couple with them. This antigen and antibody combination is known as a CIC. In a healthy person, CICs are neutralized, but in someone with a compromised immune system, they tend to accumulate in the blood where they burden the detoxification pathways or initiate an allergic reaction. If too many CICs accumulate, the kidneys and liver cannot excrete enough of them via the urine or stool. The CICs are then deposited in soft tissues, causing inflammation and bringing stress to the immune system. The overload can lead to a variety of chronic health conditions.

response. Researchers at Tampa General Hospital in Florida confirm this observation: "Parasitic infestation can induce a variety of rheumatic syndromes as a result of infiltration of musculoskeletal structures by parasites or an immune-mediated mechanism."[2] Possible parasitic infestation should be considered in all cases of arthritis.

Over the last decade, medical researchers around the world have reported on correlations between parasites and different types of arthritis. Rheumatologists at the Children's Hospital and Medical Center in Seattle, Washington, have treated children with reactive arthritis and one child with Reiter's Syndrome (a form of polyarthritis) due to *Cryptosporidium* infestation.[3] Researchers at the Children's Hospital of Eastern Ontario in Ottawa, Canada, state that reactive arthritis, synovitis (inflammation of the membrane surrounding a joint), or arthropathy (another type of joint disease) may result from an infestation by the protozoan *Giardia lamblia*. Two children (age seven and nearly two) with knee joint problems were misdiagnosed as having septic arthritis; instead, they had *Giardia* synovitis, based on the presence of *Giardia* cysts in their stools.[4] Parasitologists at the Department of Medical Research in Yangon, Myanmar, isolated amoebae of the parasite *Entamoeba histolytica* from the knee of an arthritic patient. They concluded that this parasite had caused the knee lesion, which cleared up following drug treatment for *E. histolytica*.[5]

Further confirmation of a link between parasites and arthritis comes from a Korean medical team at Inje Unversity, in Seoul, who reported a strong correlation between infection by *S. stercoralis* and a previous history of arthritis in nine patients, as evidenced by their long-term use of steroids for arthritis management. All nine patients had larvae of *S. stercoralis* in their stools. When one of the patients, a 57-year-old woman with arthritis and abdominal discomfort, was treated with conventional drugs for parasites, 220 adult parasitic organisms were found in one stool sample.[6]

Researchers in Glasgow, Scotland, have correlated a variety of musculoskeletal problems, such as arthritis and parasitic rheumatism, with different parasitic infestations. "The diagnosis of parasitic rheumatism is supported by poor response to anti-inflammatory drugs and improvement following anti-parasitic treatment."[7] In other words, the conventional approach of anti-inflammatory drugs failed to produce results, but treating the underlying cause (parasites) brought relief.

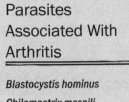

Parasites Associated With Arthritis

Blastocystis hominus

Chilomastrix mesnili

Cryptosporidia

Dientamoeba fragilus

Entamoeba histolytica

Endolimax nana

Giardia lamblia

Italian researchers report that protozoan infections in the muscles and joints are not unusual and are "directly correlated to the presence of the parasite in the organism;"[8] that is, parasites in the body lead directly to parasitic arthritis. Doctors at the University of Minnesota Hospital and Clinic, in Minneapolis, report that fungal and parasitic infections (along with tuberculosis), which afflict millions worldwide, tend to involve joints or bones and often cause rheumatologic symptoms. They predict that the incidence of arthritis and tenosynovitis (inflammation of a tendon sheath) due to parasites is likely to increase in the future.[9]

Success Story: Reversing Arthritis by Eliminating Parasites

In the following case study, you will see how treating parasitic and bacterial infections helped reverse ankylosing spondylitis, a form of arthritis that affects the spine and back.

Harold, 35, came into our office so disabled by his arthritis that he needed a cane to walk. He complained of intense pain in his lower back, neck, and hips. His arms and legs were weak and often tingled or felt numb, and the pain in his knees, relieved by orthopedic surgery several years previously, had returned. Gastrointestinal problems also afflicted Harold—he had abdominal pain and recurrent diarrhea that contributed to his incessant fatigue. He wrestled with bouts of depression, sinus infections, facial dermatitis, and toothaches brought on by bacterial infections hiding in the deep pockets of his gums. Harold was also anemic, an uncommon condition in men, although often present in arthritis patients.

As a child, Harold had asthma, hay fever, and eczema; these conditions have been linked to allergies and exposure to allergenic substances. Suspecting that food allergies contributed to his current respiratory problems, he started avoiding dairy products, coffee, cheese, and pasta and also took nutritional supplements. To relieve the pain caused by his arthritis, he tried yoga, gentle stretching, and breathing exercises three times a week, but Harold still felt that his health was worsening as his arthritis spread from his lower back to his hips and neck.

Initial laboratory tests showed that Harold had an elevated erythrocyte sedimentation rate (ESR), meaning that his red blood cells separated away from other components of the blood at an abnormally high rate. This is an indicator of chronic infection and inflammatory conditions. Harold had a history of arthritic symptoms and said that an earlier doctor had discovered that he had a genetic predisposition (the gene HLA-B27) for ankylosing spondylitis. Some bacteria, through molecular mimicry, are able to reproduce a specific pattern determined by the HLA-B27 gene and pass themselves off as legitimate parts of the body and avoid activating an immune response. Specifically, the bacteria *Klebsiella* has been implicated in triggering ankylosing spondylitis.

Ankylosing spondylitis patients (of which there are three times more men than women) typically suffer from stiffness and pain in the lower back and spine as a result of joint inflammation. Stiffness can then spread to the ribs, shoulders, hips, and knees accompanied by mild fatigue, anorexia, or anemia. Once the inflammation becomes chronic, the bone and cartilage begin to deteriorate and bone bridges (osteophytes) form; these can eventually fuse joints and parts of the spine, rendering the person immobile.

Through a stool analysis, we found that Harold had elevated levels of *Klebsiella* and *Citrobacter freundii*, intestinal bacteria believed to induce autoimmune responses through molecular mimicry. *Citrobacter* also creates antigens that are similar to those of *Salmonella* and *E. coli*, causing intestinal inflammation and, in some cases, leaky gut syndrome. Harold's stool analysis revealed dysbiosis—an unbalanced ecology of microorganisms existed in his gastrointestinal tract. Ratios of short-chain fatty acids (normally produced by "friendly" bacteria) were unbalanced. Under healthy microfloral conditions, bacteria residing in the gastrointestinal tract break down soluble fibers into short-chain fatty acids, which are then used as food by the cells of the colon. But in a dysbiotic state, pathogenic bacteria do not produce these fatty acids and instead produce toxic by-products that impair digestion. His digestive dysfunction was evidenced by decreased levels of chymotrypsin, a key enzyme secreted by the pancreas that prompts the breakdown of proteins into smaller compounds. Decreased levels of chymotrypsin in fecal samples suggest incomplete digestion and malabsorption of proteins.

Harold's stool analysis revealed high levels of *Blastocystis hominis*, a parasite commonly found in the United States that has been linked to chronic fatigue, arthritis and rheumatoid complaints, as well as more well-known parasitic symptoms such as diarrhea, abdominal cramps, nausea, and flatulence. *Blastocystis* tends to live in the intestines but can migrate (via intestinal permeability or leaky gut syndrome) to vital organs and the synovial fluid of the joints. As confirmation of this, large numbers of *Blastocystis* and yeasts normally found in the gastrointestinal tract were detected in a sample of Harold's synovial fluid, extracted and examined under darkfield microscopy. Once *Blastocystis* and other parasites have migrated outside the intestines, they can inappropriately stimulate the body's immune response, which, in the case of arthritis, turns against itself and attacks healthy cell tissues.

As *Blastocystis hominus* is not a joint organism, but an organism that infects the digestive system, we must ask how this microorganism got from the digestive system into the joint if, according to orthodox medical belief, the intestines are not permeable to intact molecules and large molecular fractions. In our estimation, this perplexing situation is resolved by assuming the following to be true: that the intestines, or gut, "leaks" these molecules across the intestinal membranes (leaky gut syndrome) and that microorganisms move (translocate) from the intestinal tract to the joints. The other bacteria detected in Harold's stool (*Citrobacter* and *Klebsiella*) both contributed to the breakdown of his intestinal membrane. *Klebsiella* is related to ankylosing spondylitis.

We started Harold on the following anti-parasitic protocol:

■ Biocidin, an herbal anti-parasite formula: ten drops, three times daily

■ AC (Anti-*Candida*) Formula: two tablets, three times daily between meals

■ AP (Anti-Parasitic) Formula: two tablets, three times daily without food

■ Enterocap: contains grapefruit seed extract and standardized berberine; two tablets, three times daily without food

We also recommended that Harold prepare an enema solution of the following ingredients: ten drops each of Biocidin and Par Qing (which contains artemesia and other herbs), three drops of grapefruit seed extract, five capsules of AP Formula and AC Formula, and ten drops each of three antimicrobial essential oils (red thyme, marjoram, and oregano). A conventional doctor that Harold also consulted prescribed metronidazole (also known as Flagyl), an antibacterial drug commonly used against amebic dysentery.

After four months on this treatment, Harold no longer experienced joint pains. We re-tested the sedimentation rate of his red blood cells and found the result to be normal (his reading was five, while the normal range is zero to 20). One month later, Harold had no further pain and we referred him to a naturopathic physician closer to his hometown for maintenance consultations. This case shows that careful microscopic analysis of the synovial fluid is *mandatory* in all cases of arthritis, especially ankylosing spondylitis and rheumatoid arthritis. Parasites and bacteria must always be considered as possible contributors to the onset of arthritis.

Diagnosing Parasite Infestations

Many doctors, hospitals, and laboratories "fail to diagnose parasitic infection because they rarely allow the time for careful analysis or multiple procedures using stool specimens collected over several days," according to Martin J. Lee, Ph.D., director of Great Smokies Diagnostic Laboratory in Asheville, North Carolina, which offers a stool analysis for parasites. Dr. Lee suggests that if you suspect you may have an intestinal parasite, make sure your physician, hospital, or laboratory follows the investigational guidelines set by the U.S. Centers for Disease Control in the *Manual of Clinical Microbiology*.[10]

Additional alternative medicine screening tools to diagnose the presence of parasites include electrodermal screening (EDS), applied kinesiology, and darkfield microscopic blood analysis (SEE QUICK DEFINITION). Regarding the latter, we have observed the presence of long tubules in the blood of many arthritis patients and contend that

Most of the remedies that we prescribed for Harold are available to practitioners only. For more information, contact: Environmental Detoxification Consultants, 413 Grassy Hill Road, Woodbury, CT 06798; tel/fax: 203-263-2970. For **Biocidin**, contact: Emerson Ecological, 18 Lomar Park, Pepperell, MA 01463; tel: 800-654-4432 or 978-433-0090; fax: 978-433-0099. For **AC and AP Formulas**, contact: Pure Encapsulations, 490 Boston Post Road, Sudbury, MA 01776; tel: 800-753-2277 or 508-443-1999; fax: 888-783-2277. For **Enterocap**, contact: Thorne Research, P.O. Box 25, Dover, ID 83825; tel: 800-228-1966 or 208-263-1337; fax: 208-265-2488. **Antimicrobial essential oils** are available at most health food stores.

these have a high positive correlation with a diagnosis of parasites.

Applied kinesiology, is the study of the relationship between muscle dysfunction (weak muscles) and related organ or gland dysfunction. Applied kinesiology employs a simple strength resistance test on a specific indicator muscle that is related to the organ or part of the body that is being tested. If the muscle tests strong (maintaining its resistance), it indicates health. If it tests weak, it can mean infection or dysfunction. When testing for parasites, the practitioner challenges a strong muscle while the patient holds a vial containing parasite specimens; the muscle will weaken if one of these parasites is causing their health problem.

Electrodermal screening (EDS) is a form of computerized information gathering which is based on physics, not chemistry. A blunt, noninvasive electric probe is placed at specific points on the patient's hands, face, or feet, corresponding to acupuncture points at the beginning or end of energy meridians. Minute electrical discharges from these points serve as information signals about the condition of the body's organs and systems, useful for the physician in evaluation and developing a treatment plan. EDS can indicate the degree of stress that is affecting an organ and can monitor the progress of therapy, avoiding trial and error and general guesswork. EDS can use a computerized list or vials containing specimens of various parasites to test the meridians of the patient; if parasites are a factor, there will be a corresponding weakened EDS reading.

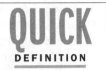

QUICK

DEFINITION

Darkfield microscopy is a way of studying living whole blood cells under a specially adapted microscope that projects the dynamic image, magnified 1,400 times, onto a video screen. The skilled physician can detect early signs of illness in the form of microorganisms in the blood known to produce disease. Relevant technical features in the blood include color, variously shaped components (such as spicules, long tubules, and roulous), and the size of certain immune cells. The amount of time the blood cell stays viable and alive indicates the overall health of the individual. Specifically, darkfield microscopy reveals distortions of red blood cells (which indicate nutritional status), possible undesirable bacterial or fungal life forms, and blood ecology patterns indicative of health or illness.

For more information about **testing for parasites**, see Chapter 3: Diagnosing Arthritis, pp. 52-77.

Natural Parasite Elimination Techniques

We recommend a period of general body detoxification (elimination, cleansing, and toning according to the protocols explained in Chapter 4: General Detoxification) prior to starting a parasite removal program. This enables the body to handle the destruction of the parasites and the liberation of toxic substances from them, which, if absorbed by the body, can lead to an unpleasant die-off (Herxheimer) reaction. This means that while, technically, your health is improving because you have destroyed and are removing toxic organisms, you feel terrible during the process, as if your illness were getting worse. Typically the die-off symptoms may include joint pains, malaise, fever, coated tongue, and gastrointestinal disturbances.

Helping your body to eliminate parasites is asking it to work harder when, under the influence of these unwanted organisms, it is probably already overworked. The combination of the extra effort asked of the body and the release of the toxic substances during the Herxheimer reaction can also cause a flare-up of pre-existing conditions, including joint pains, headaches, bloating, itching, and mood swings, just to name a few. Bear in mind that these are, in fact, good signs, indicating your body is ridding itself of the parasites.

Parasites can be difficult to eradicate, because when you begin to kill them off, they often form spores or eggs that are deposited in the body tissues. An anti-parasitic program should be undertaken with the knowledge of the typical life cycle of parasites. The eggs of many of the worms hatch every 2-3 weeks. The length of treatment is critical for successful elimination of parasites—if your program is too short, it may fail to destroy parasites at an advanced stage in their life cycle. Typically, we recommend that enemas be performed two to three times weekly for a period of four weeks, followed by an ova (egg) and parasite test, then repeat enemas and other oral anti-parasitic substances, if needed.

According to Joseph Pizzorno, N.D., author of *Total Wellness*, it is essential that you repeat your anti-parasitic program every 2-4 weeks accompanied by a parasitology test (offered by Great Smokies Diagnostic Laboratory). The ova and parasite material, collected from the patient for the test, must be derived from a purged sample or rectal swab in which saline or other laxative is administered and the purged stool is collected. This should be repeated every two months; do not consider yourself clear of parasites until you have three clearly negative results. Although self-treatment is possible, we advise you to have a knowledgeable health-care practitioner follow your progress; be sure this practitioner is familiar with parasite life cycles, testing, and cleansing procedures.

Natural Parasite Elimination Techniques

- Colon Cleansing
- Herbs for Parasites
- Dietary Changes
- Kitchen and Culinary Hygiene

Colon-Cleansing Programs

Colon cleansing is commonly recommended by natural health practitioners as an effective method for eliminating parasites. There are a number of colon-cleansing programs available to help you scrub microorganisms and other toxic materials from the intestines. Colonic irrigations and enemas, in which water or some other fluid is used to flush out the lower portion of the colon, can help restore intestinal health.

Colonic irrigation, performed in a clinic with special equipment, involves the gentle infusion of the large intestine with water or herbal tea or diluted tincture. The colonics procedure is used in many natural care practices to help rid the body of parasites. A cleansing of the colon with pure filtered water (or ozonated water or hydrogen peroxide–infused water) for 20-30 minutes is followed by the infusion of powerful botanical medicines. You then retain the herbs in the large intestine for several minutes to allow for maximum antimicrobial effect.

Parasites tend to embed themselves in the intestinal wall, but over the course of several weeks, you can flush them out by using some of these natural substances (preferably in combination): psyllium husks, agar-agar, citrus pectin, papaya extract, pumpkin seeds, flaxseeds, comfrey root, beet root, and bentonite clay (take bentonite only in combination with another substance, such as psyllium). You might also take extra amounts of vitamin C (minimum 2 g daily, but higher amounts up to individual bowel tolerance are more useful) to help flush out your intestine. Note, however, that vitamin C taken at the same time as wormwood (an anti-parasitic herb) makes wormwood ineffective.

CAUTION

Make sure to dilute hydrogen peroxide correctly as it can irritate and burn the sensitive mucosa of the intestines.

Food-grade hydrogen peroxide can be added to an enema (done at home) as an anti-parasitic agent. Add ¼ cup of peroxide per two liters of fluid. We have been successful using hydrogen peroxide (diluted before use) as an enema or in the last 5-10 minutes of a professionally administered colonic treatment. We use food-grade hydrogen peroxide because drug store brands typically contain impurities not appropriate for internal consumption. Ozonated water (SEE QUICK DEFINITION) is another safe and effective enema for treating parasites. The ozonated water destroys the parasites as well as the hard covering that surrounds their cysts or eggs, which are highly resistant to many forms of treatment.

A third approach is to perform an enema with essential oils. Combine two drops of the

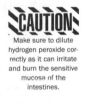

QUICK

DEFINITION

Ozone (O_3) is a less stable, more reactive form of oxygen, containing three oxygen atoms. This extra atom enables ozone to more readily oxidize other chemicals. In oxidation, the extra oxygen atom breaks off, leaving ordinary oxygen (O_2), thereby favorably increasing the oxygen content of body tissues or blood. Medical-grade ozone is used as part of oxygen therapy to increase local oxygen supply to lesions, speed wound healing, reduce infections, and stimulate metabolic processes. Ozone may be administered intravenously or by injection, or applied topically in a water- or olive oil-based solution; it may also be taken orally or rectally as ozonated water.

essential oil of thyme, two drops of oregano oil, and two drops of marjoram oil in a two-quart container of water. This will make two complete enemas utilizing a full quart bag of water. Again, we usually recommend that enemas be done 2-3 times per week for a period of four weeks, followed by a test for ova and parasites, then a repetition of the enemas and oral anti-parasitics, if necessary, in order to ensure eradication.

Herbs for Parasites

Herbs are a safe and effective alternative to drug therapies for ridding yourself of parasites. They are free of side effects and often work better than their synthetic counterparts. Purgative herbs such as pumpkin seeds act as mild intestinal cleansers. Decoctions and powders of pumpkin seeds have shown positive effects against tapeworm and other intestinal parasites in humans and in animals.[11] A typical dose consists of 10-12 seeds in the morning on an empty stomach for two weeks. If the parasites are systemic and have entered the bloodstream, antibiotic herbs such as *Coptis* (a Chinese herb high in berberine) may also be used.

Garlic—One of the least expensive yet most effective ways to deal with parasites is to use an extract of garlic (*Allium sativum*). Raw garlic and garlic extract have been shown to destroy common intestinal parasites, including roundworms and hookworms. According to Chinese research, in the treatment of 100 cases of amebic dysentery, the cure rate with garlic was 88%. The study found that purple-skinned bulbous garlic was more effective than the white-skinned variety. In another case, enemas made from tea containing garlic were used for 154 cases of pinworm in children two to nine years old; treatments were repeated on the third and seventh day after the initial treatment. After this period, tests for parasite eggs around the anus were negative (meaning no eggs were found) in 76 of the patients.[12]

In our practice, we use freshly juiced garlic (refrigerated after pressing) in the treatment of parasites, dysbiosis, *Candida albicans*, and other infectious microbes. We usually use two to three teaspoons in a two-liter bag, which is infused into the patient's colon at the end of a colonic. If a person is doing an enema at home, he can use 1-2 cloves of garlic, crush them, steep them in a tea for 10-15 minutes with a tight cover, allow this to cool to body temperature, and then put this in the enema bag. Garlic is fairly caustic and if you use too much, you can injure tissues, so it's better to use a small amount. As an oral supplement, we often recommend two cloves of fresh garlic daily; in capsule form, 500 mg, twice daily.

How to Do an Anti-Parasite Enema

- Measure two quarts of purified filtered water; don't use tap water or bottled. Bring water to a boil, then remove from heat.
- Add to the water 4 tsp of powdered goldenseal root, 4 tsp powdered thyme (a common kitchen spice), two cloves of crushed garlic juice, and 2 tsp of tea tree oil. Let solution steep and cool to body temperature for 20 minutes in a covered container.
- Make sure you empty your bowels and bladder prior to the enema. Use K-Y jelly or other common lubricants found in drug stores to lubricate the enema speculum (a small tube inserted into the anus) enabling it to easily enter the anus without abrasion. Keep a towel under your buttocks to collect run-off stools and pathogens.
- Hang enema bag above your body so that gravity assists the fluid flow.
- Assume the fetal position and lubricate your rectum, and place enema speculum into rectum. Turn/roll to position on your back with knees up. One hand keeps the speculum in, while the other controls the flow valve.
- Slowly allow the liquid to flow into your colon; stop every three seconds to allow yourself to get used to it. Allow the fluid to enter until you feel a slight cramping or discomfort.
- When your intestines are full, remove speculum, hold your sphincter muscles, get up and get to the toilet. Release bowels, and remain on the toilet seat until all the water has been evacuated.
- Repeat the enema process until you have completely used the water. Clean yourself up; soak enema speculum in bleach water; clean the area.
- Do this procedure two to three times a week for four weeks.

Goldenseal—The alkaloid berberine is found in many plants and in particularly high concentrations in goldenseal (*Hydrastis canadensis*). Berberine inhibits the growth of several common parasites that invade the intestine and vagina, including *Entamoeba histolytica*, *Giardia lamblia*, *Erwinia carotovora*, and *Leishmania donovania*. In one study, children with giardiasis were given either berberine sulfate (a standardized goldenseal extract) or the drug Flagyl. After ten days, both substances produced similar results: 90% of the berberine-treated group no longer had *Giardia* in their stools compared to 95% of the Flagyl-treated group. Unlike the Flagyl-treated group, however, those receiving berberine suffered no negative side effects.[13] Typical dosage: 500 mg, three times daily.

Thyme (*Thymus vulgaris*)—The principle chemical components of thyme are the volatile oils phenol, thymol, and carvacrol. Thymol is one of the most potent antimicrobial substances known, and even surpasses many of the strongest antibiotics.[14] Thymol's antimicrobial activity is

18 times more powerful than phenol, the major antiseptic used in commercial germicidal cleansers like Lysol®, and can destroy parasites, worms, fungi, bacteria, and many viruses.[15] We recommend a dosage of five drops of thyme essential oil diluted in a quart of pure water as an enema solution. You may also take thyme orally at the rate of two or three drops of an oil extract diluted in one cup of water, three times a day for two weeks.

Grapefruit Seed Extract—Grapefruit seed extract (GSE) offers some of the benefits of antibiotics in a natural form without the side effects. Clinical tests by the U.S. Food and Drug Administration, Pasteur Institute in Paris, and University of Georgia at Athens, have successfully treated bacterial, fungal, and viral infections, such as *Giardia*, amebic dysentery, *E. coli*, *Candida*, and herpes, with GSE.[16] Made from grapefruit seeds and pulp, the medical virtues of GSE were identified in 1964 by Florida physician Jacob Harich, M.D., and later marketed as Citricidal.

Very little is known about the active components of GSE, but it contains bioflavonoids (vitamin C enhancers) and hesperidin, a natural immune booster.[17] GSE is effective for arthritis patients with intestinal and systemic infections of candidiasis or parasites that cause joint and muscle aches, irritable bowels, and allergies. While doctors recommend a variety of dosages depending on the stubbornness of the infection, typically a few drops are taken with each meal or diluted in vegetable or fruit juice if the taste is too bitter.[18]

Worm Seed (Mexican Tea)—Epazote (*Chenopodium ambrosoides*), also called worm seed or Mexican tea, is often used in the Caribbean and Central America for worms. We have observed that among the Indians in Mexico, epazote is regularly used as a tea in the spring: a mild tea was prepared for children and a stronger one for adults, presumably as a preventive measure. When someone had a known parasitic infestation, a very thick brew of the epazote was made and taken by the spoonful. Worm seed should never be given to children under the age of six; for those ages six and older, a typical dose is 3-5 drops per day. Make a tea by steeping 3-4 teaspoons of the dried or fresh herb in one cup of water for 20 minutes; drink one cup per day. Supplement dosage: 50 mg, three times daily.

Chinese Wormwood (*Artemesia absinthium*)—*Artemesia absinthium* has a long history of use as a vermifuge or "worm expeller," hence its common name, wormwood. It was even prized by Hippocrates (460-377

B.C.) for its ability to expel worms. Similar in action to the Chinese herb *Artemesia annua*, it is especially effective against *Giardia* and other protozoa, but some caution is advised. It may initially worsen symptoms and cause some intestinal irritation. Although it may be toxic if used alone in large quantities, it is usually mixed in formulas with citrus seed extract and other anti-parasitic herbs that offset its possible toxic effects. Typical recommended dosage: 150 mg, three times daily.

Wormwood is also part of the anti-parasite protocol of naturopathic physician Hulda Regehr Clark, N.D., Ph.D. She recommends using a blend of three herbs to flush the parasites out of your system: black walnut hull tincture, wormwood capsules, and fresh ground cloves (to kill the parasites' eggs). This program should only be undertaken with professional guidance from a licensed health-care practitioner.

Ayurvedic Herbs—The traditional Indian medical science of Ayurveda (SEE QUICK DEFINITION) has several natural remedies which address specific parasite infections, according to Virender Sodhi, N.D., M.D. (Ayurveda), of Bastyr University in Seattle, Washington. For pinworms, Dr. Sodhi recommends bitter melon (*Mormordica charantia*), a cucumber-shaped fruit which is best used cut up and eaten in small pieces with other vegetables because of its bitter taste. Consuming one or two bitter melons a day for 7–10 days, then repeating this after one month, can be effective in the treatment of worms. It is easy to tell if there is any recurrent infection, says Dr. Sodhi, as thousands of little white bugs will show up in the stool the day after eating bitter melon if there is pinworm presence remaining.

The herbs *embliaribes*, *vidang*, and *kamila* are most effective for roundworms, according to Dr. Sodhi. "Take one teaspoon of the herb powder extract twice a day with sweetened water or juice to attract the parasites. Do this for seven to ten days and then check your stool. If there is still evidence of infestation, repeat the cycle until you are parasite free."

For more information about **Dr. Hulda Clark's anti-parasite program**, see *Alternative Medicine Definitive Guide to Cancer* (Future Medicine Publishing, 1997; ISBN 1-887299-01-7); to order, call 800-333-HEAL.

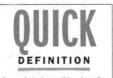

QUICK DEFINITION

Ayurveda is the traditional medicine of India, based on many centuries of empirical use. Its name means "end of the Vedas" (which were India's sacred scripts), implying that a holistic medicine may be founded on spiritual principles. Ayurveda describes three metabolic, constitutional, and body types (*doshas*), in association with the basic elements of Nature in combination. These are *vata* (air and ether, rooted in intestines), *pitta* (fire and water/stomach), and *kapha* (water and earth/lungs). Ayurvedic physicians use these categories (which also have psychological aspects) as the basis for prescribing individualized formulas of herbs, diet, massage, breathing, meditation, exercise and yoga postures, and detoxification techniques.

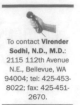

To contact **Virender Sodhi, N.D., M.D.**: 2115 112th Avenue N.E., Bellevue, WA 94004; tel: 425-453-8022; fax: 425-451-2670.

"Kamila is also effective for tapeworms," says Dr. Sodhi, "as well as betel nut, which can be chewed." The same kind of protocol as with pinworms and roundworms can be used. For *Giardia,* amoebas, *Cryptosporidium,* and other protozoal parasites, the treatment is usually longer than for worms, taking up to several months, according to Dr. Sodhi. The herbs that are most effective for these microscopic intruders are *bilva, neem,* and berberine, which can be taken in combination. Dr. Sodhi also recommends bitter melon for protozoal infestations, as well as nutritional support such as psyllium husk, turmeric, and *L. acidophilus* for the enhancement of the intestinal microflora.

Ayurvedic physicians state that when treating parasites, you must address the immune system; so various herbs and techniques for enhancing the immunity can also be utilized to support the body in its defense against the parasites. Herbs useful for this task, according to Ayurvedic medicine, include ginseng, ligustri berries, and schisandra berries.

Dietary Changes

If an intestinal parasite infection is diagnosed or suspected, we advise you to eliminate all uncooked food (which may contain parasites) from your diet and to cook all meats until well done. Soak all vegetables, including those organically grown, in salted water (one tablespoon salt for five cups of water) for at least 30 minutes before cooking to kill parasites and their eggs. Avoid coffee, sugars (including fruit and honey), and all milk and dairy products, since these substances lower immunity and make it more difficult for the body to fight off parasites. Raw goat milk is excepted because it contains IgA and IgG immunoglobulins, which help protect the intestinal lining from infectious agents.

Probiotics—Parasites can be fought with high-dosage probiotic ("friendly" bacteria) substances such as *B. bifidum* and *Lactobacillus acidophilus, bulgaricus, plantarum,* and *salvarius,* which are available as nutritional supplements. *L. plantarum* is the most effective of these in treating parasite problems. Treatment may last from eight to 12 weeks. Leon Chaitow, N.D., a British naturopath, reports an 80% success rate in cases of seriously ill people afflicted with parasites and yeast overgrowth using this method. Recolonizing the intestines with friendly bacteria can help prevent illness by depriving the pathogenic (disease-causing) bacteria of the opportunity to overgrow and flourish.

Effective Formulas for Parasites

We have found the following formulas to be effective in eliminating parasites:

- Biocidin™: This is a complex botanical formula used to destroy all types of bowel pathogens and is typically taken over the course of six to 12 weeks. Dosage is determined by the health-care practitioner.

- Tricycline: This is a combination of berberine, grapefruit seed extract, and *artemesia*, also given to destroy all types of bowel pathogens. Typical dosage (practitioner-prescribed): one pill, three times daily, but not taken with food.

- Par Qing: a combination of *artemesia*, anise, cinnamon, and marjoram, for elimination of parasites, both worms and small parasites such as amoebas. Dosage: typically two pills, three times daily, taken with meals.

- Smooth Move Tea: One tea bag can be brewed in one cup of hot water for five minutes; for children, add $\frac{1}{8}$ cup of the brewed tea to apple juice. (This commercially prepared tea is commonly available in natural food stores.)

- Epsom Salts: Known in Germany as *bittersalz*, this inexpensive but bitter-tasting salt of magnesium sulfate heptahydrate is not well-favored by children but can be tolerated by adults, when consumed orally, per directions on package.

- Worm Squirm 1 and 2: Both are encapsulated herbal formulas for ridding the body of parasites; formula 1 is for roundworms including pinworms, *Ascaris*, hookworms, and whipworms; formula 2 for tapeworms, flukes, and flatworms and both should not be taken at the same time. Worm Squirm 1 contains *Artemisia annua*, black walnut, cloves, gentian root, ginger, hyssop, mandrake root, and tansy flower; Worm Squirm 2 contains chamomile, male fern rhizome, pink root, pumpkin seeds, and senna.

- PlantiBiotic: This is an anti-parasite herbal formula (also effective against *Candida albicans*) that includes barberry (200 mg), berberine (125 mg), citrus seed extract (200 mg), thyme oil (250 mg), oregano oil (250 mg), tea tree oil (100 mg), garlic (50 mg), quassia bark (50 mg), cascara sagrada (50 mg), black walnut (50 mg), *Artemesia annua* (50 mg), epazote (50 mg), and cloves (50 mg). The dosage that we have used for ten years with greater than 90% success is three pills, three times daily with food, for two months.

For **grapefruit seed extract**, available as ProSeed™ (in liquid concentrate, Vegicaps®, Feminine Rinse, Ear Drops, Gum Cleanser, and Herbal Cleansing Spray) or a similar line called Seed-a-Sept™ (formulated for physicians), contact: Imhotep, Inc., P.O. Box 183, Ruby, NY 12475; tel: 800-677-8577. For **Biocidin**™, contact: Bio-Botanical Research, Inc., P.O. Box 1061, Soquel, CA 95073. For **Tricycline** and **Par Qing**, contact: Nutricology/Allergy Research Group, P.O. Box 55907, Hayward, CA 94544; tel: 510-487-8526 or 800-782-4274; fax: 510-487-8682; web-site: www.nutricology.com. For **Worm Squirm 1 and 2**, contact: Arise & Shine, P.O. Box 1439, Mt. Shasta, CA 96067; tel: 800-688-2444 or 530-926-0891; fax: 530-926-8866. For **PlantiBiotic**, contact: Nature's Answer, 320 Oser Avenue, Hauppauge, NY 11788; tel: 800-439-2324 or 516-231-7492; fax: 516-951-2499; website: www.naturesanswer.com.

Important Reminders During Parasite Treatment

Whatever treatment you employ to rid your body of parasites, the following recommendations can help ensure that the program is a success:

■ If you have children and/or pets, they must be treated at the same time as the adults in the household to prevent re-infection.

■ Drink more pure water (not from the tap) than usual to help the body flush out the dead parasites from your system; at least 64 ounces of water per day for a 150-pound adult.

■ Sanitize your environment. When you have almost finished treatment, wash all pajamas, bed clothes, and sheets before using them again.

■ Eat anti-parasitic foods. According to Ann Louise Gittleman, M.S., a nutrition educator in Bozeman, Montana, these include pineapple and papaya, either as fresh juice or in organic supplement form, in combination with pepsin and hydrochloric acid. Avoid all meats and dairy products for at least one week. You can also use pomegranate juice (four 4-ounce glasses daily), papaya seeds, finely ground pumpkin seeds (¼ to ½ cup daily), and two cloves of raw garlic daily. Do not drink the pomegranate juice for more than four to five days.

■ Modify your diet. For people with heavy parasitic infection, Gittleman recommends a diet comprised of 25% fat, 25% protein, and 50% complex carbohydrates. You also need a regular intake of unprocessed flaxseed, safflower, sesame, or canola oils (two tablespoons daily) and extra vitamin A. Flaxseed oil is preferable because it has much higher levels of alpha-linolenic acid (an omega-3 essential fatty acid that is commonly deficient in many people) than the other oils.

■ Recolonize your intestines. You need to reintroduce beneficial, friendly bacteria (probiotics) into your intestinal system once you have flushed out the parasites, Gittleman advises. The bacterial strains most helpful are *Lactobacillus plantarum*, *L. salvarius*, *L. acidophilus*, *L. bulgaris*, *B. bifidum*, and *Streptococcus faeceum*, which are available as nutritional supplements. *L. plantarum* is the most effective of these in resolving parasite problems.

Anti-Parasitic Foods—Certain foods inhibit parasite growth, such as garlic, onions, papaya, pineapple, pumpkin seeds, figs, pomegranate seeds, and the seeds of the rangoon creeper fruit (*Quisqualis indicae*). Since much of commercial fruit is irradiated, the amount of enzymes found in fresh pineapple and papaya, unless organic, is minimal. The enzymes are needed to break down parasites inside the body. Digestive pancreatic enzymes as well as bromelain and papain should be taken as supplements both with and between meals. When taken with meals, they aid with digestion; when taken between meals, they help to destroy parasites and other cellular debris. Pomegranate juice (four 4-

How to Avoid Parasites

There are several precautions that will help you avoid parasites:

Food

- Do not eat raw beef or pork—it can be loaded with tapeworms and other parasites.
- Do not eat raw fish or sushi—you are almost certain to get worms if you eat raw fish.
- Wash hands after handling raw meat or fish (including shrimp)—don't put your hands near your mouth without washing them first.
- Use separate cutting boards for meat and vegetables—spores from meat can seep into the board and contaminate vegetables or anything else you put on the board.
- Wash utensils thoroughly after cutting meat.
- Wash vegetables and fruit thoroughly—particularly salad items, as they often harbor parasites. Wash in one teaspoon Clorox per gallon of water. Soak for 15-20 minutes. Then soak in fresh water for 20 minutes before

refrigerating. Or substitute a few drops of grapefruit seed extract.
- Do not drink from streams and rivers.

Pets

- Do not sleep near your pets—they harbor many worms and other parasites.
- De-worm your pets regularly and keep their sleeping areas clean.
- Do not let pets lick your face.
- Do not let pets eat off your dishes.
- Do not walk barefoot around animals.

General

- Always wash your hands after using the toilet.
- Wash your hands after working in the garden—the soil can be contaminated with spores and parasites.

When Traveling

- Don't drink the water.
- Start taking herbs or other preventive medications two weeks before traveling, and continue them while you travel.

ounce glasses daily) can aid in the expulsion of worms. Wheat germ can be used to inhibit various amoebas from binding to target cells in the intestines.

Kitchen and Culinary Hygiene

Here's how to purify your raw fruits and vegetables of contaminants, including possible parasites, according to the late naturopathic physician Hazel Parcells, N.D., of the Parcells Center in Santa Fe, New Mexico. This technique will rid the food items of harmful toxins, chemicals, sprays, and poisons, reduce your chances of picking up parasites, and it will noticeably improve the flavor and shelf-life of the foods.

- Soak all fruits, eggs, meats, and vegetables in a bath of Clorox and water, at the rate of ½ teaspoon Clorox to one gallon water.

Make sure it is the old-fashioned, pure Clorox; this is hydrochloric acid, not chlorine.

■ Divide your foods into the following categories and soak no longer than the time listed: leafy vegetables (10-15 minutes), root vegetables (15-30 minutes), thin-skinned berries (10-15 minutes), heavy-skinned fruits (15-30 minutes), eggs (20-30 minutes), thawed meats (5-10 minutes per pound).

■ Prepare a fresh batch of Clorox water for each category of foods; dispose of baths after use.

■ Soak all Clorox-treated foods in a fresh water bath for 5-10 minutes before using. "This treatment has been used for the last 30 years by many families, saving them untold expenses for illness with no unfavorable reports," says Dr. Parcells.

Here are three more easy options for cleansing your foods:

■ Organiclean™: This fruit and vegetable wash contains two natural cleaning agents, sodium lauryl sulfate from coconuts and a sugar/fatty acid cleanser derived from yeast. Extracts from bilberry, sugar cane, sugar maple, orange, and lemon are included because they contain alpha-hydroxy acids. These work as emulsifiers, liquifying dirts and oils on the surface of the fruit or vegetable so they can be easily rinsed away.

■ EarthSafe™: EarthSafe is a blend of natural, food-grade cleansing agents made from vegetable, corn, and coconut extracts, as well as lemon and grapefruit extracts. It contains no artificial fragrances or dyes. Simply spray EarthSafe on fruits and vegetables and rinse off with water to remove surface residues.

■ VegiWash™: VegiWash removes up to 97% of the surface contaminants on fruits and vegetables, according to the manufacturer. VegiWash, whose main cleansing agents are also coconut-based, completely rinses away with water.

 For **naturopathic detoxification techniques**, contact: Environmental Detoxification Consultants, 413 Grassy Hill Road, Woodbury, CT 06798; tel/fax: 203-263-2970. For **natural fruit and vegetable washes**, contact: Organiclean™, 10877 Wilshire Blvd., Twelfth Floor, Los Angeles, CA 90024; tel: 888-VEG-WASH or 310-824-2508; website: www.organiclean.com. EarthSafe™, National Research & Chemical Company, 15600 New Century Drive, Gardena, CA 90248; tel: 310-515-1700; fax: 310-527-9963. VegiWash™, Consumer Health Research, Inc., P.O. Box 1718, Absecon, NJ 08201; tel: 800-282-WASH or 609-645-1110; fax: 609-645-8881; website: www.vegiwash.com.

Toxins in the body trigger inflammation

in connective tissues and contribute to the escalation

of arthritis. The body's detoxification

pathways become clogged and the immune system is

overwhelmed. Patients with rheumatoid

arthritis, ankylosing spondylitis, and other inflammatory

diseases are particularly vulnerable,

more so than osteoarthritis. But even those with

"wear and tear" arthritis (osteoarthritis)

can still have leaky gut as a contributing cause

of their disease.

CHAPTER

8 Alleviating Leaky Gut Syndrome

A HEALTHY INTESTINAL TRACT is a dual-functioning system: it must allow nutrients to pass unhindered into the body with maximum absorption while simultaneously insuring that the toxins within the tract are not absorbed and allowed to contaminate tissues, glands, and organs. But when the structural integrity of the intestines breaks down, a condition known as intestinal permeability or "leaky gut syndrome" develops, which allows undigested food proteins and other toxins to enter the bloodstream. The immune system recognizes these undigested proteins as foreign substances—it sends antibodies to attack these "invaders" and neutralize them. In leaky gut, an endless supply of toxins escape into the blood, overwhelming the immune system, and accumulating in soft tissues, joints, and elsewhere.

Toxins in the body trigger inflammation in connective tissues and contribute to the escalation of arthritis. The body's detoxification pathways become clogged and the immune system is overwhelmed. Patients with rheumatoid arthritis, ankylosing spondylitis, and other inflammatory diseases are particularly vulnerable, more so than osteoarthritis. But even those with "wear and tear" arthritis (osteoarthritis) can still have leaky gut as a contributing cause of their disease. In this chapter, we look at the causes of leaky gut and recommend dietary and lifestyle changes that have allowed many people with

In This Chapter

- Success Story: Treating Leaky Gut Reverses Arthritis
- Healthy and Unhealthy Intestines
- Causes of Leaky Gut Syndrome
- Testing for Intestinal Permeability
- Alternative Medicine Therapies for Leaky Gut Syndrome

arthritis to find sustained relief from pain without having to rely on drugs.

Success Story: Treating Leaky Gut Reverses Arthritis

Susan, 49, was diagnosed with aggressive rheumatoid arthritis and experienced pain and swelling in the joints of her neck, shoulders, wrists, feet,

---

Alternative Medicine Therapies for Leaky Gut Syndrome

- Fasting
- Dietary Guidelines
- Herbs and Botanicals
- Digestive Enzymes
- Nutritional Supplements

---

and elbows. Susan also complained of fatigue, memory and balance problems, anxiety, nausea, poor digestion, irritable bowel, bleeding gums, premenstrual syndrome (PMS), chronic sinus infections (postnasal drip, earache, and a persistent cough), difficulty breathing, and frequent urination at night.

Originally, Susan came to us because she wanted to start a supervised fasting and cleansing program, which she had previously tried at a health spa with great success for pain reduction. For many of our patients, we use fasting to reduce joint pain and correct digestive imbalances that often coincide with arthritis. But before prescribing this for a patient, we identify the most problematic imbalances and design a program to suit the individual's deficiencies.

We tested Susan for food allergies and found that she had a sensitivity to almost every food group. Such severe food allergies usually indicate leaky gut syndrome, which we confirmed in Susan through an Intestinal Permeability Assay (a test offered by Great Smokies Diagnostic Laboratory, in Asheville, North Carolina). Gaps can occur both between cells and within cells in the intestinal tract, allowing undigested food and other toxins to escape into the bloodstream. In a healthy person, these toxins would be sent to the liver, the body's chief detoxification organ, and be removed from the system without further problems or damaging effects.

But Susan's liver was not healthy. According to a Liver Detoxification Panel (another Great Smokies test), her liver was so overloaded with toxins that an important phase of detoxification (SEE QUICK DEFINITION) had effectively shut down. Susan's test results showed that her liver could adequately complete the first phase of detoxification. But a breakdown occurred in the second phase—her supplies of glutathione sulfate were depleted and high levels of inter-

QUICK
DEFINITION

mediate toxins slipped back into the bloodstream without undergoing complete detoxification. The Kupffer cells in her liver, which help with cleansing the blood, were also inactive. These toxins accumulated in the bloodstream and disturbed the connective tissue and the immune and endocrine systems, causing inflammation and illness.

A nutritional profile and hair analysis found that Susan was dangerously low in antioxidants (SEE QUICK DEFINITION). She ranked only in the 10th percentile of antioxidant levels, while the 75th percentile and greater is considered normal. She was particularly deficient in selenium (an important constituent of glutathione peroxidase), copper (necessary for healthy structural tissues, joints, and muscles), zinc (an immune-booster), vitamins B2 and B12, chromium, and calcium.

Without the liver's ability to filter the blood properly—that is, sequester the toxins caused by her leaky gut syndrome—the body used up its store of antioxidants trying to quell the free radicals caused by the deposition of toxins in her connective tissue. Her need for antioxidants soon exceeded her ability to replenish supplies. As a result, vital processes dependent upon antioxidant activities began to slow or even shut down.

Cellular energy production also depends upon a rich supply of antioxidants. Antioxidants and enzymes help carry out important phases of the Krebs cycle (SEE QUICK DEFINITION), which is the process by which the body's cells produce energy.

Susan also had very low urinary levels of the antioxidant glutathione; she scored a four on a normal scale of 15 to 70. The inability to produce cellular energy was probably the primary cause of her fatigue, while secondary factors included anemia (deficiencies in vitamin B12) and hypoglycemia (low blood sugar and deficiency in chromium, which stabilizes blood sugar production).

Susan's secondary symptoms of anxiety and premenstrual syndrome suggested imbalances of the adrenal glands caused by stress. Stress causes the adrenal glands to release cortisol, part of the body's "fight-or-flight" response. However, chronic stress and excess amounts of cortisol can cause muscle fatigue, immune dysfunction, and adversely effect metabolism and the transport of nutrients in the body. A deficiency in calcium (an essential cofactor in nerve function and energy production) further weakened Susan's adrenal system.

We started Susan on a complete program of tissue detoxification with individualized therapies focusing on the intestines, liver, connective tissues, and adrenals. To treat Susan's intestinal permeability, we prescribed the following supplements:

■ Glutamine: an essential amino acid which aids in the rebuilding of gastrointestinal cells (3,000 mg, four times daily, between meals).

■ Fiberplex: to cleanse and strengthen the intestines; contains psyllium, oat bran, pectin, guar gum, goldenseal powder, geranium, and okra powder (1 tsp dissolved in 8 oz of water followed by another 8 oz of water, taken once in the morning and once in the evening, with meals).

■ Colon-cleansing treatments: we recommended colonics that used the friendly bacteria *Lactobacillus acidophilus* during the last five minutes of therapy as an implant, in order to help reestablish healthy intestinal flora; once weekly for eight weeks.

■ Castor oil packs: to relieve joint pain or for relief of PMS symptoms; three days a week (see "How to Use Castor Oil Packs," p. 176).

Next, we worked on cleansing Susan's liver and restoring its ability to detoxify the body. We gave her lipotropic factors (SEE QUICK DEFINITION) containing the liver-detoxifying agents phosphatidyl choline, inositol, and methionine (four tablets, three times daily). Herbal lipotropics included milk thistle, chelidonium, chionathus, black radish, and beet extract. To restore vitality to her liver, we needed to increase her levels of sulfur-containing amino acids, which are integral to detoxification. So, we instructed her to drink vegetable juice (five glasses daily) containing vegetables in the cabbage family (high in sulfur), parsley, and dandelion roots and greens. Parsley and dandelion are high in sulfur and act as diuretics, helping to clear toxins from the kidneys.

DEFINITION

The **Krebs cycle** (also known as the citric acid cycle) is a metabolic process that occurs in each cell of the body in a small organelle called the mitochondria. It is an essential step in cellular respiration (the exchange of oxygen and carbon dioxide between the cell and the environment) and can be compared to the refinement of crude oil into high grade, octanerich petroleum. Foods consumed are transformed by digestion into smaller molecules of glucose, fatty acids, and amino acids; these are further converted into carbon compounds called pyruvates and acetates. In the Krebs cycle, acetates and pyruvates are converted into carbon dioxide and four pairs of electrons. It is the energy found in these electrons which is eventually stored in the molecule called adenosine triphosphate (ATP). ATP is analogous to refined gasoline and is the human fuel which provides energy to every cell.

Lipotropic factors are substances that help detoxify the liver by removing and preventing fatty deposits. Inositol (a fiber component) is considered a B vitamin and works closely with choline, especially in cases of liver disorders, diabetes, and depression; it helps remove fats from the liver, preventing stagnation of liver fats and bile. Phosphatidyl choline (a combination of two fatty acids, choline and phosphate) is needed to maintain cell membranes and to help reduce multiple liver symptoms from hepatitis and cirrhosis, and fatty liver from alcohol or diabetes. Methionine (an amino acid) helps the liver to detoxify; it is also integral to cartilage and can help improve the strength of joint tissues.

How to Use Castor Oil Packs

To prepare a castor oil pack, lightly heat enough castor oil to thoroughly wet but not soak a 10" x 12" flannel cloth. Immerse the flannel in the warm oil, then fold to make three to four layers and place against the skin. (The oil helps to draw out toxins, release tension, and improve blood circulation, especially in the lower abdomen.) Wrap a hot water bottle in a towel and place this over the pack, then cover pack and bottle with another towel to retain heat. Keep in place for one to two hours. Following the treatment, the oil-soaked flannel may be wrapped in plastic and stored in a refrigerator for later use. After the flannel has been used 20 times, discard it.

To replenish Susan's supplies of antioxidants we prescribed the following:

■ Vitamin E: anti-inflammatory action that suppresses the breakdown of cartilage while stimulating cartilage growth; 1,000 IU, three times daily with food

■ Carotenoid Complex Liquid Drops: antioxidant and anti-inflammatory; ten drops, twice daily with food (300,000 IU total)

■ Buffered vitamin C: vital for tissue repair and, when taken in combination with vitamin E, contributes to the stability of cartilage; to bowel tolerance

■ Quercetin: heals leaky gut, stabilizes gut mast cells and histamine release; 500 mg, three times daily between meals

■ Pycnogenol: contains flavonoids to strengthen tissue integrity; 150 mg daily

■ Essential fatty acids: anti-inflammatory for soothing the gastrointestinal tract; we initially recommended fish oil which was later replaced by flaxseed oil; 4 tsp daily

To improve Susan's stress level, we scheduled sessions in a flotation R.E.S.T. tank to reduce anxiety. She took several supplements to lower stress hormones and heal the adrenal glands, particularly a product called AlteraTonic, an herbal combination containing Siberian ginseng, *ashwaghandha*, *rehmannia*, *Panax ginseng*, and other botanicals. A month later she began taking *Glycyrrhiza glabra*, a solid extract of licorice root (¼ tsp, three times daily) to support her adrenal glands and liver; licorice is also a powerful anti-inflammatory. We also prescribed glucosamine sulfate (3,000 mg per day on an empty stomach) to help rebuild her joints and cartilage.

Susan undertook a fast to further detoxify her system. She then resumed a normal diet, being careful to avoid the foods that she was allergic to or that might exacerbate her arthritis symptoms. Repeat testing revealed that her leaky gut was resolved as well as the irritable bowel, PMS, and asthma. Yearly checkups showed that Susan continued to improve, but she had to maintain her arthritis-friendly diet and supplementation or inflammation would return. She walks comfortably now and no longer suffers debilitating pain in her joints.

Healthy and Unhealthy Intestines

The strength of the intestines depends on the effectiveness of the matrix that keeps its framework intact. In a healthy intestine, no unwanted molecules can penetrate the cell membranes of the small or large intestine, or escape between intestinal-wall cells because of the tight seal created by the intracellular "glue" which forms a barrier. In our clinical experience, most patients with arthritis have some degree of faulty digestive process that involves an unhealthy intestine. When this intracellular adhesive breaks down, large molecules of toxins escape into the bloodstream, where they trigger a series of harmful biochemical events.[1] Although osteoarthritis does not have as high a correlation to leaky gut as does autoimmune arthritis, we generally see intestinal problems and irritable bowel symptoms preceding the onset of many types of arthritis, especially rheumatoid arthritis.

Two facts about the intestines pertain to permeability. The small and large intestines measured together and laid flat equal about 25 feet in length. Second, the total surface area in the intestines that is capable of absorbing nutrients is about the size of a tennis court. The small intestine, which is about 21 feet long and 1" wide, absorbs about 95% of the fats and 90% of the amino acids we consume as foods. The small intestine's most important role is the absorption of nutrients. Food that has been churned in the stomach with digestive enzymes and hydrochloric acid—both are often deficient in arthritis patients and lead to incomplete digestion—is moved into and through the small intestine. That process requires contractions of the small intestine's walls, a wave-like motion called peristalsis. Absorptive projections known as villi line the intestinal walls; smaller sub-projections, or microvilli, also line the walls. Microvilli provide a twentyfold increase in the absorptive surface area of the small intestines.

In healthy intestines, all of the semi-digested food stays inside the intestines, which is also lined with a protective mucus layer (glycocalyx). The only substances that are absorbed are digested

For more information on **FiberPlex**, contact: Tyler Encapsulations, 2204-8 N.W. Birdsdale, Gresham, OR 97030; tel: 800-869-9705 or 503-661-5401; fax; 503-666-4913. For **Carotenoid Complex Liquid Drops, quercetin, and pycnogenol**, contact: Environmental Detoxification Consultants, 413 Grassy Hill Road, Woodbury, CT 06798; tel/fax: 203-263-2970. For **Altera–Tonic**, contact: Nature's Answer, 320 User Avenue, Hauppauge, NY 11788; tel: 800-439-2324 or 516-231-7492; fax; 516-231-8391; website: www.naturesanswer.com.

For more on **fasting**, see Chapter 4: General Detoxification, pp. 78-100. For **dietary recommendations for arthritis**, see Chapter 12: The Arthritis Diet, pp. 250-278.

Most patients with arthritis have some degree of faulty digestive process that involves an unhealthy intestine. Although osteoarthritis does not have as high a correlation to leaky gut as does autoimmune arthritis, we generally see intestinal problems and irritable bowel symptoms preceding the onset of many types of arthritis, especially rheumatoid arthritis.

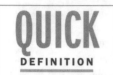

QUICK
DEFINITION

Circulating immune complexes (CICs) form in the body when poor digestion results in undigested food proteins "leaking" through the intestinal wall and into the bloodstream. The immune system treats these foreign substances or antigens as invaders, causing antibodies to form and couple with them. This antigen and antibody combination is known as a CIC. In a healthy person, CICs are neutralized, but in someone with a compromised immune system, they tend to accumulate in the blood where they burden the detoxification pathways or initiate an allergic reaction. If too many CICs accumulate, the kidneys and liver cannot excrete enough of them via the urine or stool. The CICs are then stored in soft tissues, causing inflammation and bringing stress to the immune system. The overload can lead to a variety of chronic health conditions.

nutrients in molecular form, which are absorbed by the microvilli. In the leaky gut, however, larger molecules of incompletely digested foods are able to escape through the damaged intestinal cell membranes. These particles are recognized by the immune system as invaders and become circulating immune complexes (SEE QUICK DEFINITION), which initiate inflammation throughout the body when deposited in unwanted areas.

The average transit time through the small intestine is two hours, although one to six hours is the range. Digested food then passes through the ileocecal valve from the small intestine to the large intestine (which is, on average, five feet long and 2½" wide). At that point the food is in a semi-fluid state. Once in the large intestine, or colon, water is reabsorbed from the digested food and the remaining contents form the feces; this consists of indigestible cellulose fibers, friendly and unfriendly microbes (yeast and bacteria common to the intestine and representing about 30% of fecal weight), and potentially harmful bile that contains the liver's processed toxins. Average transit time through a healthy large intestine is 12 hours.

We estimate that at least 80% of patients in our practice have some degree of abnormally increased intestinal permeability or leaky gut syndrome—a far greater incidence than the conservative 11%-21% cited by the Arthritis Foundation. Research reported in the *Journal of Rheumatology* and elsewhere supports the connection between arthritis and the passage of microorganisms or other substances capable of causing disease (pathogens) through the intestinal wall.[2]

Causes of Leaky Gut Syndrome

Common causes of leaky gut syndrome include a diet high in fried foods, processed foods, inorganic meat products, and simple carbohydrates, as well as excessive alcohol intake. Ironically, medications such as NSAIDs used to relieve symptoms of discomfort associated with arthritis also cause severe leaky gut.

NSAIDs—NSAIDs (nonsteroidal, anti-inflammatory drugs) are conventional drugs given to reduce inflammation, pain, and joint stiffness associated with osteoarthritis and rheumatoid arthritis, lupus, and other similar conditions. Side effects commonly associated with NSAIDs include rash, edema, vertigo, nausea, vomiting, and potentially fatal gastrointestinal hemorrhages. NSAIDs may cause gastrointestinal malfunction and irritation, which are leading contributors to leaky gut syndrome. They have been known to "burn holes" through the gastrointestinal wall, particularly the stomach, even at normal therapeutic doses in some individuals. When the intestines are irritated and duodenal lesions occur, brought on by NSAID toxicity, the stage is set for leaky gut syndrome.[3]

Habitual Alcohol Use—In 1984, research published in *The Lancet* looked at the effect of alcohol on the gut and found that all alcoholics in the study had increased leaky gut, which lasted up to several weeks after the cessation of drinking. Study subjects who abstained from alcohol for less than four days "almost invariably" had a higher level of intestinal permeability than those not drinking at all.[4] To reduce the risk of leaky gut syndrome, it is advisable for patients with arthritis to abstain from alcohol consumption.

Lectins—Lectins are protein fragments of incompletely digested foods that bind with specific sugars on the surface of all cells of the body. They tend to stick like Velcro® to the lining of the gastrointestinal tract, where they irritate the tissues and can destroy cell membranes. Further, lectins can cause the intestinal villi to die.

One treatment that can help patients deal with lectins is the use of decoy sugars.

Causes of Leaky Gut Syndrome

- Aspirin and Other NSAIDs
- Lectins (Harmful Protein Fragments) in Foods
- Alcohol
- Toxins
- Viruses
- Standard American Diet (SAD)
- *Candida* and Parasites

Decoy sugars (a term coined by Dr. Zampieron) act by attracting and neutralizing dietary lectins before the lectin can attach itself to the intestinal lining (where it can cause impaired absorption, poor digestion, and leaky gut syndrome). Choosing the correct decoy sugar ("decoy" because it "tricks" the lectins into moving away from the gut lining) depends on the person's blood type: for instance, the supplement NAG (N-acetyl-glucosamine) is useful for type A, while the sugar fucose (from the herb bladderwrack) works well for blood type O. Both are readily obtainable in health food stores. (The prevalence of autoimmune arthritis is higher for people with type O blood than any other type.)

Toxins—In a recent study, Jeffrey Bland, Ph.D., author of *Genetic Nutritioneering*, found that when gastrointestinal mucus cells were exposed to various toxins, the tight junctures between them expanded and allowed for the absorption of larger molecules. These molecules translocated from the gut and migrated to other areas of the body, causing inflammation.[5] Toxins produced in the intestines can exert another harmful effect, says Dr. Bland. They can stimulate a particular enzyme that leads to the depletion of the cell's primary energy molecule, called ATP; this enzyme can also impair the movement of nutrients across their membranes. For the tissues of the gastrointestinal system to rapidly regenerate, they need high levels of nutrients such as amino acids. This regeneration requires ample supplies of ATP, but in patients with abnormal bowel flora or intestinal imbalance, there is a decrease in ATP levels, which curtails efficient cell regeneration; this can then contribute to increased leaky gut syndrome and degenerative changes throughout the body.

Viruses—Many studies suggest that increased gut permeability in ankylosing spondylitis and rheumatoid arthritis cases may exist prior to the start of arthritic symptoms and that it is a factor in the development of these illnesses.[6] Viruses may be implicated in the development of many cases of rheumatoid arthritis. Patients often report that their arthritis began after a prolonged flu-like illness, which either slowly or never resolved. Often, the influenza-like disorder severely affected their digestive system. More research is still needed to determine if viruses are the "missing link" in arthritis.

For more on *Candida*'s role in arthritis, see Chapter 6: Eradicating Bacteria and Yeast, pp. 130-151.

Yeast Infections—*Candida* and other opportunistic yeast organisms, as well as parasites, can grow on the inside of the intestines. There, they send out structures called hyphae (roots) that puncture the intestinal lining, causing leaky gut syndrome to develop. An overgrowth of *Candida* and translocation of the yeast into distant parts of the body causes many arthritis-like symptoms, such as joint pain and stiffness, inflammation, and loss of energy, as well as allergies, headaches, immune suppression, and liver dysfunction.

Alternative Medicine Therapies for Leaky Gut Syndrome

Treating leaky gut requires an approach using multiple therapies. Underlying causes, such as diet, medications, alcohol use, viruses, or *Candida*, should be the first issues to address. Fasting and dietary changes can help ease the stress on the digestive system and begin the healing process. Herbs, enzymes, and nutrients can then help tonify and soothe inflamed tissues and normalize digestion.

Fasting

Fasting has been shown in scientific studies to be beneficial in treating leaky gut syndrome. It is an inexpensive, rapid, effective therapy for elim-

Testing for Intestinal Permeability

There is a specific laboratory test that can measure the degree to which leaky gut is present called the Intestinal Permeability Assay. In this test, the patient drinks a liquid which contains a combination of two large sugar molecules, mannitol and lactulose. A majority of these sugars are not absorbed through the intestine and pass through the colon and are excreted in the stool. However, if the person has leaky gut syndrome, some of these large sugar molecules "leak" through the intestines and into the blood. They are then filtered out by the kidneys and exit the body through the urine. According to John Furlong, N.D., of Great Smokies Diagnostic Laboratory, the specific lactulose/mannitol ratio is used as a diagnostic "gold standard," providing a reliable assessment of the intestinal wall's condition. Elevated levels of both sugars in the urine can indicate increased permeability.

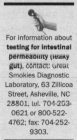

For information about **testing for intestinal permeability (leaky gut)**, contact: Great Smokies Diagnostic Laboratory, 63 Zillicoa Street, Asheville, NC 28801, tel. 704-253-0621 or 800-522-4762; fax: 704-252-9303.

inating poisons from the body and not as difficult as it may seem at first. Fasting reduces gut permeability by allowing the damaged intestines to heal when the offending foods are removed.[7] Fasting can help the body excrete stored toxins and, at the same time, decrease the intake of new toxins. Also, by decreasing the amount of food allergens and dietary lectins, the gut has time to regenerate. Fasting allows ener-

For a **complete guide to detoxification and fasting,** see Chapter 4: General Detoxification, pp. 78-100.

gy and nutrients to be diverted to other metabolic processes. By cutting off the supply of circulating immune complexes entering the bloodstream from the gut, fasting affords the body time to divert its energy toward detoxification. Those CICs deposited in the connective tissue are digested by white blood cells whose activity has been shown to increase with fasting.[8]

Dietary Tips to Reduce Leaky Gut Syndrome

Here are two key adjustments you can prudently incorporate in your dietary habits that can make a significant difference in the operation of your intestines:

■ Avoid alcohol, foods containing antibiotic residues (animal proteins, including dairy products, except those designated organic and free-range) and artificial substances (which can irritate the intestinal lining), foods known to be allergenic to you, sources of dietary lectins, sugars, and refined foods. Instead, use organically grown foods whenever possible. While completely abstaining from alcohol and sugar may seem unrealistically austere, even a substantial reduction of these substances in your diet will produce beneficial results.

■ Eat with awareness. Eat and chew slowly, chew thoroughly until the food is liquified, and try to be more conscious of the fact you are consuming foods. Begin the digestive process in a state of calm with appreciation of the sensory qualities of the foods. Consider using chopsticks instead of a knife and fork; the chopsticks will slow you down and induce a more contemplative approach to eating. If you eat with your right hand, switch to your left. Put down your fork between bites and take smaller bites. When you're eating, do nothing else—don't watch TV, don't read the newspaper—eat with purpose to heal your arthritis. We also recommend drinking only a small volume of liquid with meals, because large amounts of liquid dilute digestive juices, rendering digestion less effective.

Tonify the Digestive System

Naturopathic physicians and other holistically oriented doctors use various approaches to strengthen the digestive and enzymatic functions of the intestines, including the use of bitter herbs and digestive enzymes.

■ Bitter Herbs—Chemicals present in bitter-tasting herbs stimulate the central nervous system (via nerves in the tongue); a message is then sent to the gut to activate a powerful digestive hormone, gastrin.[9] Bitters stimulate the production of hydrochloric acid, increase the liver's production of bile, and stimulate the appetite. Bitters can also

promote saliva and gastric juices and accelerate the emptying of the stomach, thus triggering the pancreas to begin to
release digestive enzymes. Bitters are useful for sluggish
digestion, heartburn, dyspepsia, bowel tension, flatulence,
and bloating.

For more **dietary rec-
ommendations help-
ful for arthritis,** see
Chapter 12: The
Arthritis Diet,
pp. 250-278.

While bitters have been used for thousands of years as a
digestive tonic in many traditional cultures, most
Americans shun them and have not, like many Europeans and Asians,
become accustomed to their taste. We suggest an excellent, pleasant-
tasting bitters formula: brew one teaspoon each of gentian, dandelion,
goldenseal, rue, *artemesia*, and prickly ash in six cups of boiling water
to make a tea. Add a few drops of peppermint oil. Bitters need to be
sipped and tasted, because they work through the slow stimulation of
the tongue.

A bitters salad can be made with dandelion leaves, escarole, endive,
and other bitter salad greens. These can be combined with romaine,
green leaf and red leaf lettuce, and some olive oil, flaxseed oil, spices,
and lemon juice. This salad triggers the entire digestive system to
function more effectively. Bitters are available commercially as
"Swedish Bitters" in health food stores and as Italian Fernet Brancha
in any liquor store. Be aware that Swedish Bitters contains camphor,
which can sabotage the effectiveness of homeopathic remedies.

■ Digestive Enzymes—Arthritis patients have deficiencies in
digestive enzymes. Papain from papaya and bromelain from pineapples are effective digestive enzymes when taken along with food.
These same enzymes can be used for their anti-inflammatory action
when taken without food. Pancreatic enzyme supplements aid in the
body's production of enzymes. The pancreas can recycle and recircu-
late pancreatic enzyme extracts, so not only do they support digestion
while it's occurring in the small intestine, but they also support future
digestion and tonify the pancreas and small intestine. People with
arthritis and leaky gut syndrome desperately need this digestive toni-
fication. Tonifying the digestive system breaks down large food molecules, decreases the amount of food allergies, inactivates dietary
lectins, stimulates digestion, and halts or alters the growth of dysbiotic microorganisms in the gut. In essence, it arrests the processes
responsible for arthritis.

Demulcent Herbs and Foods
Demulcent is a term used by herbalists to describe an herb which has
a protective effect on the mucous membranes. Most of the herbs that

contain demulcents have large amounts of mucilaginous materials—gummy, slimy chemicals that have a direct action on the lining of the intestines, soothing irritations. In general, all mucilage-containing demulcents minimize irritation down the whole length of the bowel, reducing the sensitivity of the digestive system to gastric acids, relaxing painful spasms, and decreasing leaky gut and digestive inflammation and ulceration.[10]

Marshmallow (*Althea officinalis*)—Marshmallow root contains 25% to 35% mucilage. The root of the plant is used by herbalists for any inflammation of the gastrointestinal system. It is usually taken as a tea: take several teaspoons of the root or leaves, cover with boiling water, and steep for 20-30 minutes to extract all the medicinal components. Six cups of this tea a day can be useful in severe cases of leaky gut.

Slippery Elm Bark (*Ulmus fulva*)—Slippery elm, obtained by removing the bark from the branches of the slippery elm tree, has been used as a demulcent for the respiratory and gastrointestinal systems. Its traditional use is in ulcers, colitis, irritable bowel, infections, and diarrhea.[11] Slippery elm is available as a tincture or capsules, or a decoction can also be made: simmer the bark very gently, one part of the bark to eight quarts of water; bring to a boil and let it brew for 20-30 minutes; drink 2-3 cups a day.

Cabbage Juice—Raw, green, organic cabbage juice contains high amounts of glutamine, an essential amino acid that aids in the metabolism of gastrointestinal cells. Cabbage juice can be made in combination with other vegetables that are effective in reconstructing a healthy gut mucosa, such as chickweed and plantain banana. Put them together to make an excellent healing juice; 4-8 ounces a day is advisable.

Okra (*Hibiscus esculentus*)—Okra, a mucilaginous vegetable that is under-utilized as a food source, contains ingredients that soothe and restore the irritated gastrointestinal tract. It is included in several commercial herbal formulas, such as GastroGuard (from Nature's Answer) and Robert's Formula (from Phyto-Pharmica).

Fenugreek—Crushed fenugreek seeds contain 28% mucilin and make an excellent demulcent. The use of this medicinal plant dates back to the Egyptians and the Greek physician Hippocrates. Fenugreek seeds can be steeped as a tea or used in capsules. To make tea, use one teaspoon of fenugreek to one cup of water. In supplement form: one capsule (250 mg) 2-3 times daily, with hot water.

Anti-Inflammatory and Astringent Herbs

Anti-inflammatory herbs help to reduce localized tissue swelling and inflammation in the gut. Astringent herbs tighten and tonify tissues, thus sealing the permeable intestines.

Ginkgo biloba—The ginkgo tree is one of the oldest living trees on earth. Its leaves contain biochemical compounds responsible for ginkgo's healing properties.[12] Clinical and laboratory tests have shown that standardized *Ginkgo biloba* extract (standardized to 24% ginkgo flavoglycosides) has significant benefit in the treatment of increased intestinal permeability, as well as many other health problems associated with inadequate blood supply. Ginkgo protects the intestines by reducing the oxidative damage in the intestinal lining due to free-radical activity. Recommended dosage: 300 mg, two times daily.

Khella (*Ammi visnaga*)—Khella is a relatively unknown herb in the treatment of leaky gut syndrome. The use of khella was part of Bedouin folk medicine for centuries. Khellin, the chief active component of khella, inhibits the release of histamine, which otherwise induces an inflammatory response, and also has anti-spasmodic properties.[13] The allopathic antihistamine drug Intal® is based on this ancient remedy.

Chinese Skullcap or Scute (*Scutellaria baicalensis*)—Japanese research has yielded new information that Chinese skullcap has significant anti-allergenic and antioxidant properties.[14] The active ingredient, baicalin, is responsible for its anti-inflammatory action. Chinese skullcap has been shown to block highly inflammatory end products of the arachidonic acid cascade (SEE QUICK DEFINITION).

Licorice Root (*Glycyrrhiza glabra*)—Licorice is a traditional herbal remedy with an ancient history. Modern research has shown that it has beneficial effects on the endocrine system, adrenal glands, and liver; it is also a systemic anti-inflammatory.[15] The anti-irritant effect on the gastrointestinal sys-

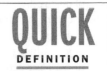

DEFINITION

The **arachidonic acid cascade** is a chemical reaction occuring in cell membranes that results in the production of molecules such as prostaglandins and leukotrienes that cause many negative physiological reactions. These include bronchial constriction (in asthmatics), intestinal permeability or leakiness, water retention and swelling, allergies, inflammation, and, ultimately, tissue destruction. Arachidonic acid is a fatty acid found primarily in animal foods such as meat, poultry, and dairy products. When the diet is abundant with arachidonic acids, these are stored in cell membranes; an enzyme transforms these stored fatty acids into chemical messengers called prostaglandins and leukotrienes that instigate inflammation.

tem is thought to be due to flavonoid derivatives of licorice called steroidal saponin glycosides, which exert a protective effect. Licorice root is used internationally for its antiulcer and healing effects on the gastrointestinal system.[16] Licorice root has also been shown to reduce the gastric bleeding caused by the use of NSAIDs. If the use of NSAIDs is necessary, gastric mucus damage has been reduced by giving simultaneous dosages of 500 mg of deglycerinated licorice.

Meadowsweet (*Filipendulia ulmaria*)—Meadowsweet contains anti-inflammatory glycosides, tannins, mucilage, and flavonoids. The anti-inflammatory properties in combination with other effects makes meadowsweet one of the prime herbs in the treatment of ulcers or other problems with the gastrointestinal system. Its astringent properties allow this herb to strengthen the connective tissue bonds between the cells of the gastrointestinal tract, thus solidifying the protective barrier and helping to decrease leaky gut. Meadowsweet is a powerful astringent and can actually help stop bleeding in the digestive tract. Recommended dosage: 250 mg, twice daily.

Chamomile (*Matricaria chamomilia*)—The flower of the chamomile plant produces a calming effect, easing anxiety and reducing tension.[17] It can be helpful with overall anxiety, sleep disorders, and muscle tension, and its calming properties have a beneficial effect on the gastrointestinal system as well. In addition, it stimulates digestive secretions, so it can improve digestive function. In Europe, chamomile is recognized as a digestive aid, a mild sedative, and an anti-inflammatory, notably in antibacterial oral hygiene and skin preparations.[18] Its anti-inflammatory properties also reduce allergic responses. In Germany, chamomile is licensed as an over-the-counter drug for internal use against gastrointestinal spasms and inflammatory diseases of the intestinal tract (two of its constituents, azulene and bisboline, are powerful anti-inflammatories). Chamomile's Latin name, *Matricaria chamomilia*, means "mother of the gut." Recommended dosage: 250 mg, 2-3 times daily.

Goldenseal (*Hydrastis canadensis*)—One of the most widely used American herbs, goldenseal is considered to be a tonic remedy that stimulates immune response and is a germ destroyer as well. In addition, because of its astringent effects, goldenseal can help in many digestive problems, from peptic ulcers to colitis.[19] It also promotes the production and secretion of digestive juices. Goldenseal's germ-fighting properties are due to berberine, which is effective against bacteria, protozoa, and fungi, including *Staphylococcus, Streptococcus, Candida,* and *Giardia lamblia.*[20] Berberine has also been shown to increase immune function by activating the white blood cells that digest cell debris and other waste matter in the blood.[21] We often recommend the use of berberine-rich substitutes for goldenseal (such as barberry), because over-harvesting is a major problem with this herb. Goldenseal also contains alkaloids and tannins that support the intestinal barrier and is considered a major herb for treating chronic gastrointestinal inflammatory conditions. Recommended dosage: 250 mg, 2-3 times daily.

Other Nutrients for Leaky Gut

■ Quercetin—Quercetin is a naturally occurring bioflavonoid (vitamin C helper) found in many species of plants, including the oak, onion, and blue-green algae. As a bioflavonoid, it has powerful antioxidant and anti-inflammatory properties and has been used by alternative practitioners for many years in the treatment of arthritis, autoimmune diseases, asthma, and cataracts. Quercetin blocks inflammation that can otherwise lead to leaky gut syndrome. Quercetin has an excellent affinity for the gut and, in the treatment of leaky gut syndrome, it represents one of nature's most perfect medicines. By decreasing the rapid opening of mast cells and basophils—white blood cells which release histamines—quercetin stabilizes the gut and decreases permeability. Recommended dosage: 200 mg, 2-3 times daily between meals.

■ Glutamine—The amino acid glutamine is an important nutrient for the intestinal mucosa. An increase of L-glutamine in the diet has been shown to support gastrointestinal mucus integrity.[22] Glutamine reduces unwanted movement of bacterial forms through the permeable intestinal wall and into general circulation, where they can often end up in the joints and instigate or aggravate arthritis.[23] Glutamine is used in the synthesis of an important nutrient known as N-acetyl-D-glucosamine (NAG), which is fundamental to the production of the protective mucus lining the digestive and respiratory tracts and the first line of defense against leaky gut syndrome. Glutamine supplementation also enhances glutathione, an important antioxidant.[24] Typical recommended dosage for patients with leaky gut syndrome: 3,000-10,000 mg per day, in divided doses between meals.

Chinese Herbal Combination for Leaky Gut

Our favorite herbal remedy for leaky gut is to combine ginkgo, quercetin, scutellaria, khella, and okra with any of the Chinese patent medicines mentioned below. These formulas work well in combination with herbs; especially good pre-formulated combinations include GastroGuard from Nature's Answer and Robert's Formula from Phyto-Pharmica. In Chinese medicine, there are several excellent patent formulas that have a soothing effect on the digestive system:

Pill Curing Formula—Pill Curing Formula, helps cramping, abdominal pain, diarrhea, irritation, and mucousy stools. It is made up of many ingredients, including coix seed, atractylodes, chrysanthemum flowers, and citrus peel.

Chinese patent medicines are available in most Chinese pharmacies. For information about the patent medicines mentioned here, contact: Lin's Sister, 4 Bowery Street, New York, NY 10013; tel: 212-962-5417. For Gastro-Guard, contact: Nature's Answer, 320 Oser Avenue, Hauppauge, NY 11788; tel: 800-439-2324 or 516-231-7492; fax: 516-231-8391; website: www.naturesanswer.com. For Robert's Formula, contact: Phyto-Pharmica, P.O. Box 1745, Green Bay, WI 54305; tel: 800-558-7372 or 920-469-9099; fax: 920-469-4418.

Shenling Baizhupian—Shenling Baizhupian is a classic patent medicine formula for digestion, erratic loose stools, and symptoms of irritable bowel. It includes codonopsis, wild yam root, citrus peel, and licorice root (*Glycyrrhiza glabra*).

Yunnan Paiyao—Yunnan Paiyao is a valuable first-aid remedy for internal and external bleeding; studies indicate that it can cause blood to clot 33% faster. The main ingredient is pseudo ginseng root. When taken internally, Yunnan Paiyao has been shown to stop internal bleeding in the gastrointestinal system and is used for the treatment of gastrointestinal inflammation. Recommended dosage: 200 mg, twice daily on an empty stomach.

■ Glutathione—Glutathione is a tri-peptide, a small protein consisting of three amino acids, that functions as a principle antioxidant, scavenging free radicals and toxins that would otherwise damage and destroy cells. Further, glutathione regulates the activities of other antioxidants, such as vitamins A, C, and E. Vitamin C can also help increase glutathione levels.[25] When the body is overrun by free radicals, supplies of glutathione become depleted. This condition, known as oxidative stress, negatively affects the musculoskeletal, nervous, immune, and endocrine systems and may underlie many of the symptoms associated with arthritis. Glutathione exerts another protective and scavenging role in concert with the liver, the body's primary organ of detoxification and internal cleansing. In the liver, glutathione combines with toxins, carcinogens, and waste products as a way of neutralizing them and then more effectively securing their elimination from the body. In addition, glutathione helps red blood cell membranes retain their structure, and must be present for white blood cells to perform their function of immune regulation. Although taking glutathione directly as a supplement may be beneficial, some studies have shown that the absorption of oral glutathione supplements is limited.[26] The best way of increasing the availability of glutathione is by increasing the precursors that the body needs to manufacture glutathione, including foods in the cabbage family as well as onions and garlic.

■ N-Acetyl-D-Glucosamine—N-acetyl-D-glucosamine (NAG) is a sugar that is important to the formation of a type of mucus, glycocalyx, that protects the delicate intestinal tissues and acts as a first line of defense against bacteria, fungi, and viruses. These disease-causing microorganisms attempt to adhere to the cell surface and invade the intestinal walls. NAG also functions as a decoy sugar, attracting and binding dietary lectins, which then prevents them from attaching to the gut. People with a compromised gastrointestinal lining are more likely to experience the irritation caused by food allergies, dietary lectins, and bacterial, fungal, and viral organisms. Also, they are more susceptible to the damage due to aspirin, NSAIDs, and the contents of their own intestines, such as bile acid.[27] Again, elevated levels of circulating immune complexes are the end result, which cause inflammation and create serious problems for arthritis sufferers. NAG promotes the growth of friendly bacteria and is quickly digested by healthy intestinal bacteria. Recommended dosage: 500 mg, three times daily on an empty stomach.

■ Essential Fatty Acids—The kind of fats and oils that we take into our bodies are of paramount importance in determining the amount of inflammation we experience. A significant reduction in lab indicators of inflammation after using omega-3 fatty acids has been verified in clinical studies.[28] These fatty acids are found in fish oils and certain vegetable oils, such as flaxseed and hemp seed oil. Those with arthritis should consume at least 4-6 tablespoons of these oils daily, along with a significant decrease in consumption of the "bad oils" found in commercially raised meat products, butter, hydrogenated oils from commercial baked goods, and margarine. In addition to omega-3 fatty acids, borage seed oil and evening primrose oil, which contain large amounts of gamma-linolenic acid (GLA), an omega-6 oil, cause clinical improvement in tissue inflammation associated with rheumatoid arthritis.[29] Joint Lubrication, from Alternative Therapy, contains a therapeutic combination of "good oils."

For more information on **Joint Lubrication**, contact: Alternative Therapy, Inc., 1664 Fairlawn Avenue, San Jose, CA 95125; tel: 800-311-7922.

For more on **herbs and nutrients helpful in treating arthritis**, see Chapter 13: Supplements for Arthritis, pp. 280-313.

■ Vitamins and Minerals—The nutrients zinc, selenium, ascorbic acid, vitamin E, beta carotene, and vitamin A, the enzymes superoxide dismutase (SOD) and catalase, and the amino acid N-acetyl-L-cysteine have been shown to quench various types of free radicals. Some intestinal lining damage is due to free radicals, so neutralizing free radicals is beneficial. Not only do the antioxidants help the gut in preventing intestinal damage due to oxidation, but these antioxidants also help to decrease inflammation systemically, particularly in the joints and connective tissues associated arthritis.

■ Probiotics and FOS—The human body contains an estimated several trillion beneficial bacteria comprising over 400 species, all necessary for health. Many of these "friendly" bacteria, also called probiotics, reside in the intestines, where they are essential for proper nutrient assimilation. Among the more well-known of these are *Lactobacillus acidophilus* and *Bifidobacteria*.[30] Prior to 1945 and the introduction of mass market foods and chemical agriculture, North Americans normally obtained adequate amounts of probiotics from fresh vegetables. Now, supplements may be necessary if you do not consume a diet filled with vegetables and fruits.

Another option you may have heard of is FOS (fructo-oligosaccharides), known popularly as "fast food for probiotics." FOS is a natural sugar found in food sources such as Jerusalem artichokes, onions, barley, honey, asparagus, and garlic. It provides a growth medium for beneficial bacteria in the intestines. There is a continuing debate in the medical community over the use of FOS as a supplement. We have observed that FOS tends to enhance the unwanted presence of harmful bacteria and fungi, and do not recommend its use. To increase the amount of FOS in your system, eat more fresh fruits and vegetables.

Allergies, intestinal dysfunction,

and painful inflammation seem to operate in a

loop—one triggers the next—and, until

the loop is permanently disrupted, the cycle repeats

itself with increasingly more serious

and painful consequences for arthritis sufferers.

Fortunately, alternative medicine

offers safe, effective, and natural therapies to

get out of the allergy loop and

obtain lasting relief.

CHAPTER

9

Allergies and Arthritis

ALLERGIES PLAY A SIGNIFICANT ROLE in the onset of inflammation and arthritis. Both rheumatoid (autoimmune) arthritis and the inflammation in osteoarthritis can be caused by chemical allergies (sensitivities to environmental pollutants) and food allergies. Allergies can disrupt normal digestive function, leading to intestinal permeability and an increase in inflammation throughout the body. Allergies, intestinal dysfunction, and painful inflammation seem to operate in a loop—one triggers the next—and, until the loop is permanently disrupted, the cycle repeats itself with increasingly more serious and painful consequences for arthritis sufferers. Fortunately, alternative medicine offers safe, effective, and natural therapies to get out of the allergy loop and obtain lasting relief.

In This Chapter

Success Story: Eliminating Food Allergies and Arthritis

The following brief case study from our patient files shows the linkage among foods consumed, allergies, and arthritis symptoms. Morton, 32, complained of minor muscle and joint pain affecting his neck, fingers, and wrists. For most of the year, Morton followed a healthy, semi-vegetarian diet and took nutritional supplements and was free from joint pain. He also followed a rotational diet, in which foods are eaten in a four-day cycle, to reduce allergic reactions. But, once a year (every St. Patrick's Day in mid-March), he attended a family gathering and would drink a large amount of stout beer. The following day, Morton did not wake up with a hangover; instead, he had severe and disabling arthritis pain unlike his usual symptoms of mild

> ### Natural Therapies for Allergies
>
> ■ Dietary Recommendations
> ■ Applied Kinesiology
> ■ Supplements and Herbs

muscle aches. "Is there a possible connection between drinking beer and arthritis?" he asked us.

In addition to standard blood tests, we ran a food allergy test that showed the following: Morton had minor allergies to eggs, green beans, kidney beans, yellow wax beans, oysters, and sesame seeds, and major allergies to brewer's yeast (an ingredient in beer) and baker's yeast. Clearly, Morton was allergic to beer and the increase in beer consumption during this once-yearly family celebration was making his arthritis worse.

More precisely, Morton was allergic to the yeast in beer; yeast is found in many foods, including vinegar, breads, pickles, ketchup, mustard, mayonnaise, salad dressing, sauerkraut, and certain cheeses. Not only did Morton like his beer, but his diet included large quantities of bread and he was fond of salad dressings and condiments like pickles. In essence, Morton craved foods that worsened his arthritis and that continually toxified his system. The St. Patrick's Day bash was the proverbial "straw that broke the camel's back," but his over-indulgence also provided us with a striking clue to the nature of his arthritis.

To address Morton's allergies, we recommended that he limit his consumption of the foods that aggravated his symptoms. We also gave him homeopathic Yeast and Mold Drops (15 drops, twice daily, for six months) from Professional Health Products. By the time St. Patrick's Day rolled around again, Morton was able to indulge (slightly) in the festivities with much less aggravation of his arthritis symptoms.

For information on **Yeast and Mold Drops**, contact: Professional Health Products, Nutritional Specialties, P.O. Box 5897, Pittsburgh, PA 15209; tel: 800-245-1313 or 412-821-0520; fax: 412-821-0529.

The Allergy Connection

A reliable sign of long-term undischarged toxicity is the emergence of allergic symptoms. In fact, it usually surprises our arthritis patients to learn that both rheumatoid arthritis

A Primer on Allergies

An allergy is an adverse immune system reaction—sometimes mild, sometimes severe—to a substance that other people find harmless. Quite often, an allergen (a substance provoking an allergy symptom) is a protein that the body judges to be foreign and dangerous. The adverse reaction that follows is called an allergic response. Common manifestations of this allergic response include fatigue, headaches, sneezing, watery eyes, and stuffy sinuses following exposure to an allergen. Allergies fall into two categories, those caused by environmental factors and those caused by food. The most common source of environmental allergies is the pollen of plants, particularly trees, weeds, and grasses. The most common culprits in food allergies are yeast, wheat, corn, milk and other dairy products, egg whites, tomatoes, soy, shellfish, peanuts, chocolate, and food dyes and additives.

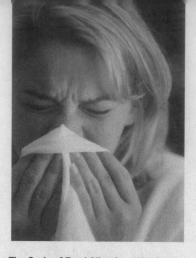

Common Symptoms of a Typical Allergic Reaction—Breathing congestion, inflamed, bloodshot, or scratchy eyes, watery eye, tears, sneezing, coughing, itching, nosebleeds, puffy face, flushing of the cheeks, dark circles under the eyes, runny nose, swelling, hives, vomiting, stomachache, intestinal irritation or swelling.

Common Health Problems Partly Caused by Allergens—Acne, allergic rhinitis (inflammation of mucous lining of nose), bedwetting, diarrhea, asthma, ear infections, eczema, fatigue, arthritis, chronic runny nose, headache, irritability, hay fever, concentration problems, hyperactivity, attention deficit disorder.

The Cycle of Food Allergies—With food allergies, there is a strange paradox: often a person becomes addicted to a food that produces an allergic response. When a person stops eating an allergy-producing food to which their body is "addicted," such as coffee or chocolate, there is a three-day period in which they experience unpleasant withdrawal symptoms, such as fatigue; eating more of this addictive substance can actually improve the situation by suppressing these withdrawal symptoms. This becomes an unhealthy cycle of addiction, craving, and fulfillment that eventually leads to more serious health problems. Allergy experts call this suppression of symptoms by an allergenic food *masking*, because it masks or disguises the true allergic symptoms.

What Happens in an Allergic Response—The typical allergic reactions people have to foods, dust, pollen, and other substances are the body's way of fending off the intrusion of toxins that disrupt the body's equilibrium. Allergens enter the body through breathing, absorption through the skin, by eating or drinking foods, or by injection, such as insect bites or vaccinations. Because the body judges the substances to be dangerous to its health, the immune system identifies them as antigens. Antigens trigger an allergic inflammatory response. The mobilized immune system then releases specific forms of protein called antibodies to deactivate the allergenic antigens, setting in motion a complex series of events involving many biochemicals. These chemicals then produce the inflammation or other typical symptoms of an allergy response. The antibody most commonly involved in the allergic response to pollens and environmentals is IgE, one of five immunoglobulins, or specially designed antibody proteins, involved in the immune system's defense response to foreign substances. The main types of immunoglobulins, grouped according to their concentration in the blood, are: IgG (80%), IgA (10%-15%), IgM (5%-10%), IgD (less than 0.1%), and IgE (less than 0.01%). Mast cells, which produce the allergic response and are found throughout the body's tissues, next come into play; they tend to be concentrated in the skin, nose, and lung linings, gastrointestinal tract, and reproductive organs. When the IgE antibody senses an allergen, it triggers the mast cells to release histamine and 28 other chemicals and the allergic response flares into action. The IgE molecules also attach themselves, like a key fitting a lock, to the allergens.

Immediate vs. Delayed Allergic Reactions—The most common allergic reactions occur immediately after exposure to a certain substance (peanuts, pollen, bee stings, or cats). These reactions are typically caused by IgE immunoglobulins, resulting in a runny nose, watery eyes, itching, and skin rashes; more severe reactions include constriction of the bronchial tubes and difficulty breathing. Delayed allergies are

another type of allergic reaction, which can manifest symptoms up to 72 hours after exposure to a triggering substance. These can commonly appear as seemingly unrelated illnesses or disorders such as lethargy, attention deficit disorder, fatigue, hyperactivity, acne, itchy skin, mood swings, insomnia, and arthritis inflammation. Many of these reactions are caused by IgG immunoglobulins. Up to 80 different medical conditions—from arthritis, asthma, and autism to insomnia, psoriasis, and diabetes—have been clinically associated with IgG food allergy reactions. Many patients display little or no immediate sensitivity reactions (produced by IgE), but instead show moderate to severe delayed reactions (produced by IgG).

Chemicals Released During an Allergic Response—

■ Histamine: This substance causes the blood vessels to widen, enabling more fluid to pass into body tissues, resulting in swelling; it also triggers the smooth involuntary muscles in the lungs, blood vessels, heart, stomach, intestines, and bladder to contract. Histamine gives us runny noses, red itchy eyes, hot, tender, or swollen body parts, flushing, and the other symptoms associated with allergic reactions. In general, the allergic response, in the form of an inflammation, swelling, or tenderness, is the body's attempt to heal itself from the affect of the allergen. These responses are normal ways the body takes care of itself, albeit in the process they can make us feel miserable. However, if they continue unchecked for too long, your health will suffer.
■ Heparin: Increases blood flow to the site of inflammation or swelling.
■ Platelet-Activating Factor: Causes blood platelets to group together so

continued on next page

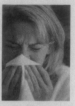

that they release chemicals to change the diameter of blood vessels, thereby affecting blood pressure.

■ Serotonin: A brain chemical known as a neurotransmitter, found in the mucous membrane cells of the gastrointestinal tract, and involved in the allergic response to foods.

■ Lymphokines: Produced by white blood cells (lymphocytes) and involved in communications among cells.

■ Leukotrienes: Found in cell membranes and involved in making the lung muscles contract and the lungs to retain more air, as in the bronchial spasm of asthma.

■ Prostaglandins: Hormone-like substances that help dilate blood vessels, affect smooth muscle contraction, increase pain in affected areas, and heat up inflamed tissues.

■ Thromboxanes: These chemicals contract blood vessels and bronchial tubes.

■ Bradykinin: Supports the cascade of inflammatory symptoms set in motion by the mast cells.

■ Interleukins: Antibodies involved in the activity of lymphocytes.

■ Interferons: Produced by lymphocytes to regulate the speed of immune responses.

QUICK
DEFINITION

Circulating immune complexes (CICs) form in the body when poor digestion results in undigested food proteins "leaking" through the intestinal wall and into the bloodstream. The immune system treats these foreign substances or antigens as invaders, causing antibodies to form and couple with them. This antigen and antibody combination is known as a CIC. In a healthy person, CICs are neutralized, but in someone with a compromised immune system, they tend to accumulate in the blood where they burden the detoxification pathways or initiate an allergic reaction. If too many CICs accumulate, the kidneys and liver cannot excrete enough of them via the urine or stool. The CICs are then stored in soft tissues, causing inflammation and bringing stress to the immune system. The overload can lead to a variety of chronic health conditions.

and the inflammation in osteoarthritis are caused to some degree by a combination of sensitivities to environmental pollutants, food sensitivities, and/or food toxic reactions.[1] There is ample evidence that food antigens (foreign substances) can cross the gastrointestinal membrane, enter the bloodstream, and circulate as injurious immune complexes (SEE QUICK DEFINITION). High levels of immune complexes have been found in both the blood serum and the fluid around the joints of arthritis patients.[2]

In a research study conducted by Marshall Mandell, M.D., author of *Dr. Mandell's Lifetime Arthritis Relief System*, sublingual drops of common allergy-producing foods and chemicals were used to invoke arthritis symptoms. In 87.5% of the cases receiving these drops, the following symptoms were experienced: joint and muscle pain, stiffness, swelling, limited motion of joints, and fatigue. The patients who received placebo drops experienced no reactions.[3]

Evidence is gradually mounting that strongly links arthritis and allergies. One study tracked the medical history and progress of a 52-year-old woman who had suffered from inflammatory arthritis for 11 years to see if her symptoms were linked with food sensitivities. The researchers were especially concerned to study her reactions to milk, meat, and beans. First they evaluated her while on her regular diet, then while fasting, and then while being "challenged" with foods known to provoke allergies. When she was given eight ounces of milk four times a day, this produced 30 minutes of morning stiffness, 14 tender joints, and four swollen joints 24-48 hours later. She also experienced morning stiffness during her normal diet period. In contrast, when the woman fasted for three days, she had no morning stiffness, no swollen joints, and only one tender joint. This study clearly showed that food sensitivities were associated with arthritic symptoms in this patient.[4]

Researchers at the Asthma and Allergy Research Center at Sahlgren's University Hospital in Göteborg, Sweden, also reported strong correlations between milk consumption and arthritis. Of 58 patients who came to the hospital with food-related gastrointestinal symptoms, 41% (24 patients) had joint swelling and 71% (41 patients) had joint pain (arthralgia).[5] In another study, researchers at the All India Institute of Medical

Allergies play a significant role in the onset of inflammation and arthritis. Both rheumatoid arthritis and the inflammation in osteoarthritis can be caused by sensitivities to environmental pollutants and food allergies.

Sciences examined 14 patients with rheumatoid arthritis. These patients abstained from grains, cereals, milk, and non-vegetarian protein foods for two weeks; 71% showed "significant clinical improvement" as a result of eliminating these foods from their daily intake. The researchers concluded that dietary factors may influence inflammatory response in rheumatoid arthritis.[6]

What Causes Allergies?

One of the primary causes of allergies is an overactivated immune system, which substantially increases the risk of allergic reactions. "This occurs when the immune system becomes stressed due to an overload of toxins," says Charles Gableman, M.D., a former practitioner of environmental medicine (SEE QUICK DEFINITION), now living in Lake Forest, California. Many alternative practitioners agree. In researching allergies, Leon Chaitow, N.D., D.O., based in London, England, has found that a number of factors have a negative impact on the

For more on **leaky gut syndrome and arthritis**, see Chapter 8: Alleviating Leaky Gut Syndrome, pp. 172-190.

immune system, including pollution, vaccinations and immunizations, and an over-reliance on steroids, birth control pills, and antibiotics. "Antibiotics further add to the confusion the immune system is facing," states Fuller Royal, M.D., of Las Vegas, Nevada, "until the immune system is no longer able to tell friend from foe. When that happens, it starts reacting to all sorts of things which are not foes, that then become treated as allergens." Allergies can cause immuno-aggression against everything, including healthy tissue (like joint tissue in rheumatoid arthritis). Dr. Royal contends that the immune system may also be weakened by hereditary problems.

"A repetitive diet can contribute greatly to the development of allergies," says Dr. Mandell. The diets of allergy patients normally consist of 30 foods or less, which they eat repeatedly. "These 30 foods then become the basis for the most common food intolerances," says Dr. Mandell. "If someone eats wheat bread every day, for instance, he could easily develop a wheat allergy due to the immune system's continuous exposure to it." Leaky gut syndrome, or excessive permeability in the digestive tract, is another major factor that can lead to allergies. Among the causes of leaky gut syndrome are poor digestion, viral and bacterial infections, parasites, nutrient deficiencies, excessive stress, antibiotics, and *Candida*, all of which can also be factors in arthritis.

Foods That Create Arthritic Problems

Although any food can theoretically trigger an allergic reaction in an individual, this list includes the most common food allergens of arthritis patients:

- Dairy products
- Wheat
- Eggs
- Oranges
- Nuts (especially peanuts)
- Green beans
- Beef
- Yeast (both baker's and brewer's)
- Chocolate
- Sugar
- Corn
- Yellow wax beans
- Nightshades (eggplants, Irish potatoes, green and red peppers, paprika, tomatoes, tobacco)

The Wheat Connection

Wheat is well-known as a food that triggers arthritic conditions. One study focused on a 15-year-old girl who suffered with synovitis (SEE QUICK DEFINITION) of the knees and ankles for three years. The researchers determined that she had an intestinal disease brought about by wheat-gluten sensitivity. When she eliminated wheat gluten (a lectin) entirely from her diet, the synovitis symptoms disappeared, leading researchers to conclude that her arthritis was associated with the bowel disorder produced by wheat allergies.[7]

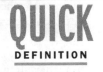

DEFINITION

Synovitis results in painful swelling and inflammation of the membrane (the synovium) surrounding joints; it weakens the bone and joint tissues, destroys cushioning cartilage, and is commonly associated with rheumatoid arthritis. In an advanced stage, it also kills off healthy red blood cells.

The most common causes of allergies are often molecular sub-fractions (such as proteins) found in the food, not the whole food itself. According to James Braly, M.D., medical director of Immuno Laboratories in Fort Lauderdale, Florida, and author of *Dr. Braly's Food Allergy & Nutrition Revolution*, often testing for sensitivities to whole foods will miss the true allergenic substances. "The point here is simple but vivid," says Dr. Braly. "If you test for whole-grain wheat antigens alone, you may miss food allergies to gliadin, which is only a part of the wheat kernel. The test may read negative for an allergy to wheat, while the person is actually desperately reactive to wheat gliadin."[8] Standard food-allergy testing (assessing the whole food) means that a small percentage of people (about 5%) who are allergic to a subfraction of wheat go undiagnosed.

The principal allergically offending component of wheat (also rye and, to a lesser extent, oats and barley) is gluten, the protein-carbohydrate combination that enables wheat flour to bind when baking. A protein substance called gliadin (which includes the amino acid glutamine) is the prime allergen within the gluten. It initiates an immune response that can lead to inflammation and swelling. According to a recent study, 18 different medical conditions have been directly linked to gliadin sensitivity and additional studies have supported these findings.[9] Medical researchers at the Federico II University in Naples, Italy, correlated the incidence of arthritis and intestinal wheat-gluten intolerance or celiac disease (a severe type of leaky gut caused by gluten) in 200 adults with high gluten intake in their diets. They found that 26% had signs of arthritis compared to 7.5% of control subjects. Of these patients with symptoms, almost twice as many patients (41%) who maintained their regular diet continued to have arthritic symptoms compared to those put on a gluten-free diet (21.6%).[10]

The Milk Connection

Dr. Braly's research has also found similar results in allergies to dairy products. Dairy milk contains about 25 different proteins; of these, four have been consistently linked with food allergies. Dr. Braly found that out of 45 patients tested for milk proteins, two were not allergic to whole milk yet allergic to a milk sub-fraction. Dr. Braly's research shows that out of 53 patients whose blood samples tested allergic to cow's milk, 82% also tested positive to the following proteins in milk: casein, bovine serum albumin, beta lactoglobulin, and alpha lactalbumin.

The Nightshade Vegetable Connection

Vegetables in the nightshade family are strongly and consistently linked with arthritis. The nightshade family includes such common vegetables as potatoes, eggplant, peppers (both green and hot), paprika, tomatoes, and tobacco. The necessity for avoiding the nightshades in certain forms of arthritis was popularized by Norman Childers, Ph.D., author of *A Diet to Stop Arthritis*. Childers worked with over 5,000 osteoarthritis and rheumatoid arthritis patients who agreed to eliminate nightshade vegetables from their diet. The patients were then tested for both subjective and objective measurements of pain and inflammation. The result was a 70% remission from aches and pains, simply due to avoidance of nightshades.[11] Dr. Childers theorizes that chemical alkaloids contained in nightshades are deposited in the connective tissue and stimulate inflammation as well as inhibit the formation of normal cartilage. As a result, cartilage begins to break down and is not replaced by healthy, new cartilage cells.

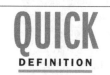

For more on **dietary factors in arthritis**, see Chapter 12: The Arthritis Diet, pp. 250-278.

Many patients who don't show any nightshade allergies in laboratory tests still tend to report a decrease in pain after eliminating nightshades from their diet. One theory to explain this phenomenon suggests that lectins (SEE QUICK DEFINITION) in tomatoes and other nightshades may persist in the body and initiate the formation of circulating immune complexes. Immune complexes are deposited in soft tissues if the detoxification pathways are overburdened, causing an inflammatory response, joint swelling, and pain.

QUICK
DEFINITION

Lectins are protein fragments of incompletely digested foods that bind with specific sugars on the surface of all cells of the body. They tend to stick to the lining of the gastrointestinal tract, where they irritate the tissues and can destroy cell membranes. Lectins also cause food allergies and toxic reactions of the mucosal membranes in the intestines, leading to intestinal permeability (leaky gut syndrome). Most dietary lectins are derived from beans, grains, soy, and wheat.

Testing For Allergies

The problem with diagnosing a food allergy is that reactions are often varied, inconsistent, and may take several days to develop after eating an allergy-causing food. How much or how often you eat an allergenic food or how it is cooked may be factors in whether or not you have a reaction. Or the allergy may be caused by an additive or ingredient rather than the food itself.[12] In addition, more than one food is frequently involved in causing the reaction, and, as explained earlier, symptoms are often "masked" by regular consumption of the foods.

Do You Suffer From Food Allergies?

The following questionnaire, developed by osteopathic physician and naturopath Leon Chaitow, N.D., D.O., can help determine if you have a food allergy. If your answer is "no" or "never" to any question, give yourself a score of zero for that particular question; the other scores are provided with each question.

■ Do you suffer from unnatural fatigue? (Score 1 if occasionally, 2 if regularly—three times a week or more.)

■ Do you sometimes experience weight fluctuations of four or more pounds in a single day, accompanied by puffiness of the face, ankles, or fingers? (Score 1 if infrequently, 2 if frequently—more than once a month.)

■ Do you have hot flashes (apart from menopause) or find yourself sweating for no obvious reason? (Score 1 if infrequently, 2 if several times a week or more.)

■ Does your pulse race or your heart pound strongly for no obvious reason? (Score 1 if infrequently, 2 if several times a week or more.)

■ Do you have a history of food intolerance, causing any symptoms at all? (Score 2 if your answer is yes.)

■ Do you crave bread, sugary foods, milk, chocolate, coffee, or tea? (Score 2 if your answer is yes.)

■ Do you suffer from migraine or severe headaches, irritable bowel syndrome, eczema, depression, asthma, or muscle aches? (Score 2 if your answer is yes.)

The most anyone could score on this test would be 14, explains Dr. Chaitow. "If your score is five or higher, there is a strong likelihood that allergies are part of your symptom picture."

For more on **tests to detect allergies**, see Chapter 3: Diagnosing Arthritis, pp. 52-77.

The Elimination Diet

Despite the name, this is not really a diet in the conventional sense, but a test procedure to help you identify your allergy foods. It involves three steps: 1) eliminating the possible allergic foods from your diet for ten to 14 days; 2) carefully observing any changes in your symptoms; and 3) testing the eliminated foods by bringing them back into your diet, one by one, and noting any return of symptoms. The foods you choose to eliminate should be from those that you eat every day or nearly every day, ones that you crave, or foods that make you feel weak. It is important to eliminate all of the suspected foods on your list, as multiple allergies are quite common and, if all are not eliminated, it could skew your testing results. Also, read the ingredients on any packaged foods very carefully to ensure you do not inadvertently consume whatever it is you are trying to eliminate (for example, sugar or the flavor-enhancer monosodium glutamate). Remember that delayed food allergies can take as long as 72 hours to exhibit symptoms. If you experience symptoms such as irritability, fatigue, headaches, and intense cravings during the elimination period, you may be going through withdrawal, which is a sure sign that you have been suffering from an allergy.

Blood Test

The ELISA (enzyme-linked immunoserological assay) test is a blood test considered by many alternative medicine practitioners to be among the most sensitive and useful in detecting food allergies. For example, Immuno Laboratories in Fort Lauderdale, Florida, offers a bloodprint assay to test for delayed food allergies. They use a small blood sample from the patient, then process it so as to collect the IgG antibodies. A drop of this serum is placed in a holding container or "well" (there are 102 wells in each laboratory testing plate) containing antigens from potentially allergenic foods. If the patient is allergic to a certain food, the serum placed into the well containing the offending substance will coagulate (clot). The results are automatically processed and an analysis of the individual's food allergies is generated. Based on this analysis, the patient is advised which foods should be avoided.

Success Story: Treating Allergies Relieves Painful Joints

Leonard, 47, had suffered with joint and muscle pains for several months, particularly in his hands and wrists, elbows, knees and ankles, back, and neck. His medical history included childhood environmental allergies—he was still extremely sensitive to pollutants and chemicals—and sarcoids (tumor-like growths) in his lungs (most likely from working around asbestos and chemicals for many years). Leonard was also a recovering alcoholic.

We found that Leonard's diet was generally not a very healthy one. He rarely cooked at home, preferring to eat out at fast food establishments and restaurants. His diet consisted predominantly of chicken, shellfish, eggs, whole milk and cheese, French fries, and wheat bread. In addition, Leonard was fond of sodas (9-11 cans per week), sweet desserts, and chocolate. He ate few salads or vegetables and 6-8 servings of fruit per week. Leonard also exercised only infrequently.

There was a history of rheumatoid arthritis in Leonard's family, perhaps indicating a genetic predisposition for the condition. Leonard had numerous physical complaints other than his arthritis symptoms, including itchy eyes and ears, stuffy nose, gastrointestinal problems (gas, bloating, infrequent bowel movements), frequent urination, and periodic bouts of acne.

We did a food allergy test (IgG ELISA blood test) and found that Leonard had many food sensitivities: almonds, bananas, green beans, kidney beans, yellow wax beans, cheese, eggs, garlic, limes, milk, mustard, oysters, rye and wheat, spinach, yeast (baker's and brewer's), and zucchini. Leonard immediately began working with our nutritionist to change his diet to deal with his sensitivities and improve his nutrient intake.

We also used the Herbal Crystallization Analysis (a simple saliva test) to determine which herbs would be most beneficial for Leonard. Based on the results, we gave him an individualized botanical extract containing the following:

- Barberry (*Berberis vulgaris*) root bark: digestive tonic, liver stimulant, antibacterial, anti-fungal
- Bayberry (*Myrica seriphera*) root bark: tonic for the respiratory system; helpful for hay fever, sinus congestion, and colds and flu
- *Panax ginseng*: adaptogenic herb that enhances the overall constitution; strengthens the endocrine glands
- Dandelion (*Taraxacum officinale*) root and leaf: a blood purifier, liver and gallbladder tonic, balances blood sugar, laxative
- Burdock (*Arctium lappa*) root: a blood purifier
- Yellowdock (*Rumex crispus*) root: liver tonic, blood purifier, helps skin problems; contains high levels of botanical iron

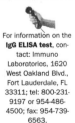

For information on the **IgG ELISA test**, contact: Immuno Laboratories, 1620 West Oakland Blvd., Fort Lauderdale, FL 33311; tel: 800-231-9197 or 954-486-4500; fax: 954-739-6563.

Inside the Sick Building Syndrome

In the early 1980s, physicians began using the term "sick building syndrome" (SBS) to refer to a host of symptoms produced by low-grade toxic environmental conditions found in living, work, or office spaces. SBS symptoms are numerous: mucous membrane irritation of the eyes, nose, and throat, chest tightness, skin complaints (dryness, itching, abnormal redness), headaches, fatigue, lethargy, coughing, asthma, wheezing, chronic nasal stuffiness, temporary weight loss, infections, and emotional irritability. All of these depress the immune system, rendering the individual susceptible to long-term chronic illness.

"Indoor air pollution in residences, offices, schools, and other buildings is widely recognized as a serious environmental risk to human health," explains Michael Hodgson, M.D., M.P.H., of the School of Medicine at the University of Connecticut Health Center in Farmington. Dr. Hodgson notes that most people in industrialized nations spend more than 90% of their time indoors, that indoor concentrations of pollutants (including toxic chemicals) are often "substantially" higher than found outdoors, and that small children, the elderly, and the infirm are likely to spend all of their time indoors, leading to a permanent chronic exposure to low-grade toxic factors.

In most cases, problems with a building's engineering, construction, and ventilation system are the causes. Studies suggest that symptoms occur 50% more frequently in buildings with mechanical ventilation systems. Among 2,000 office workers in Germany with work-related symptoms, there was a 50% higher than average rate of upper respiratory tract infections that were directly traceable to problems with mechanically ventilated buildings, reports Dr. Hodgson. A U.S. study found that 20% of office workers had job-related SBS symptoms, including a subjective sense of being less productive in their work.

Besides ventilation problems, other sources of indoor toxic pollution include volatile organic compounds released from particleboard desks, furniture, carpets, glues, paints, office machine toners, and perfumes. All contribute to "a complex mixture of very low levels of individual pollutants," states Dr. Hodgson. Bioaerosols are also indoor contaminants and originate as biological agents from mold spores, allergy-producing microbes, mites, or animal danders; then they are distributed through an indoor space by ventilation, heating, or air conditioning systems.

Of buildings classified as sources of SBS, one study showed that 70% have inadequate flow of fresh outside air. It also found that 50% to 70% of such buildings have poor distribution of air within the occupied space; 60% have poor filtration of outdoor pollutants; 60% have standing water that fosters biological growths; and 20% have malfunctioning humidifiers.[13]

For more on **environmental illness**, see *Alternative Medicine Guide to Chronic Fatigue, Fibromyalgia, and Environmental Illness* (Future Medicine Publishing, 1998; ISBN 1-887299-11-4); to order, call 800-333-HEAL.

For information on the **health effects of sick building syndrome**, contact: Environmental Detoxification Consultants, 413 Grassy Hill Road, Woodbury, CT 06798; tel/fax: 203-263-2970.

■ Juniper (*Juniperus communis*): kidney and adrenal tonic, diuretic; helpful for gout, diabetes, and hypoglycemia

We prepared this formula as a non-alcoholic standardized extract, which Leonard took for four months (one teaspoon, three times daily).

To encourage the detoxification process, we instructed Leonard on the proper way to fast. Regular fasting eases the stress on the gastrointestinal system and allows the body to purge itself of its toxic load. We also had Leonard undergo regular sauna sessions in order to "sweat out" additional toxins from his body.

After four months on this program, Leonard was completely pain-free, with no stiffness or limitation of movement. His gastrointestinal difficulties were greatly improved as well and he vowed to continue with his healthier eating habits. Leonard reported that his environmental allergies were also much better—he was able to withstand greater exposure to pollution or other toxins without it sending him "over the edge."

For information on **fasting**, see Chapter 4: General Detoxification, pp. 78-100. For more on **saunas and other detoxification therapies**, see Chapter 14: Exercises and Physical Therapies, pp. 314-359.

Alternative Medicine Therapies for Allergies

Once you have identified the foods you are allergic to, the next step is to eliminate them from your diet. Initially, you should completely refrain from eating all allergenic foods for 60 to 90 days. After this period, you can begin to slowly reintroduce them into your diet. You should also vary the foods that you eat on a daily basis to avoid developing new allergies. You are likely to find that, as you reintroduce the foods to which you were once sensitive, your old symptoms will not reappear. This is because most food allergies can be cured through abstinence.

Although there is great therapeutic benefit in avoiding foods and chemicals that trigger allergies, rarely is it entirely possible. Below you will find a summary of treatments we have used to reduce our patients' allergies and arthritic pain. We often use fasting to reduce allergic reactions and the corresponding arthritic symptoms. During a fast, a person typically eats only high-nutrient soups, water, and/or vegetable juices. Following this type of diet for four to six weeks decreases the amount of immune complexes (substances formed when antibodies attach to antigens) circulating in the blood.

Ways to Halt an Allergic Reaction

If you are experiencing an allergic reaction, there are also safe and effective ways to halt it before it escalates.

■ Alkaline Salts: You can make your own alkaline salts by combining one part potassium bicarbonate (available at any pharmacy) and two parts sodium bicarbonate (or baking soda). Take one teaspoon of mixture in a 12-ounce glass of filtered water. Repeat this dose every hour for three hours in the case of an acute allergic reaction or several times per day if you are on an elimination diet and reintroducing offending foods into your daily meals. Or use commercial brands of alkaline salts (such as Alka Seltzer Gold™): dissolve one tablet in 6-8 ounces of water and consume it; after ten minutes, repeat. If necessary, repeat every hour for up to three hours.

■ Vitamin C: Use buffered vitamin C because it does not upset the stomach. The buffering action is due to the alkaline salts sodium, potassium, or magnesium ascorbate. Take two teaspoons in water every 15-20 minutes during an acute situation; during a detoxification period, take vitamin C to bowel tolerance (the amount that makes your system produce loose stools).

■ Anti-Allergy Nutrient Cocktail: Take the following formula two to three times per day for relief of allergic reactions: powdered and buffered vitamin C (2,000 mg in eight ounces of water), bioflavonoids (liquid form, 250 mg), calcium (capsule form, 1,000 mg), magnesium (capsule form, 1,000 mg), and vitamin B6 (capsule form, 250 mg).

See the **non-aller-genic recipes** in Chapter 12: The Arthritis Diet, pp. 250-278.

Applied Kinesiology

Applied kinesiology, first developed by George Goodheart, D.C., of Detroit, Michigan, is the study of the relationship between muscle dysfunction (weak muscles) and related organ or gland dysfunction. Applied kinesiology employs a simple strength resistance test on a specific indicator muscle related to the organ or part of the body that is being tested. If the muscle tests strong (maintaining its resistance), it indicates health. If it tests weak, it can mean infection or dysfunction.

A special application that uses kinesiology to detect food allergies is the Nambudripad Allergy Elimination Technique (NAET). Developed by Devi Nambudripad, D.C., L.Ac., R.N., Ph.D., this method also helps to eliminate allergies by using acupuncture (or acupressure) and chiropractic. After determining the allergy-inducing substances through muscle testing, the patient again holds the offending substance while the NAET practitioner uses acupuncture or acupressure to reprogram the way the body responds to the substance, thereby removing the allergic charge.

Supplements and Herbs

Quercetin-bromelain is one of the most effective supplements available to treat a food allergy. Quercetin is a natural bioflavonoid (SEE QUICK DEFINITION) derived from plants, such as blueberries, cranberries, cherries, or onions. It enhances the body's ability to use vitamin C, increasing its absorption by the liver, kidneys, and adrenal glands. Bromelain, a digestive enzyme derived from pineapple, enhances the absorption of quercetin. Taken together, quercetin and bromelain strengthen the membranes of the body's cells so that they are less likely to be damaged in the presence of an allergen. This, in turn, lessens the severity and reduces the symptoms of an allergy. Typical recommended dose: 500 mg, three times daily.

You can reduce the reaction of the digestive system to offending foods by using the appropriate enzyme supplements: protease digests protein, lipase digests fats, amylase digests carbohydrates, lactase digests dairy products, and disaccharidases digest sugars. Typical dose: 500 mg with meals. Supplementing with betaine hydrochloric acid (500-1,000 mg with meals), the dietary form of the primary acid in the stomach, may also help digestive function. As digestion improves, the allergic reactions should be minimized or eliminated.

Other nutrients and herbs useful for enhancing tissue repair and regenerating the digestive system include the amino acid L-glutamine, vitamin E, chlorophyll, aloe vera, papaya, slippery elm, and marshmallow root. Probiotics (friendly bacteria) can also help heal the digestive system.

For **Devi Nambudripad, D.C., L.Ac., R.N., Ph.D.** (for appointments or referrals), contact: Pain Clinic, 6714 Beach Blvd., Buena Park, CA 90621; tel: 714-523-0800. Dr. Nambudripad's book about NAET, *Say Goodbye to Illness*, is available from her clinic.

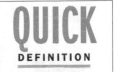

QUICK
DEFINITION

A **bioflavonoid** is a pigment within plants and fruits that acts as an antioxidant to protect the body against damage from free radicals and excess oxygen. In the body, bioflavonoids enhance the beneficial activities of vitamin C, and they are often formulated with this vitamin in supplements. Originally called vitamin P, these vitamin C "helper" substances include citrin, hesperidin, catechin, rutin, and quercetin. When taken with vitamin C, bioflavonoids increase the absorption of vitamin C in the liver, kidneys, and adrenal glands. As antioxidants, they also protect vitamin C from destruction by free radicals.

Desensitize the Autoimmune Reaction

THE AUTOIMMUNE DISEASES (rheumatoid arthritis, ankylosing spondylitis, juvenile rheumatoid arthritis, and lupus) involve destruction of healthy cells by the body's own defensive mechanism, the immune system. For people with rheumatoid arthritis, normal cartilage cells that line the joints and ensure smooth motion become the target of repeated attacks by the immune system, eventually eroding the cartilage and causing joint deformities and disabilities. The immune system fails to recognize its error and the disease progresses to the heart, lungs, and other vital organs.

Just why the immune system turns on the body is not entirely clear. Heavy metal toxicity, leaky gut syndrome, infections of bacteria and parasites, and nutritional imbalances can weaken the body so that the immune system becomes overloaded and confused. But what mechanism fails within the immune system, making it suspect the body's own healthy tissues as possible invaders, is still the subject of intense research. In this chapter, we discuss the components of the immune system and how these parts interact to fight infections. Then we explain what is known about the abnormal action of the immune system in autoimmune diseases. We also address natural therapies that can regulate the immune system's aggressive behavior, without suppressing or altering its necessary defenses.

In This Chapter

- Protecting the Body: The Immune System
- Uncontrolled Inflammation: The Autoimmune Response
- Measuring the Autoimmune Reaction
- Natural Therapies for Calming the Immune System

Protecting the Body: The Immune System

The immune system, through protein and chemical components in the blood and tissues, surveys the body looking for pathogens (foreign, "non-self" substances such as cancerous cells, bacteria, viruses, and parasites). During a normal immune response, leukotrienes and prostaglandins (hormone-like members of the immune system) dilate blood vessels so that white blood cells and other immune components can quickly travel to the injury. Increased blood flow to an area is what causes swelling, redness, and heat. Another wave of pro-inflammatories (causing inflammation) known as chemotactic factors activate the white blood cells so they can begin digesting damaged cells and circulating immune complexes, and attacking pathogens.

As pathogens are destroyed, their cell walls and internal components leak out, triggering still another phase of the immune defense. In this offensive, B cells are triggered to produce antibodies specific to the pathogen or cell under attack. B cells also alert other immune cells (macrophages) to the presence of pathogens, who then join the attack.[1]

The oxidizing chemicals used by white blood cells to destroy pathogens can inadvertently affect surrounding cells. The healthy cells surrounding an inflammatory response secrete their own chemicals to protect themselves. Specifically, they secrete anti-inflammatory prostaglandins against pro-inflammatory prostaglandins, antioxidants against inflammatory chemicals, anti-chemotactic chemicals to halt the progression of white blood cells, and enzymes to counter the digestive enzymes released by white blood cells.[2]

In a body that is functioning normally, as the disease-causing agents are destroyed and their cell fragments removed, the pro-inflammatory chemicals are soon suppressed by the anti-inflammatory chemicals secreted by neighboring cells. The inflammatory response subsides: suppressor T cells stop the production of antibodies, blood vessels return to their normal size, and the repair process begins to mend damaged tissues.

Natural Therapies for Calming the Immune System

- Oral Tolerization
- Urine Therapy
- Auto-Sanguis Dilution Therapy
- Herbal Medicine

The Major Players in Your Immune System

The immune system is made up of millions of "workers" that have specific roles in guarding the body from opportunistic organisms. The most abundant and varied workers are the white blood cells, comprised of neutrophils, eosinophils, basophils, macrophages, and lymphocytes.

Neutrophils, or granulocytes, make up 50% to 70% of the white blood cells circulating in the bloodstream. They engulf invading particles, especially bacteria and fungi.

Eosinophils make up about 5% of all the white blood cells and are involved in allergic reactions and the suppression of parasites.

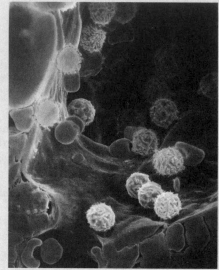

Basophils account for less than 1% of the white blood cells. Basophils that reside in body tissues are called mast cells, which combat specific parasites and fungi. They are also involved in histamine release caused by allergic reactions.

Macrophages swallow foreign proteins, then release an enzyme that chemically damages, kills, or neutralizes whatever is ingested. Macrophages are the "vacuum cleaners" of the immune system, ingesting antigens and the by-products of inflammation (damaged cells and tissue debris). They comprise 5% of the circulating white blood cells.

Lymphocytes make up 20%-40% of the white blood cells and serve as the immune system's security guards, migrating between the blood and tissues. Lymphocytes can live up to 20 years and have two subsets, T and B cells. About 70% of the lymphocytes are T cells, which specialize their function to become helper, suppressor, or natural killer cells. Helper T cells organize the immune system's function; they facilitate the production of antibodies by the B cells, direct other defender cells to an area, and monitor the attack. Suppressor T cells suppress the production of antibodies by B cells so that an attack does not get out of control. Natural killer cells are nonspecific, free-ranging cells that are armed with 100 different biochemical poisons to kill foreign proteins upon first encounter. T cells also function as the immune system's memory. They remember foreign substances and alert other immune components upon future exposure to the substance.

B cells, which account for 10%-15% of all lymphocytes, produce antibodies to neutralize specific foreign cells (this is known as humoral immunity). B cells do not survey the body for foreign invaders as do the T cells; instead they wait for the T cells to signal for the production of a particular antibody. Antibodies are protein molecules (containing about 20,000 atoms) made from amino acids by B cells and set in motion by the immune system against a specific antigen (foreign and potentially dangerous protein). An antibody is also referred to as an immunoglobulin and may be found in the blood, lymph, colostrum, saliva, and the gastrointestinal and urinary tracts, usually within three days after the first encounter with an antigen. The antibody binds tightly with the invader as a preliminary for removing it from the system or destroying it. There are five main types of immunoglobulins: IgG, IgA, IgM, IgD, and IgE.

Other chemical components of the immune system prepare the body for an upcoming attack on a foreign substance. Cytokines are hormone-like substances, such as interleukins and interferons, that are responsible for "heightening" an immune response. They trigger the production of necessary chemicals and allow certain cells involved in inflammation to proliferate. Prostaglandins are hormone-like complex fatty acids that affect inflammatory processes and constriction and dilation of blood vessels, particularly in the lungs and intestines. Essential fatty acids (EFAs-SEE QUICK DEFINITION) in the diet (both omega-3s and omega-6s) provide the raw material for prostaglandin production. Once ingested, these essential fatty acids can be converted to prostaglandins by nearly any cell in the body. Omega-6-derived prostaglandins (the most common type) can have either pro-inflammatory or anti-inflammatory properties, while most prostaglandins converted from omega-3 sources help reduce pain and inflammation.

The complement system, made up of 28 proteins, is dormant until activated by a series of enzymatic reactions intiated by circulating immune complexes (antibodies mixed with antigens) or certain bacteria and viruses. Once activated, the complement system stimulates the release of inflammation-enhancing chemicals, clears away immune complexes, and kills bacteria. The complement system is very powerful and is carefully controlled by inhibitors to keep it from damaging the body.

Autoimmune diseases involve the destruction of healthy cells by the immune system. In rheumatoid arthritis, normal cartilage cells become the target of repeated immune attacks.

Uncontrolled Inflammation: The Autoimmune Response

In the case of an autoimmune disease, the immune system never recognizes when the danger of infection has passed and the immune response continues unabated. Researchers have yet to determine the sequence of events that leads to the immune system turning against the body, but they have identified the following suspects: pro-inflammatory agents including prostaglandins (hormone-like substances that cause inflammation), autoantibodies (immune cells produced by lymphocytes that attack body cells), and defective suppressor T cells (see "The Major Players in Your Immune System," pp. 210-211).

Patients with rheumatoid arthritis often have elevated concentrations of pro-inflammatory prostaglandins. While prostaglandins are part of the normal immune response, an excessive amount causes swelling and pain. In effect, the immune system is eager for an attack, although the threat may be insignificant or nonexistent. In addition, defective suppressor T cells, which regulate the immune system's response and normally stop the production of antibodies, fail to suppress a heightened response.

Defective lymphocytes, for unknown reasons, promote production of antibodies that attack the body's own cells, called autoantibodies (against "self"). There are different types of autoantibodies, produced by B cells, that attack specific body cells or cell parts. Autoantibodies that target the nucleus (control center of a cell) are called antinuclear antibodies (ANAs). The destruction of healthy cells can trigger further autoimmune response. When healthy cell membranes are torn apart, the cell's internal components leak out. Since the immune system is only familiar with the cell's outer membranes—patterns on the membrane are how the immune system determines friend from foe—these internal components are viewed as foreign bodies and attacked (see "Know Thyself," p. 213). An autoimmune disease may be the result, as the immune system becomes confused and begins to attack healthy body tissues.

For **other factors and causes in immune system dysfunction,** see Chapter 2: What is Arthritis?, pp. 30-51.

Know Thyself

How does the immune system "recognize" friend from foe? All cells have cell membranes containing chains of glycoproteins (sugar-protein complexes) that coat the membranes like the fuzz on a tennis ball. These glycoproteins are configured in various patterns that identify their function and type. Joint cells display a certain pattern that differs from that of the heart or other organ tissues. Similarly, some bacteria and viruses have specific protein patterns that identify them as "foreigners" in the body.

In the set of human chromosomes, we inherit genetic markers that determine the cellular (glycoprotein) pattern of our cell membranes. These markers, known as the major histocompatibility complex or HLA (Human Leukocyte Antigen) complex, are divided into three classes which are expressed, respectively, on all cells with a nucleus, certain immune cells, and structural genes typically involved in autoimmune diseases. In 1973, it was discovered that ankylosing spondylitis (a type of arthritis that affects the spine) frequently occurred in individuals with the genetic marker HLA-B27. Further research determined that over 100 diverse types of diseases are associated with specific types of HLA markers. Researchers have theorized that HLA-associated diseases, particularly autoimmune diseases, are induced by "molecular mimicry," in which bacteria and viruses are able to cloak themselves in a cellular pattern similar to one in normal body tissues and escape detection by the immune system. Once the invader is detected, a vigorous immune response ensues against the invader as well as the normal body cells with the similar cellular pattern.

Genetic testing can ascertain the presence of particular genetic markers, such as HLA-DR4 (associated with rheumatoid arthritis) and HLA B27 (associated with ankylosing spondylitis).[3] However, these diseases also occur in individuals without these markers.

Measuring the Autoimmune Reaction

Standard blood tests can determine the activity of different immune components, which may indicate abnormal inflammation or an infection of a bacteria, virus, or parasite. By looking at the number of white blood cells and other factors in the blood, doctors can determine the presence and severity of an autoimmune disease. They can also use these tests to measure the effect of certain therapies at reducing inflammation and disease activity.

■ Erythrocyte Sedimentation Rate (ESR) measures blood levels of fibrinogen, a protein that makes the red blood cells clump together. The level of fibrinogen varies with the degree of inflammation in the body, with an elevated ESR indicating inflammation. Rheumatoid arthritis patients typically have elevated ESR.

Unlike conventional methods, the natural therapies that we use to balance the immune system do not suppress or block normal immune function. Instead, they promote and encourage the immune system's own regulating components to turn off the abnormal autoimmune response.

■ Anti-Nuclear Antibodies (ANAs) are antibodies that attack the nucleus of one's own cells; they are often present in autoimmune diseases. Under the microscope, blood samples will have a speckled pattern of ANAs if rheumatoid arthritis is present.[4]

■ C-reactive protein is another marker of inflammation produced in the liver and involved in stimulating white blood cell activity. It is often elevated in rheumatoid arthritis patients.

■ Another diagnostic marker is rheumatoid factor (RF), an autoantibody usually present in 70% of rheumatoid arthritis cases, but they also appear in the blood of patients with tuberculosis, parasitic infections, leukemia, or connective tissue disorders. In some cases, RF enhances the degree of joint inflammation and thus renders joints more susceptible to damage by other immune cells.

Natural Therapies for Calming the Immune System

The most common (and short-sighted) allopathic treatment for autoimmune diseases is immunosuppressant drugs (prednisone, methotrexate, Plaquenil®, and cyclophosphamide), which inhibit the formation of white blood cells in an attempt to suppress the immune system's destruction of healthy cells. Like many conventional drugs, their immediate result is favorable and swift: they quickly mask the immune system's aggressive behavior by killing off its fundamental components. But their inhibiting effects are not specific or localized to rheumatic joints. If used for long periods of time, they affect all cells throughout the body that reproduce rapidly—specifically, the cells located in the gastrointestinal tract, reproductive organs, and bone marrow, as well as white blood cells. Prolonged use has deleterious results, including gastrointestinal problems, increased susceptibility to infection, sterility, and injury to the kidneys, liver, spleen, and bone marrow.[5]

Unlike conventional methods, the natural therapies that we use to balance the immune system do not suppress or block normal immune function. Instead, they promote and encourage the immune system's own regulating components to turn off the abnormal autoimmune response, so that this vital function can regain normalcy. These therapies include auto-sanguis dilution therapy, oral tolerization, urine therapy, and herbal remedies.

Several of these therapies are based upon homeopathy's (SEE QUICK DEFINITION) main principle of "like cures like," meaning that a substance which causes particular symptoms in large doses can cure those symptoms when given in small doses. Examples of this principle can be found in modern immunization, which uses trace amounts of infectious agents to invoke the body's immune defenses, and in the treatment of allergies, which uses minute levels of the suspected allergy-provoking substance to bolster the body tolerance of the allergen. When treating rheumatoid arthritis, the body's immune response can be modulated through therapies drawing upon homeopathic principles.

Equally important is homeopathy's holistic model, which treats illness as a unique experience for each individual. A homeopathic practitioner carefully reviews all symptoms of the patient—seemingly unrelated complaints build an individual profile that can then be matched to a remedy specifically suited for that profile. When treating the autoimmune response of rheumatoid arthritis, the practitioner's job is simplified because the patient's own bodily fluids (blood or urine) contain the causes and agents involved in the disease and are therefore perfectly suited to the patient's specific profile.

For most of our rheumatoid arthritis patients, we first focus on decreasing pain and swelling by using nontoxic pain-relieving and anti-inflammatory treatments and modalities as well as identifying and treating the underlying causes (intestinal imbalances, nutritional deficiencies, toxicity, allergies, etc.). After relieving discomfort through the use of natural pain relievers, and beginning to reverse the disease process by addressing the underlying disorders, patients (with the consent of their rheumatologists) are often able to decrease or discontinue their prescription drugs. Then, immune-regulating therapies are pursued after the patient stops taking all conventional pain medications.

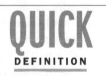

DEFINITION

Homeopathy was founded in the early 1800s by German physician Samuel Hahnemann. Today, an estimated 500 million people worldwide receive homeopathic treatment; in Britain, homeopathy enjoys royal patronage. Homeopathy is now practiced according to two differing concepts. In classical homeopathy, only one single-component remedy is prescribed at a time, in a potency specifically adjusted to the patient; the physician waits to see the results before prescribing anything further. In complex homeopathy, typified by *Hepar compositum*, a prescription involves multiple substances given at the same time, usually in low potencies.

For more on the **connection between allergies and arthritis**, see Chapter 9: Allergies and Arthritis, pp. 192-207.

For information on **Arthred**, contact: Source Naturals, Threshold Enterprises, 23 Janis Way, Scotts Valley, CA 95066; tel: 800-777-5677 or 831-438-1144. For **products containing shark cartilage**, contact: Futurebiotics, 145 Ricefield Lane, Hauppauge, NY 11788; tel: 800-FOR-LIFE (367-5433) or 516-273-6300.

Oral Tolerization

Oral tolerization is an adaptation of a common immunological procedure, in which a highly allergic person is exposed (usually through injections) to the substances causing the allergies. But in oral tolerization, the offending substance is ingested rather than injected. A specific type of collagen cell, the most abundant protein in cartilage, is considered to be the allergenic (cause of the allergic reaction) substance in autoimmune diseases.

Oral tolerization is "a form of vaccination via the intestinal tract—it stimulates the immune system in a way that helps the host suppress autoimmune disease," according to Howard Weiner, M.D., an immunologist at Mount Sinai Hospital and Brigham and Women's Hospital in Boston, Massachusetts. Researchers at Harvard Medical School gave oral doses of this type of collagen (derived from chickens) to ten patients with rheumatoid arthritis for one month. They found that six out of the ten patients showed a substantial response: improvement of swollen and tender joints, less morning stiffness, better grip strength, and a reduction of inflammatory indicators in their blood. One patient experienced complete remission of the disease for two years. There were no adverse reactions reported.[6] But researchers have yet to determine why ingesting allergens creates beneficial results. They suspect that orally ingesting collagen may alter or re-program T-cell function, either by desensitizing T cells to collagen antigens or by triggering the production of suppressor T cells that migrate to joints and block T cell–mediated inflammation.

Cartilage derived from bovine and shark sources has demonstrated similar immune-modulating effects. Both bovine and shark cartilage are available as nutritional supplements. At the recommended dosage, shark cartilage can be quite expensive, so we usually recommend alternatives such as Arthred, which contains hydrolyzed collagen from bovine cartilage along with 19 amino acids, which are the building-blocks for joint cartilage. Evidence suggests that consuming these very small collagen molecules can be helpful with arthritis.[7]

Auto-Sanguis Dilution Therapy

In auto-sanguis dilution therapy, small doses of the patient's blood are prepared as a homeopathic remedy and administered to the patient. The effectiveness of this therapy relies on the homeopathic principle that small doses of a substance that in large doses causes disease symptoms can help to reverse the disease. People who suffer from an autoimmune disease have elevated levels of pro-inflammatory agents (certain types of prostaglandins and leukotrienes), antibodies, and circulating immune complexes in their bloodstream, which are all involved in the abnormal immune response. A homeopathic mixture containing minute traces of these substances can reduce or even completely eliminate the autoimmune response as exemplified by the following case history:

Success Story: Auto-Sanguis Therapy Calms the Autoimmune Reaction—

Yvonne, 13, developed symptoms of juvenile rheumatoid arthritis shortly after a visit to the dentist. We performed our standard diagnostic tests, which included screening for infectious organisms (viruses, bacteria, and parasites). The results of the Streptozyme Titer (a test measuring specific antibodies to *Streptococcus* bacteria) were very high, indicating an immune response against *Streptococcus* (commonly referred to as strep).

She also had the genetic marker HLA-DR4 commonly associated with rheumatoid arthritis. This means that the structure of Yvonne's cell membranes exhibited a pattern easily mistaken for the *Streptococcus* bacteria. Through "molecular mimicry," strep has evolved a cell membrane pattern so similar to the body's own cell membranes (in those with the HLA-DR4 marker) that the immune system treats the "invader" as a "native cell." But once the invading bacteria are dis-

Sulfur and the Immune System

Two sulfur-containing substances, dimethylsulfoxide (DMSO, derived from wood pulp, garlic oil, or as a by-product of petroleum) and methylsulfonylmethane (MSM, a sister compound derived from food sources), may have immune-modulating actions, according to a study conducted at Oregon Health Sciences University. The researchers fed DMSO and MSM to mice prone to develop illnesses similar to autoimmune diseases in humans. The mice typically suffered from anemia, lupus-like kidney disease, and enlarged lymph nodes, spleen, and thymus gland, and had a lifespan of five-and-a-half months. After 39 weeks, every animal in the control group, which received no supplements, died, while 80% of the mice that were fed DMSO or MSM were still alive. The mice exhibited a reduction of their autoimmune symptoms and, on average, lived for ten months, nearly double their projected lifespan. A follow-up study confirmed the initial study's results that DMSO and MSM could extend the lifespan of the animals. Researchers also found a reduction in the levels of certain autoantibodies that attack the kidneys. "Although we are not sure about the mechanism of action, DMSO and MSM may act by decreasing inflammatory responses and the production of autoantibodies and immune complexes," the researchers stated. [8]

covered, the immune system attacks all (bacterial and healthy) cells with this pattern and an autoimmune response ensues.

In order to reverse Yvonne's arthritis, we had to eradicate her strep infection and modify her autoimmune response. This was acheived through two autoimmune therapies: auto-sanguis oral nosode therapy and injectible auto-sanguis dilution therapy. First, we prescribed the homeopathic remedy *Streptococcinum* 200C at three sublingual pellets, once a day between meals, for one month. We also prepared an oral auto-sanguis nosode (SEE QUICK DEFINITION) through the following method: an extraction of a small amount of Yvonne's blood was placed in a centrifuge for 20 minutes; then, one part serum was mixed with nine parts Willard's Water (SEE QUICK DEFINITION); the mixture was shaken vigorously 100 times. This process produces a homeopathic nosode at 1X potency. To increase the potency of the nosode, the process was repeated six times, rendering the remedy at a potency of 6X; we added 15% ethyl alcohol to stabilize the solution. We instructed Yvonne to place ten drops of this solution under her tongue three times a day. Upon her second visit, we increased the potency of the original nosode to 12X potency; her third visit to 30X potency; and finally to 60X potency.

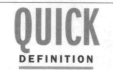

DEFINITION

A **nosode** is a super-diluted and percussed remedy made as an energy imprint from a disease product, such as bacteria, tuberculosis, measles, bowel infection, influenza, and about 200 other substances. The nosode, which contains no physical trace of the disease, stimulates the body to remove all "taints" or residues it holds of a particular disease, whether it was inherited or contracted. Only qualified practitioners may administer a nosode.

Willard's Water, which claims 21 U.S. patents, is water into which a catalyst has been introduced, changing the water's molecular structure and thereby its properties, according to its manufacturer. It is called "catalyst altered water," based on a catalyst (called a "micelle," comprising tiny electrically charged particles) discovered by John W. Willard, Ph.D., Professor Emeritus at South Dakota School of Mines and Technology, in Rapid City.

In addition, she was treated with an auto-sanguis injectible dilution by extracting 3 cc (cubic centimeters) of her blood and emptying the syringe until only a microscopic film of blood remained in the cartridge. We then mixed into the same syringe 1 cc of the homeopathic nosodes *Streptococcus viridans-injeel* and *Streptococcus haemolyticus-injeel*, and 1 cc of the homeopathic remedies Traumeel and ZEEL (indicated for inflammation and degenerative processes). The mixture was agitated 20 times rendering a solution at 1X potency and was injected into her buttock. The process was repeated to produce a remedy of 2X potency and injected as well. Yvonne returned for treatment once a week for one month. During this time, injections reached a potency of 4X.

Two weeks after Yvonne's last treatment, we repeated all initial blood tests and found that her body was no longer producing *Streptococcus* antibodies. She also no longer had positive blood factors (RF and ANA) for autoimmune reactions and she experienced complete relief of her arthritis symptoms. We suspected that Yvonne's recent visit to the dentist may explain how she was infected by the strep bacteria. During the routine dental cleaning, strep cell fragments in the teeth or gums translocated to other regions of the body, prompting an immune response, leading to autoimmunity. We suggested that, in the future, Yvonne should receive preventive homeopathic treatment with *Streptococcinum* 200C before visiting the dentist.

Urine Therapy

It may seem a hard fact to swallow, but urine has a broad spectrum of health benefits. We normally think of it only as a waste product that is unhealthy and unclean. But in actuality, healthy urine is completely sterile and rich in nutrients when it is first passed from the body. Modern drug manufacturers long ago discovered that many important chemical compounds are contained in urine. Urine is routinely collected from humans, horses, and other animals for the purpose of isolating and condensing desirable components. Premarin®, for instance, a type of estrogen used for hormone replacement therapy, is derived from the urine of pregnant mares.[9] Urokinase, a drug commonly used to treat patients with advanced atherosclerosis (fatty calcified deposits on the arterial walls), is manufactured from urine collected from portable toilets. Most shampoos and cosmetics contain a component of urine, urea, or its synthetic counterpart known as carbamide.

Urine is composed of water, urea (a breakdown product of proteins and amino acids), hormones, enzymes, minerals, and salts, which are specific to the individual. The chemical components of a person's urine reflect the individual's health profile. This physiological "fingerprint" contains evidence of infectious agents, specific types of antibodies used to combat them, circulating immune complexes (antibodies that have attached themselves to antigens or foreign bodies), substances that have initiated an immune response, hormones and other natural chemicals used to regulate and control the body's functions, and synthesized vitamins and other nutritive substances.[10]

In the case of autoimmune diseases, in which the immune system is overactive, urine's precise mechanism of action is still not completely clear, but researchers hypothesize that the person's urine con-

Auto-sanguis (oral or injectible) dilution therapy can be administered only by a licensed physician (practitioners can contact Dr. Eugene Zampieron at 203-263-2970). For information about **Streptococcinum 200C** (available to licensed practitioners only), contact: BOIRON, 6 Campus Boulevard, Building A, Newtown Square, PA 19073; tel: 800-264-7661 or 610-325-7464. For **Traumeel and ZEEL**, contact: Heel/BHI, Inc., 11600 Cochiti Road Southeast, Albuquerque, NM 87123-3376; tel: 800-621-7644 or 505-293-3843.

For more on homeopathic remedies for arthritis, see Chapter 13: Supplements for Arthritis, pp. 280-313.

tains autoantibodies involved in the aggressive allergic response, along with the offending allergens. These antibodies and other substances are biotransformed into powerful, effective medicinals when reintroduced to the body through drinking or injecting one's own urine. The concentration of these agents in urine is so diluted that they are rendered ineffective in posing a threat to the body. Instead, these minute traces of substances act like a self-vaccine or a homeopathic remedy, triggering the body to regulate its immune system and stop the autoimmune response.[11]

Many doctors have used urine therapy as an injection, but it can also be very effective if taken orally. People with an aversion to drinking their own urine can start off very slowly following this procedure: in the morning, catch a small amount of urine in a clean cup, have another cup of filtered water available. Then, use a clean glass eyedropper and add just two drops of urine to the cup of water. Every few days, increase the amount of urine by one drop; go slowly, adding a little bit more urine each morning. The ideal dosage is ten drops of urine to one glass of water. Once this amount is reached, maintain it indefinitely. Urine tastes like salty water, but you can add a drop of peppermint oil to disguise the taste, if needed. Research has suggested that a person's ability to taste their own urine decreases as the therapeutic dose is reached.[12]

Herbs for Autoimmune Disease

Immunological researchers have discovered several important plants whose pharmacological actions seem to dampen the aggressive autoimmune response. These plants include *Tripterygium wilfordii*, Indian Sarsaparilla, and Lithospermum.

***Tripterygium wilfordii* (Chinese Thunder God Vine)**—The *Tripterygium wilfordii* (TW) vine grows wild in remote areas of southern China and has been used in traditional Chinese medicine for 2,000 years. Recently, clinical trials have found that TW is effective in treating autoimmune diseases (rheumatoid arthritis and ankylosing spondylitis) and other types of arthritis. TW contains chemical components called glycosides, which have immune-suppressing, anti-inflammatory, and analgesic properties.

In one Chinese study, 144 rheumatoid arthritis patients were treated with extracts of TW. The study found that 93.3% of the patients experienced overall improvement in their physical symptoms, while laboratory blood analysis confirmed that inflammatory and autoimmune markers in these patients had decreased. The majority of these patients noticed improvements within the first two weeks of treatment. For 37.5% of the patients, TW extracts produced relief from joint pain, recovery of joint motion and function, and reduced inflammatory indicators—erythrocyte sedimentation rate became normal and rheumatoid factor became negative. A complete remission of all symptoms occurred in 17.6% of patients.

CAUTION:
Because of the possible side effects of *Tripterygium wilfordii*, use this herb only under the care of a licensed health-care professional.

While the results of this and other studies are promising, there are related side effects with TW. The patients tested in the study above reported skin rashes, dry mouth, poor appetite, menstrual disturbances in women, and hormonal disturbances in men.[13] Researchers have also found that TW causes a temporary reduction of sperm count in men and have begun to develop a male contraceptive drug from the plant's active ingredients. However, fertility is restored upon cessation of use.[14] Additional Chinese studies have found that the side effects of TW are reduced when administered in combination with other Chinese herbs.[15]

Indian Sarsaparilla Vine (*Hemidesmus indicus*)—Indian sarsaparilla vine is not a true sarsaparilla, but is actually a close family member to American milkweed and European pleurisy root. It is traditionally used for snakebites, chronic skin diseases, and in autoimmune diseases such as rheumatoid arthritis.[16] Research published in the *Journal of Ethnopharmacology* revealed that Indian sarsaparilla vine is mildly immunosuppressive, yet is very safe and non-toxic.[17] The active chemical components, coumarins and triterpenoid saponins, work like immuno-suppressing drugs without the side effects, regulating the activity of pro-inflammatory agents (interferons, interleukins, prostaglandins) and other immune cells (T and B cells, antibodies, cytokines) involved in the inflammatory process.

Lithospermum 15—An excellent Chinese herbal formula, Lithospermum 15, combined with other alternative medicine therapies has yielded measurable reductions in inflammation and autoimmune activity, as well as RF (rheumatoid factor—SEE QUICK DEFINITION) and anemia. The herbs in this formula include lithospermum, astragalus, smilax, and red peony.

Herbs for Inflammation

Chronic or excessive inflammation in the joint area is a preliminary stage in what can develop into the autoimmune response. High levels

For more information about **Lithospermum 15** (for practitioners only), contact: Institute for Traditional Medicine and Preventive Health Care, 2017 Southeast Hawthorne, Portland, OR 97215; tel: 800-544-7504 or 503-233-4907; fax: 503-233-1012.

For more information on *Boswellia serrata*, see "An Herbal Aid for Arthritis and Inflammation," *Alternative Medicine* 24 (June/July 1998), pp. 67-68; www.alternativemedicine.com.

of inflammatory agents spur the immune system into constant activity, initially against foreign substances but later against the body's own tissues. Herbs that reduce inflammation by digesting proteins that trigger an immune response can help calm the immune system.

***Boswellia serrata*—**Known as Indian frankincense, the *Boswellia serrata* tree grows in the arid and mountainous regions of India. The tree's gum resin has been used for centuries in Ayurvedic medicine as a tonic for a variety of health conditions. The medicinally active extract of this resin is now available in supplement form as a natural anti-inflammatory, particularly helpful for osteoarthritis and rheumatoid arthritis. According to research, *Boswellia serrata* promises a safe and effective alternative to most conventional arthritis drugs and their considerable side effects.

One study involved 175 patients with rheumatoid arthritis and ankylosing spondylitis (inflammation and deterioration of joints, cartilage, and bone): all of the patients had suffered from their condition for one to five years and received little relief from conventional NSAIDs (nonsteroidal, anti-inflammatory drugs). They were given *Boswellia serrata* extract at a dose of 200 mg, three times daily. After four weeks of this therapy, 122 (70%) reported complete relief from morning stiffness in their joints; another 20% reported some degree of relief. Overall, 97% of the patients reported some level of improvement with *Boswellia* with no side effects. An animal study showed that *Boswellia* extract "significantly reduced" the inflammatory response to arthritis in rabbits. In particular, it limited the infiltration of leukocytes (white blood cells which are part of the immune system's response to infection) into the arthritic joint by as much as 50%.

Boswellic acid, the biologically active component of *Boswellia* extract, reduces the number of leukotrienes by inhibiting the activity of the enzyme needed for their formation. In arthritis, leukotrienes are the predominant mechanism leading to inflammation. The standardized compound is marketed as Boswellin® and is found in a variety of products, including both oral supplements and topical creams which can be applied directly to stiff or sore joints. The typical recommended dose for the oral supplement is three tablets daily (about 600 mg total), taken at meal times.

Ginger (*Zingiber officinale*)—Ginger's high concentration of proteolytic enzymes (which break down proteins) is responsible for its ability to subdue pain and inflammation. Proteolytic enzymes block the action of several inflammatory substances, including prostaglandins and leukotrienes.[19] In one study, arthritis patients (many of them with mixed rheumatoid arthritis, osteoarthritis, and fibromyalgia) were given supplements of ginger over two-and-a-half years. In 89% of rheumatoid arthritis patients and 88% of osteoarthritis patients, ginger brought about relief from pain and swelling.[20]

Michael Murray, N.D., author of *The Healing Power of Herbs*, suggests juicing ⅔ ounce or 20 g per day of ginger, equivalent to a half-inch slice of the fresh root.[21] Ginger can also be used as a hot compress: grate fresh ginger root and place it on a warm wash cloth, then apply the wash cloth to sore muscles or joints; keep the cloth warm by using a hot water bottle. Try this on a small area to observe your skin's reactions; fresh ginger may irritate delicate skin. Powdered ginger can also be effective in a compress. Another way of enjoying the health benefits of ginger is to make a cup of tea. Add one teaspoon of grated fresh ginger root to one cup of boiling water, cover to prevent the escape of important essential oils and ingredients, and steep 15 minutes; add honey or stevia, if desired.

A Spot of Tea for Arthritis

Add to green tea's list of health benefits a recent finding by researchers at Case Western Reserve University in Cleveland, Ohio—they found that green tea contains antioxidants that can successfully regulate the immune system and reduce inflammation. After isolating compounds known as polyphenols from green tea, the researchers mixed them into the drinking water of mice that were later injected with a substance that invokes a condition similar to rheumatoid arthritis. A control group received the same injection but were not given extracts of green tea. Most (94%) of the mice in the control group developed swelling, redness, and reduced mobility of their two front paws, while only 44% of the mice that drank green tea extract developed arthritis symptoms (which were isolated to one paw and milder than the control group's symptoms). Biopsies of the affected joints revealed that immune cells and key enzymes that promote inflammation were significantly reduced in the mice drinking green tea. The tea-drinking mice experienced little or no cartilage damage.[18]

For more **herbs helpful for Inflammation**, see Chapter 13: Supplements for Arthritis, pp. 280-313.

Turmeric (*Curcuma longa*)—Turmeric is a bright yellow spice used in Indian cooking, but it also has powerful anti-inflammatory properties, which are credited to the chemical component curcumin. Curcumin was found to be better at reducing acute inflammation than either cortisone or phenylbutazone, two commonly prescribed drugs.[22] Use turmeric in combination with ginger as a flavorful food seasoning and enjoy an inexpensive and accessible addition to your arthritis treatment. Turmeric can also be used as a poultice for aching joints.

Cayenne Pepper (*Capsicum anuum*)—Cayenne pepper contains capsaicin, a chemical component useful for pain relief. Capsaicin depletes body reserves of substance P, which is believed to be responsible for intensifying and prolonging muscle and joint inflammation and pain.[23] Substance P is a group of several amino acids bonded together that is normally present in minute amounts in the nervous system and intestines. Typically involved in the pain response, substance P expands and contracts smooth muscles in the intestines and other tissues. In patients with fibromyalgia (chronic muscle pain), substance P has been found in abnormally high levels and is regarded as one of the most potent compounds affecting smooth muscle contraction and inflammation.

Products containing *Boswellia serrata* extract are available in health food stores. For more information, contact: Nature's Herbs, 600 East Quality Drive, American Fork, UT 84003; tel: 801-763-0700 or 800-437-2257; fax: 801-763-0789; website: www.naturesherbs.com. Natural Organics, 548 Broad Hollow Road, Melville, NY 11747; tel: 800-532-0100 or 516-293-0030; fax: 516-293-0349; website: www.natplus.com. America's Finest Inc., 140 Ethel Road West, Suite S & T, Piscataway, NJ 08854; tel:800-350-3305 or 908-985-9899; fax: 908-985-9851. For the manufacturer of **Boswellin***, contact: Sabinsa Corporation, 121 Ethel Road West, Unit 6, Piscataway, NJ 08854; tel: 732-777-1111; fax: 732-777-1443. For **products containing turmeric, licorice root, ginger, or cayenne**, contact: Nature's Plus, 548 Broadhollow Road, Melville, NY 11747-3708; tel: 800-645-9500 or 516-293-0030. WGI, 35008 Emerald Coast Parkway, 5th Floor, Destin, FL 32541; tel: 800-854-8353 or 850-654-4744. BioDynamax, 6525 Gunpark Drive #150-507, Boulder, CO 80301; tel: 800-926-7525 or 303-530-4665. Nature's Answer, 320 Oser Avenue, Hauppauge, NY 11788; tel: 800-439-2324 or 516-231-7492; fax: 516-231-8391; website: www.naturesanswer.com.

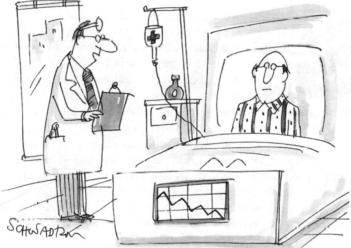

" THE GOOD NEWS IS WE CAN CURE YOU. THE BAD NEWS
IS THE CURE IS WORSE THAN THE DISEASE.

CHAPTER 11

Mind/Body Approaches to Arthritis

STRESS IS A COMMON PART of everyday life, but it can become harmful to the body when it is prolonged or chronic. It affects the body in very real, physical ways by influencing the immune and hormonal systems. For arthritis sufferers, this can mean an increase in pain and inflammation. A basic premise of mind/body medicine is that chronic stress contributes to illness and that relaxation techniques and learning positive ways of coping with stress will improve your health. In this chapter, we examine how stress, suppressed emotions, and lifestyle choices can contribute to arthritis. We also explore a number of therapies that can help you reprogram negative thought patterns into more healthful ones, deal with stress in a positive way, and incorporate habits for relaxation into your life.

Success Story: Mind/Body Therapies for Rheumatoid Arthritis

Prue, 42, developed rheumatoid arthritis seemingly overnight. The pain and stiffness hit her feet first, then spread to her wrists and hands, and finally to her neck and back. Synovial cysts had formed on the carpal bones (connecting the wrist to the hands) aggravated by the repetitive motion of typing required for her job. Like many of our arthritis patients, Prue first pursued a conventional medical treatment through rheumatologists, who pre-scribed prednisone, Plaquenil®, and other nonsteroidal, anti-inflammatory drugs or NSAIDs. After two years on these drugs, Prue experienced very little pain relief and later developed gastrointestinal problems (irritable bowel, occult blood in the stool indicating gastrointestinal bleeding, gas, and bloating). To offset the pain caused by her pain medication, Prue took an average of 12 aspirin per day, which caused yet more side effects. Frustrated and feeling hopeless, Prue came to see us six years after the onset of her arthritis.

We ran a battery of tests on Prue that showed a number of underlying physical problems contributing to her arthritis:

> ## Mind/Body Therapies for Arthritis
>
> ■ Meditation
> ■ Cognitive Therapy
> ■ Neuro-Linguistic Programming
> ■ Biofeedback
> ■ Hypnotherapy
> ■ Guided Imagery/ Visualization
> ■ Restricted Environmental Stimulation Therapy (R.E.S.T.)
> ■ Flower Remedies
> ■ Aromatherapy

■ Intestinal permeability or "leaky gut syndrome"—Intestinal permeability means that toxins leak into the bloodstream through the intestinal lining. Once bowel toxins enter the bloodstream or get absorbed by connective tissues, they can trigger inflammation.

For more information on **tests for diagnosing arthritis**, see Chapter 3: Diagnosing Arthritis, pp. 52-77.

■ An overburdened liver—Prue's liver was over-whelmed by the increased levels of toxins entering the bloodstream from the intestines. It was unable to filter these toxins and they re-entered the bloodstream where they were absorbed into tissues, leading to inflammation and putting additional stress on the immune system.

■ Bacterial infection—A harmful bacteria called *Enterobacter taylorae* present in Prue's stool sample contributed to her maldigestion and intestinal permeability. Harmful bacteria can alter the pH of the stomach, which shuts down the sequential phases of digestion; food is not properly digested and nutrients are not absorbed.

■ Mineral deficiencies—Hair mineral analysis found that Prue had inadequate levels of calcium, magnesium, zinc, and chromium, as well as selenium, germanium, and molybdenum, which are important nutrients in liver detoxification. Her copper level was in excess.

■ Food allergies—Prue had sensitivities to bananas, beans (green, kidney, and yellow wax), cheese, eggs, cow's milk, mushrooms, black and white pepper, sugar cane, wheat, and baker's and brewer's yeast.

Stress is a common part of everyday life, but it can become harmful to the body when it is prolonged or chronic. It affects the body in very real, physical ways by influencing the immune and hormonal systems. For arthritis sufferers, this can mean an increase in pain and inflammation.

Our first goal was to help Prue solve these underlying problems and achieve better control of pain and inflammation without depending on prescription drugs. We initiated a program of dietary changes, vitamin and mineral supplements, and other therapies to alleviate her condition.

Once this was accomplished, Prue wanted to focus on the psychological and emotional elements of her arthritis. She was frustrated at work because she found it difficult to say "no" to additional work loads, even if she was too busy to handle these requests. People, especially her immediate supervisor, took advantage of her pleasant and good-natured disposition, and never considered the physical limitations of her arthritis. Hiding behind an artificial smile, Prue felt angry at herself for not expressing her true feelings. Her silence toward her co-workers eventually grew into resentment and jealousy. She was jealous of their self-confidence, a quality that she didn't possess but compensated for by trying to please everyone. Prue's silence didn't help to improve her self-esteem; instead it only fed her unexpressed anger and diminished her ability to stand up for herself.

We pointed out to her the psychological effects of holding in anger, as expressed in her body by the "freezing up" of her joint mobility. The effects of suppressed emotions can extend beyond the psyche and into the physiological realm, where the body responds to pent-up anger by slowly breaking down. Prue turned all of her frustrations in on herself, contributing to the onset of a self-destructive disease such as arthritis.

We often see emotional problems such as anger in correlation with liver imbalances. This connection is clearly elucidated in traditional Chinese medicine, which recognizes areas of the body that correspond to different emotional states. In Prue's case, this connection was the major contributor for her onset of arthritis. The problem that Prue described to us about her co-workers was not an isolated incident, but an example of a pattern of behavior that contributed to a history of chronic illness. Another effect of Prue's internalized anger and subsequent low self-esteem could be found in her poor lifestyle choices, which worked to undermine her health. Prue had uncontrollable chocolate cravings that she succumbed to daily. The amount of sweets (pies, ice cream, and cookies) that she ate in a week outnumbered the amount of fruits or vegetables. In addition, she rarely exercised. These are lapses that even conventional doctors would not condone for a rheumatoid arthritis patient.

To support Prue's recovery, we had to redirect the way she perceived herself and her emotions and help her make wiser choices in behavior and health. We used a technique called Neuro-Linguistic Programming (NLP), a question-and-answer exchange that detects unconscious patterns of thought and behavior and provides ways to alter those negative patterns. We asked Prue about her identity, personal beliefs, and life goals. She considered her disease part of her identity, as if without arthritis she would cease being herself. Based on this first NLP session, we designed affirmation tapes that would help her regain control of her identity. She listened to these tapes during hydrotherapy in the flotation R.E.S.T. (restricted environmental stimulation therapy) tank, which we recommended to reduce her stress levels.

In NLP, the patient envisions being healthy and happy. If Prue could imagine herself healthy, then her body could respond to this positive stimulus by triggering the necessary immunological responses for healing. Without positive visualizations of health, Prue might have dutifully taken the supplements that we prescribed yet not believed that it would make a difference. She would be stuck thinking that she was not worthy of being healthy. Her body would have believed her defeated attitude and she would have remained sick.

We also used visual imagery sessions to teach Prue how to relax in stressful situations. We asked Prue to hold in her mind a picture of a distressing or emotion-provoking situation (such as a conflict with a co-worker or supervisor) and focus on relaxing her body in that situation. Imagery is like a dress rehearsal, so that the patient can learn to feel more relaxed when a stressful real-life situation occurs.

After 12 weeks on this program, Prue was pleased by her improved physical health. She no longer suffered stiffness and pain in her joints and her digestive problems had cleared up shortly after discontinuing conventional drugs and changing her diet. The cysts along her wrists were no longer painful, but an MRI scan showed evidence of fluid in the synovial sheaths (membranes lining the cavity of a bone through which a tendon moves). Examination by an orthopedic surgeon determined that aggressive surgery to remove the fluid was not necessary since Prue had no pain from the increased fluid and had not lost

For more information on **Neuro-Linguistic Programming**, see this chapter, pp. 239-241.

strength in her grip. And Prue found that she had more self-confidence as well. She actually said "no" to a co-worker's request to take on an additional project and felt like that response generated a more respectful attitude from that co-worker.

Stressed Out— A Pervasive Problem

Although the concept of stress—being "stressed out" or "under constant stress"—may be commonly discussed today, its role as a contributing factor in many diseases is underappreciated. Estimates suggest that as much as 70% to 80% of all visits to physicians' offices are for stress-related problems.[1] Chronic stress directly affects the immune system and, if not effectively dealt with, can seriously compromise health.

Stress is a pervasive problem among Americans, according to a 1996 poll of corporate executives. For example, 44% of employees polled said their work load is excessive compared to 37% in 1988; 43% are bothered by excessive job pressure; 55% worry considerably about their company's future; 25% of both men and women feel stressed out at work every day, another 12% feel it almost every day, and another 38% feel it once to several days a week.[2]

Stress can be defined as a reaction (to any stimulus or interference) that upsets normal functioning and disturbs mental or physical health. It can be brought on by internal conditions such as illness, pain, emotional conflict, or psychological problems, or by external circumstances, such as bereavement, financial problems, loss of job or spouse, relocation, food allergies, and electromagnetic fields. Stress, when it becomes chronic, is often unrecognized by the person whose body is experiencing it; one begins to accept it as a fact of life, without being aware of how it is actually compromising all bodily functions and preparing the foundation for illness.

More specifically, research confirms that high levels of emotional stress increase one's susceptibility to illness. Unrelieved, chronic stress begins taxing and eventually weakening or even suppressing the immune system. Stress can also lead to hormonal imbalances, which, in turn, interfere with immune function. Of all the body's systems, stress damages immune function the most. It does so by overly activating the sympathetic part of the autonomic nervous system, the part that controls the "fight-or-flight" response and initiates adrenaline and cortisol release.

Research in psychoneuroimmunology, or PNI, has shown that the immune and nervous systems are linked by extensive networks of nerve endings in the spleen, bone marrow, lymph nodes, and thymus gland (a primary source of T cells). At the same time, receptors for a variety of chemical messengers—catecholamines, prostaglandins, thyroid hormone, growth hormone, sex hormones, serotonin, and endorphins—have been found on the surfaces of white blood cells. Such connections serve to integrate the activities of the immune, hormonal, and nervous systems, enabling the mind and emotional states to influence the body's resistance to disease.[3]

Fight-or-Flight Response

Pioneering stress researcher Hans Selye, M.D., a Canadian physiologist, noted a consistent pattern of response to stress and termed this the general adaptation syndrome (GAS), commonly referred to as the "fight-or-flight" response. The GAS occurs in three stages: the alarm reaction, the stage of resistance, and the stage of exhaustion.

Initially, the body's biochemistry tends to react to stress in an orderly fashion. Stimulation of the sympathetic nervous system (part of the autonomic nervous system) activates the secretion of hormones from the endocrine glands and constricts both the blood vessels and the involuntary muscles of the body. When the endocrine glands (pancreas, thyroid, pituitary, sex glands, and par-

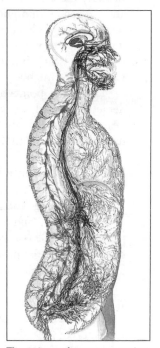

The autonomic nervous system (ANS) can be likened to your body's automatic pilot. It keeps you alive through breathing, heart rate, and digestion, without your being aware of it or participating in its activities. The ANS has two divisions: the sympathetic, which expends body energy; and the parasympathetic, which conserves body energy. The sympathetic nervous system is associated with arousal and stress; it prepares us physically when we perceive a threat or challenge by increasing our heart rate, blood pressure, and muscle tension. The parasympathetic nervous system slows heart rate and increases intestinal and most gland activity.

ticularly the adrenals) are stimulated, heart rate, glucose metabolism, and oxygen consumption increase. The parasympathetic nervous system is also stimulated, which begins a process of relaxation. The pituitary gland responds by releasing a variety of hormones throughout the body, which influence the defensive and adaptive mechanisms. Endorphins, the body's own natural painkillers, are also released.

Dr. Selye points out, however, that eventually chronic stress depletes the body's resources and its ability to adapt. If stress continues and remains unattenuated for a long period, coping functions will be compromised and illness will result.[4]

Stress, the Adrenal Glands, and Arthritis

The adrenal glands, part of the body's endocrine system, are located atop the kidneys. The glands are composed of two types of tissue: the adrenal medulla and the adrenal cortex. The adrenal medulla, comprising 10%-20% of the gland, is located in the interior portion and is responsible for the production of the hormones epinephrine (adrenaline) and norepinephrine (noradrenaline). These hormones are released in direct response to the sympathetic nervous system, which is responsible for the fight-or-flight response to stress or physical threats. The adrenal cortex, the outer layer, surrounds the medulla and accounts for 80%-90% of the gland. It is responsible for the production of corticosteroids (also called adrenal steroids). Over 30 different steroids have been isolated from the adrenal cortex, including cortisol and cortisone.

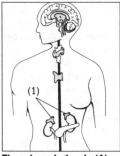

The adrenal glands (1) are two triangular-shaped glands above the kidneys. They release adrenaline and other hormones in the fight-or-flight response to stress.

Cortisol secretion (as well as the adrenal gland's other steroids, DHEA, adrenaline, and aldosterone) occurs in daily cycles, peaking in the morning and having the lowest values at night. Cortisol promotes protein building, regulates insulin and glycogen synthesis, and helps produce prostaglandins (hormone-like fatty acids involved in inflammatory processes). Under conditions of stress, high amounts of cortisol are released. Imbalances in cortisol secretion are linked with low energy, inflammation, muscle dysfunction, impaired bone repair, thyroid dysfunction, immune system depression, sleep disorders, and poor skin regeneration.

In a prolonged stressful state, chronic pain sets in as supplies of cortisol and other adrenal hormones plummet and eventually run out as the adrenals become exhausted. One function of cortisol is to act as a potent anti-inflammatory hormone. If you have arthritis, the pain and inflammation in your joints will worsen as your adrenal glands stop producing cortisol. This results in fatigue, muscle weakness, depression, and a magnification of arthritic symptoms.

Based on our clinical experience with hundreds of patients, we find that arthritis sufferers, both osteoarthritis and rheumatoid arthritis, are typically in a moderate to advanced state of adrenal exhaustion. Researchers are also beginning to find evidence of a connection between stress and arthritis. A recent study found that in 86% of cases, the onset of rheumatoid arthritis was preceded by stressful events in the patients' lives. In addition, there was a correlation between arthritis flare-ups and stressful events in 60% of patients.[5] When people with psoriatic arthritis are questioned, there will often be a correlation between a stressful life event (divorce, loss of job) and the initial onset of the condition.

For someone in this situation, conventional medicine typically prescribes pharmaceutical drugs similar to cortisol (corticosteroids) for the pain and inflammation; prednisone, for example, is 30 times as potent as endogenous cortisol.[6] Many practitioners of natural medicine feel that, while the judicious use of corticosteroids is helpful for a short period of time to stabilize the patient, the long-term use and reliance on these powerful drugs is devastating. These drugs can suppress immunity, interfere with sleep cycles, and increase bone and collagen breakdown as well as suppress the proper function and production of the adrenal hormones and further diminish the functioning of the adrenal glands.

The Arthritis Personality

The most critical aspect of stress is not the event itself, but your response or interpretation of the situation. Do you respond with hope or despair? With helplessness or commitment to resolve the situation? With pent-up anger or tranquility? How you respond, to some degree, reflects your personality type.

Human behavioral patterns are commonly broken down into two basic personality types, Type As and Type Bs. Type A personalities are described as aggressive and competitive, easily angered, always in a hurry, and hostile. Type Bs do not exhibit these characteristics, but are more deliberate, thinking through a situation and formulating a plan of action. Beginning in the 1960s, studies began to show that personality type can have a profound influence on your health. One study fol-

The arthritis personality, due to their critical nature, wants things to be different, but the impulse to change is constantly suppressed by an unwillingness to change. Stiffness and rigidity are the dominant states of mind and the dominant conditions of an arthritic joint.

lowed 3,000 middle-aged men over an eight-and-a-half year period and found that Type As were twice as likely to develop heart disease as Type Bs.[7] A recent study of air traffic controllers found that Type As had three-and-a-half times more job-related injuries and 38% more illnesses overall than Type Bs.[8]

We have repeatedly seen certain common personality characteristics exhibited by those with arthritis. One of our observations matches that of Louise Hay, author of *Heal Your Life*, who notes that arthritis is a disease seen frequently in men and women who develop a constant pattern of criticism of themselves and others.[9] We've also noted that the critical tendency does not always have to be overt: it might be completely internal, a type of inner voice that keeps telling the person that things are not 'OK', that they could be better.

However, it is generally not in the nature of the arthritis personality to express their feelings or to attempt to creatively change the situation that disturbs them. This is the second trait of the arthritis personality: they are more likely to appear to accept it, but have an internal resistance to change. Researchers at Ohio State University, in Columbus, conducted a study to evaluate the personality traits of rheumatoid disease sufferers. Their findings indicate that "patients with rheumatoid diseases are likely to be excessively conscientious, fearful of criticism yet critical of themselves and others, frequently depressed, and have a poor self-image." The study group exhibited characteristics that led them to try to be overly nice to other people at the expense of their own well-being, to be stoic, and to conceal their emotions (especially anger). "Many rheumatic disease sufferers have a situation of long-standing tension or anger in their lives, yet would assert when questioned that everything was 'OK', even though it was furthest from the truth. They were remarkably conforming to these traits, which seemed to precede their disease, not be caused as a result of it."[10]

In these individuals, unfulfilled expectations lead to a sense of increased frustration and even anger that they keep to themselves, perhaps eventually turning the immune system against itself.[11] From this perspective, arthritis can be seen as a form of frozen impulse. The arthritis personality, due to their critical nature, wants things to be different, but the impulse to change is constantly suppressed by an unwillingness or inability to change. Biochemically, this may manifest itself by the accumulation of stress hormones in the body, particularly in the joints, the area of the body representing the greatest flexibility and mobility. Stiffness and rigidity are the dominant states of mind and they are also the dominant conditions of an arthritic joint.

Those traits seem related to a third one we have noted in our work with arthritis sufferers: a pronounced tendency to cling to the status quo. They tend to be very rigid and structured in their dietary routines, sedentary or overly active lifestyle, and even dependence on medications. We have found it extremely difficult to persuade arthritis patients to adopt the lifestyle changes needed for recovery, sometimes even if they were experiencing severe pain.

Are You Stressed Out?

If you answer "yes" to more than five of the questions below, it indicates that you have too much stress in your life. In parentheses after each question are some potential underlying causes for the problem.

■ Do you often grind your teeth? (digestive dysfunction, parasites)

■ Is your breath shallow and irregular? (low metabolic energy, food allergies)

■ Are your hands and feet cold? (hormonal imbalance, adrenal/thyroid weakness)

■ Do you have trouble sleeping or tend to wake up tired? (liver dysfunction, food allergies)

Emotional Tissues

According to Louise Hay, the particular area of the body affected by arthritis reveals emotional issues related to it:

■ The arms represent the capacity to embrace life.

■ Old emotions are stored in the joints.

■ Elbows represent flexibility in changing directions.

■ Legs represent the ability to move ahead in positive directions.

■ Joints represent changes and directions in life and the ease of these movements.

■ Inflammation indicates suppressed anger and frustration.

■ Swelling represents clogging and stagnation in emotional thinking.

■ Stiffness in the body represents stiffness in the mind—inflexible attitudes and beliefs, feeling stuck or trapped, repressed anger, and other strong emotions.[12]

■ Do you often have an upset stomach? (food allergies)

■ Do you get mad or irritated easily? (liver dysfunction)

■ Do you feel worthless? (low metabolic energy, chronic fatigue)

■ Do you constantly worry? (hormonal imbalance)

■ Do you have problems concentrating and articulating your

For the **Adrenal Stress Index test**, contact: Diagnos-Tech, Inc., 6620 South 192nd Place, J-2204, Kent, WA 96032; tel: 800-878-3787 or 425-251-0596; fax: 425-251-0637.

thoughts? (low metabolic energy, digestive or hormonal imbalance)

■ Do you frequently fidget, chew your fingers, or bite your nails? (food allergies, digestive disturbances)

■ Do you have high blood pressure? (food allergies, digestive disturbances)

■ Do you eat, drink, or smoke excessively? (low metabolic energy, poor diet)

■ Do you sometimes turn to recreational drugs just to get away? (low metabolic energy, poor diet)

Are Your Adrenal Glands Stressed?

The Adrenal Stress Index (ASI) can pinpoint whether an imbalance in the adrenal glands might be contributing to stress and arthritis. This test evaluates how well one's adrenal glands are functioning by tracking hormone levels over a 24-hour cycle (circadian rhythm). Four saliva samples taken at intervals throughout the day are used to reconstruct the adrenal rhythm in the laboratory. Saliva has been shown to closely mirror blood levels of hormones and a saliva test is also less invasive. These samples are used to determine whether two main stress hormones (cortisol and DHEA) are being secreted in proper proportion to each other, and at the right times. Based on the results, a physician can prescribe the appropriate treatment to restore the balance of hormones and correct the circadian rhythm.

Mind/Body Therapies for Arthritis

According to Hans Selye, M.D., whether a person experiences stress as a positive motivational force or as a negative detrimental one depends on their perception of the stress.[13] People who perceive that they are in control of their lives and generally feel good about themselves (referred to as an "inner locus of control") will use life's stressors in a positive fashion. However, those who feel that their life circumstances are controlled by outside forces and other people ("outer locus of control") tend to react negatively to stress. The locus of control can be consciously shifted by deliberately "reprogramming" the mind, with positive instead of negative thoughts, through meditation, cognitive therapy, and Neuro-Linguistic Programming. Relaxation therapies, such as biofeedback, hypnotherapy, guided imagery, flower remedies, and aromatherapy, can help reduce your stress levels and relieve arthritis pain.

Meditation

Meditation is a safe and simple way to balance a person's physical, emotional, and mental states. It is easy to learn and can be useful both for treating stress and in pain management. Meditation, in the broadest sense, is any activity that keeps the attention focused in the present. When the mind is calm and focused in the present, it is neither reacting to past events or preoccupied with future plans, two major sources of chronic stress. There are many forms of meditation, but they can be categorized into two main approaches, concentration meditation and mindfulness meditation.

Concentration meditation focuses the "lens of the mind" on one object, sound (mantra), the breath, an image, or thought, to still the mind and allow greater awareness or clarity to emerge. The breath is one of the most popular objects of focus in

According to Hans Selye, M.D., whether a person experiences stress as a positive motivational force or as a negative detrimental one depends on their perception of the stress.

this type of meditation. As the person focuses on the ebb and flow of their breath, the mind is absorbed in the rhythm and becomes more placid, tranquil, and still. Mindfulness-based meditation entails bringing the mind to a still point, tuning out the world and bringing the mind to a halt as much as possible. Mindfulness meditation helps you practice non-judgment. The meditator sits quietly and simply witnesses whatever goes through the mind, not reacting or becoming involved with thoughts, memories, worries, or images. This helps the person gain a more calm, clear, and non-reactive state of mind.

Transcendental Meditation™ (TM), a popular form of concentration meditation, is the most well-documented regarding the physiological effects of meditation, with over 500 clinical studies conducted to date.[14] Research shows that, during TM practice, the body gains a deeper state of relaxation than during ordinary rest or sleep.[15] Brain wave changes indicate a state of enhanced awareness and coherence and TM has been found to increase intelligence, creativity, and perceptual ability and reduce blood pressure and rates of illness by 50%.[16]

A Simple Meditation Exercise

The first step to practicing meditation is learning to breathe in a manner that facilitates a state of calmness and awareness. Dr. Jon Kabat-Zinn recommends the following exercise for achieving a sense of calmness—find a quiet place where you will not be disturbed and practice for several minutes each day:

■ Assume a comfortable posture lying on your back or sitting. If you are sitting, keep the spine straight and let your shoulders drop.

■ Close your eyes if it feels comfortable.

■ Bring your attention to your belly, feeling it rise or expand gently on the in-breath and fall or recede on the out-breath. Keep the focus on your breathing.

■ When your mind wanders off the breath, notice what it was that took you away and then gently bring your attention back to your belly and the feeling of the breath moving in and out. If your mind wanders away from the breath, your "job" is simply to bring it back to the breath every time, no matter what it has become preoccupied with.

Practice this exercise for 15 minutes every day, whether you feel like it or not, for one week and see how it feels to incorporate a disciplined meditation practice into your life.

TM also causes decreased blood levels of cortisol, a hormone responsible for many of the deleterious physiological changes seen with stress.[17] By reducing cortisol levels, the adrenal glands are allowed to heal, which positively influences pain and inflammation.

A direct effect of meditation in arthritis is the reduction of pain. "Chronic pain can erode the quality of life," says Jon Kabat-Zinn, Ph.D., founder and director of the Stress Reduction Clinic at the University of Massachusetts Medical Center, and author of *Wherever You Go, There You Are*. In one study performed by Dr. Kabat-Zinn, 72% of the patients with chronic pain achieved at least a 33% reduction in pain after participating in an eight-week period of mindfulness meditation, while 61% of the patients achieved at least a 50% reduction in pain and perceived their bodies as being less problematic (suggesting an improvement in self-esteem).[18]

Cognitive Therapy

It has been estimated that the average human being has around 50,000 thoughts per day, according to Dr. Richard Carlson, author of *Don't Sweat The Small Stuff...And It's All Small Stuff*. Unfortunately, he reminds us, many of them are also going to be negative—angry, fearful, pessimistic, or worrisome. Up to 85% of the thinking we regularly engage in is negative and self-defeating.[19]

The basis of cognitive therapy is to identify—through maintaining a journal and by introspection—the negative, self-defeating inner dialogue of thoughts (what cognitive therapists refer to as "automatic thoughts"). Positive, coping thoughts can then be used to counter the negative thoughts. The goal is to pull yourself out of reflexive self-destructive mental behavior that may be exacerbating your illness and to bolster the positive, self-reliant aspect of your personality.

Cognitive therapy does not focus on the root causes of psychological problems, rather it seeks to support health by interrupting the flow of negative thoughts. Countering each negative thought on paper with a list of positive responses to the same problem enables the mind to reframe the situation. For arthritis sufferers, replacing negative thoughts with positive ones can help facilitate healing. Cognitive therapy may also be helpful for dealing with pain. The intensity of pain is partly determined by how you perceive it—if you "catastrophize" the pain, you may actually make it worse. Cognitive therapy can be used to gain control of your thought processes and allow you to alter your perception of pain.

Neuro-Linguistic Programming

A technique similar to cognitive therapy, Neuro-Linguistic Programming (NLP) helps people detect unconscious patterns of thought, behavior, and attitudes that contribute to their illness. These unconscious patterns are then reprogrammed in order to alter psychological responses and facilitate the healing process. *Neuro* refers to the way the brain works and how thinking demonstrates consistent and detectable patterns; *linguistic* refers to the verbal and nonverbal expressions of thinking patterns; *programming* refers to how these patterns are recognized and understood by the mind and how they can be altered.

NLP was developed in the early 1970s by a professor of linguistics and a student of psychology and mathematics, both at the University

How to Stop a Thought Attack

One technique to stop a 'thought attack' is to keep a rubber band around your wrist. When you are aware of a negative thought, snap the rubber band in order to "snap" your consciousness out of its negative pattern. Then replace the negative thought with a positive affirmation that means something to you personally. "I am making progress in treating myself as a friend," for instance. This coping technique helps you to become aware of your automatic thoughts and begin to change them consciously.

For more information on **cognitive therapy**, contact: University of Pennsylvania Center for Cognitive Therapy, 3600 Market Street, 8th Floor, Philadelphia, PA 19104, tel: 215-898-4100; fax: 215-898-1865. The American Institute for Cognitive Therapy, 136 E. 57th Street, Suite 1101, New York, NY 10022; tel: 212-308-2440.

Success Story: Cognitive Therapy Relieves Stress-Induced Arthritis

Ray came to the office suffering extreme pain due to chronic psoriatic and gouty arthritis. It was clear that he had a very stressful life—he was in bankruptcy, contemplating divorce, had very low self-esteem, and had problems with his teenage children. He was so depressed that he had even contemplated suicide. Not surprisingly, he felt like he was caught in a downward spiral, with little he could do.

The first thing we realized about this patient is that his sense of hope was low and helplessness was high. Ray's team of rheumatologists offered little else but higher doses of medication and opiates to control his pain. We explained to Ray that chronic pain is a complicated mixture of physical, perceptual, cognitive, emotional, environmental, and other factors. Pain is actually an individual experience and is real, regardless of whether or not an organic cause can be found.

We stabilized Ray's depression with a combination of kava-kava (*Piper methysticum*), Botanodyne (from Nature's Answer), DL-phenylalanine (an amino acid helpful in pain management), and cognitive therapy. We made a list of his negative thoughts and brainstormed with him on a list of positive, coping thoughts to replace them. Every time Ray would catch himself in the act of a negative thought, he would snap the rubber band kept around his wrist as a reminder, then repeat his coping thoughts in the form of a present tense, personal, and positive affirmation.

The combination of naturopathic arthritis treatment, diet changes, and cognitive therapy helped tremendously. Ray began to transform himself into a positive thinker; he became less critical of himself and others. He felt strong enough emotionally to be able to manage his pain and cure himself of arthritis. He ended his dysfunctional marriage (a major component of his constant stress) and was able to begin to work from his home again. He smiled more and became angered less frequently. He occasionally would slip back to his old habit of worrying, but when he became conscious of doing it, he would snap the rubber band, then go for a walk or, in some way, interrupt his downward spiraling vortex of negative thoughts. After ten months, Ray was not only "completely out of pain," but also in possession of a different self-image. "Not only is my arthritis better, but I've learned to manage my emotions, and become a better, happier person," he said.

of California at Santa Cruz. They studied the thinking processes, language patterns, and behavioral patterns of several accomplished individuals. They found that body cues—eye movement, posture, voice tone, and breathing patterns—coincided with certain unconscious patterns of a person's emotional state. Based on their findings, they developed the NLP technique to help people with emotional problems.

People who have difficulty recovering from physical illness have often adopted negative beliefs about their recovery. They perceive themselves as helpless, hopeless, or worthless, expressed in statements like "I can't get healthy" or "There's no hope." NLP tries to move the person from their present state of discomfort to a desired state of health by helping reprogram these beliefs about healing.

NLP practitioners ask questions to discover how the person relates to issues of identity, personal beliefs, life goals, and their health, then observe the person's language patterns, eye movements, postures, muscle tension, and gestures. These relay information about how the person relates to their condition in both conscious and unconscious ways, revealing what limiting beliefs may exist. These belief structures can then be altered using NLP. The practitioner will ask the person to see herself in a state of health. By doing so, an outcome is set that facilitates the healing process. The brain's natural response is to duplicate whatever images or beliefs are created about getting better.[20] The brain then triggers the necessary immunological responses to guide the body toward health. NLP has proved successful in treating people with chronic illnesses, such as AIDs, cancer, allergies, and arthritis.

Biofeedback

Biofeedback training is a method of learning how to consciously regulate normally unconscious bodily functions (such as breathing, heart rate, and blood pressure) through the use of simple electronic devices. Biofeedback is particularly useful for learning to reduce stress, eliminate headaches, reduce muscle spasms, and relieve pain.

Stress Management Helps Rheumatoid Arthritis

A study at the Harry S. Truman Memorial Veterans Hospital, in Columbia, Missouri, showed that stress management techniques produced clinical benefits for rheumatoid arthritis patients. In the study of 141 patients, one group received stress management training while the other received standard medical care without additional psychological counseling. The training consisted of a ten-week course on stress management techniques followed by a 15-month maintenance phase. At the end of this period, the researchers found that the stress management group showed statistically significant improvements in measures of self-efficacy, coping, feelings of helplessness, pain, and overall health status.[21]

For more information on **Neuro-Linguistic Programming**, contact: NLP University/ Dynamic Learning Center, P.O. Box 1112, Ben Lomond, CA 95005; tel: 408-336-3457; fax: 408-336-5854; website: www.nlpu.com. NLP Comprehensive, 5695 Yukon Street, Arvada, CO 80002; tel: 800-233-1657 or 303-940-8888; fax 303-940-8889; website: www.nlpcomprehensive.com. NLP Seminars Group International, P.O. Box 424, Hopatcong, NJ 07843; tel: 201-770-1084; website: www.purenlp.com.

Biofeedback can help arthritis sufferers by relaxing tight muscles, correcting muscular imbalances, and providing muscular re-education, which can prevent and correct abnormal joint biomechanics. It can also intercept a chronic fight-or-flight response and aid in revitalizing adrenal gland functions. By teaching patients both relaxation techniques and control over their muscle spasms, biofeedback helps them reduce or eliminate pain.[22]

Biofeedback devices give immediate "feedback" or information about the biological system of the person being monitored, so that he or she can learn to consciously influence that system. For example, a person seeking to regulate their heart rate would train with a biofeedback device set up to transmit one blinking light or one audible beep per heartbeat. Electrodes are placed on the skin (a simple, painless process). The patient is then instructed to use various techniques such as meditation, relaxation, and visualization to effect the desired response (muscle relaxation, lowered heart rate, or lowered temperature). The biofeedback device reports the person's progress by a change in the speed of the beeps or flashes. By learning to alter the rate of the flashes or beeps, the person would be subtly programmed to control the heart rate.

For more information on **biofeedback** or for referrals, contact: The Association for Applied Biofeedback and Physiopsychology, 10200 W. 44th Avenue, Suite 304, Wheat Ridge, CO 80033; tel: 800-477-8892 or 303-422-8436; fax: 303-422-8894.

"Central for a person in pain is the need to begin to take some degree of control of the situation, to feel empowered to influence the processes at work and not to feel himself or herself to be a mere object. When a person suffering pain understands the causes, nature, mechanisms, and role of the pain or illness, a vital step has been taken in the successful handling of the problem," according to Leon Chaitow, N.D., D.O., of London, England.[23] Biofeedback helps a person take this critical step in controlling arthritis pain.

Hypnotherapy

Hypnotherapy has therapeutic applications for both psychological and physical disorders. A skilled hypnotherapist can facilitate profound changes in respiration and relaxation to create positive shifts in behavior and an enhanced sense of well-being. A physiological shift can be observed in a hypnotic state, as can greater control of autonomic nervous system functions normally considered to be beyond one's ability to control. Stress reduction is a common occurrence as is a lowering of blood pressure.

Hypnosis can be used to alleviate many varieties of pain, such as back, abdominal, and joint pain, as well as headaches and migraines. It works by accessing the unconscious mind and training it to react in a positive way to the experience of pain, such as inducing an immediate sense of relaxation. Hypnotherapy can be a nurturing and highly relaxing experience. Certified hypnotherapists do not attempt to control your mind or take you into a state so deep that you do not have control over yourself. Most people are aware of everything that transpires during a hypnotherapy session, yet they are able to mobilize deeper levels of their mind to facilitate healing.

Hypnotherapy is currently taught in several allopathic medical programs and has been approved by the American Medical Association as a clinical adjunct in the management of chronic pain.[24] Some states certify the profession of hypnotherapy by requiring a certain level of training. Other types of practitioners, such as psychotherapists and bodyworkers, may also use hypnosis as a tool to help their patients relax.

For information and referrals for **hypnotherapy**, contact: Bryan Knight, The International Registry of Professional Hypnotherapists, 7306 Sherbrooke Street West, Montreal, Quebec, Canada H4B 1R7; tel: 514-489-6733; fax: 514-485-3828; website: www.hypnosis.org.

Guided Imagery/Visualization

Using the power of the mind to evoke a positive physical response, guided imagery and visualization can modulate the immune system and reduce pain. Guided imagery uses the imagination to elicit positive physiological responses. By directly accessing emotions, imagery can help an individual understand the needs that may be represented by an illness and can help develop ways to meet those needs. Imagery is also one of the quickest and most direct ways to become aware of emotions and their effects on health, both positive and negative.

Imagery is simply a flow of thoughts that one can see, hear, feel, smell, taste, or experience. According to Martin L. Rossman, M.D., of the Academy for Guided Imagery, in Mill Valley, California, while the sensory phenomenon which is being experienced in the mind may or may not represent external reality, it always depicts internal reality. What Dr. Rossman means is that the sensations in the body that imagery creates are very real phenomena that can be measured via laboratory devices. Research using brain scans indicates that imagery activates parts of the cerebral cortex and centers of the primitive brain. During visualization, the visual (optic) cortex is active, and when sounds are imagined, the auditory cortex is active. It appears that the cortex can create imaginary realities and the lower centers (and perhaps every cell in the body) respond to this information.

"If you are a good worrier," states Dr., Rossman, "and especially if you ever 'worry yourself sick', you may be an especially good can-

For information on **guided imagery**, contact: Academy for Guided Imagery, P.O. Box 2070, Mill Valley, CA 94942; tel: 800-726-2070 or 415-389-9325; fax: 415-389-9342; website: www.healthy.net/agi.

didate for learning how to positively affect your health with imagery, as the internal process involved in worrying yourself sick and 'imagining yourself well' are quite similar."[25] Imagery is a proven method for pain relief, helps people tolerate medical procedures, reduces side effects of treatments, and stimulates the body to heal.

William Lowe Mundy, M.D., has used imagery to treat individuals with autoimmune arthritis as well as systemic lupus. Studies show that depression and other psychiatric symptoms often precede the development of lupus and rheumatoid arthritis.[26] In order to reverse the disease, the patient must access, and reverse, the recurrent, negative thought patterns. In one case, Dr. Mundy instructed a patient to use two sets of visual images to rid herself of rheumatoid arthritis, which had developed after a life of depression and destructive self-criticism. He first instructed her to visualize and compare the difference between what a bacteria looked like and what normal cells looked like, in order to inform her immune system of the difference between "self and non-self" and the mistake her immune cells were making in killing normal cells. He also suggested she develop different imagery to relieve her arthritic symptoms: she pictured little dragons carrying ice to put out the arthritic "fire" in her joints. In less than three weeks, 75% of her arthritic pain was gone and she was able to discontinue medication.[27]

Restricted Environmental Stimulation Therapy (R.E.S.T.)

Restricted environmental stimulation therapy (R.E.S.T.), a therapeutic tool that has been researched for over 35 years, is known to aid individuals in relaxation. The principle behind this therapy is the isolation of the person from sensory input from the external environment, accomplished by using a flotation tank.

You customarily float for one hour in a small, shallow flotation tank or pool. The water is 18 inches deep and supersaturated with 1,000-1,500 pounds of Epsom salts (magnesium sulfate). This makes the water so buoyant that it is impossible to sink. One just floats effortlessly on the surface and experiences something that only astronauts usually experience—the feeling of weightlessness. In addition, the environment of the flotation tank is specifically designed to reduce the perception of all external stimuli ("sensory deprivation"), which can lead to powerful healing effects on the body and mind. The water and air temperature is kept constant at 93°-94° F; this

For more information on **flotation tanks**, contact: The Floatation Tank Association, P.O. Box 1396, Grass Valley, CA 95945-1396; tel: 916-432-4502; fax: 916-432-3794.

allows the patient to lose the ability to discern where the body ends and the outer environment begins.

Flotation provides the most reliable induction of deep relaxation attainable without medication or years of training in meditation or biofeedback. R.E.S.T. has been scientifically documented to produce a myriad of psychological and physiological responses the are conducive to relaxation. The following are particularly beneficial to those with arthritis: a decrease in pain,[28] diminished response to stress,[29] a decline in cortisol levels in the blood,[30] and an increase in magnesium levels.[31] Magnesium is important because it helps muscles to relax and low levels of magnesium can contribute to muscle spasms; arthritis patients often have a deficiency of magnesium.

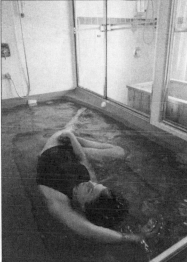

One person with arthritis who used flotation described it this way: "My health status followed my mind. If I can use computer jargon to illustrate the point, flotation helped me

Flotation provides the most reliable induction of deep relaxation attainable without medication or years of training in meditation or biofeedback.

erase my old mental software and reinstall new mental software. This enabled me to 'print-out' a new, disease-free prototype of my body. The pain is completely gone and all lab tests that were previously positive for arthritis indicators have now been normal for five years. I am truly cured of arthritis."[32]

Flower Remedies

Flower remedies directly address a person's emotional state in order to facilitate both psychological and physiological well-being. By balancing negative feelings and stress, flower remedies can effectively remove the emotional barriers to health and recovery. Flower remedies comprise subtle liquid preparations made from the fresh blossoms of flowers, plants, bushes, even trees, to address emotional, psychological, and spiritual issues underlying physical and medical problems. The approach was pioneered by British physician Edward Bach in the 1930s, when he introduced the 38 Bach Flower Remedies, based on English plants.

The Spiritual Connection to Healing

Spirituality and a feeling of connection to a divine presence can cultivate a hopeful attitude and a sense of meaning in one's life, which may help promote healing and recovery even with an illness as serious as arthritis. The particular way this is expressed, through a specific religious practice or time spent in nature, for instance, is not the important issue. Prayer (of any kind or denomination) has been proven to be a health-giving practice in over 250 studies and can be used as an effective means of aiding with physical wellness and healing.[33]

A recent study at the University of Michigan, in Ann Arbor, found that people who regularly attended religious services (at least once per month) lived significantly longer than those who did not. The national survey followed 3,617 Americans over a seven-year period. The non-churchgoers were about one-third more likely to die over the study period. Churchgoers tended to be more physically active, at a healthy weight, and non-smokers. Even eliminating these healthier lifestyle factors, the non-churchgoers still had a 25% greater likelihood of dying. Researchers speculated that the community involvement and religious rituals might promote feelings of hope, serenity, and optimism, all helpful in prolonging life. Attending religious services "extends the life span about as much as moderate exercise or not smoking," the researchers concluded.[34]

The placebo effect—the surprising healing results of inert substances due to the patient's belief that these will be healing—is often ridiculed or marginalized. But the insightful physician understands that the power of the mind—call it placebo effect, faith, spirituality, or the mind/body connection—when marshaled for its positive aspects, can be a potent healing force.

Two new studies show how this works. One survey of 300 HMO executives showed that 94% believe that personal prayer, meditation, or other spiritual practices can assist a medical treatment and speed up the healing process. This study of the beliefs of members of the American Association of Health Plans was sponsored by the John Templeton Foundation, founded in 1987 in Radnor, Pennsylvania, to support the teaching of spirituality in medical schools.

In fact, the Templeton study directly asked its HMO participants if they were familiar with the placebo effect. They were: 95% said they knew about it, 83% said they believe it works, 76% believe it can speed or assist in medical treatment, while 92% contend that belief of any kind can have a healing effect. The Templeton poll also noted that 74% of the HMO executives consulted believe the positive effects of spirituality on medical care could reduce health-care costs. However, they are reluctant to test this in actual policy changes. The HMO executives said they would need "direct evidence of clinical effectiveness" (76%), cost savings (65%), and patient satisfaction (62%) before they incorporated spirituality practices into their policies.

The Templeton study also reported that 89% of HMO executives said the policies of their organization's health plans do not yet take into account the research regarding spirituality and healing. Yet these execu-

Today, an estimated 20 different brands of flower remedies, based on plants native to many landscapes, from Australia to India to Alaska, offer about 1,500 different blends for a diverse range of psychological conditions. Each flower remedy addresses a particular emotional issue: for example, Vine helps to increase feelings of self-worth, Impatiens is recommended for feelings of impatience with others and yourself, and Aspen is for feelings of fear. An individual formula can be made by combining four to six of the remedies and taking them orally or rubbing them into the skin. They can be taken for a short time to cope with a crisis or for a period of months.

Amanda, 52, came to the office in severe pain. Her arthritis was "out of control," as she put it. Her joints were swollen and stiff, she was suffering from chronic fatigue, and she felt hopeless. After a blood test for laboratory and food allergy assessment, we reviewed her life situation with her. She had been through a "terrible divorce" over the past year and her arthritis symptoms had increased during that same time. Along with initial dietary changes (the Arthritis Diet), we put together a Bach flower remedy combination to help with her emotional issues: Cherry Plum (for feeling a loss of control), Crabapple (for cleansing), Rock Rose (for terror), and Water Violet (for more self-reliance). Amanda was instructed to take ½ teaspoon of this combination four times daily. "I can't believe it," she said after three days on the therapy. "The feeling of hopelessness has lifted. It feels like a veil of confu-

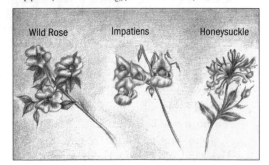

Wild Rose   Impatiens   Honeysuckle

Aromatherapy to Soothe Arthritis Pain

Place two ounces of almond oil in a small bowl, then add four drops each of lavender, birch, cypress, and juniper oils. Mix together and apply the oil to any painful or tense joint or muscle area. Place some of the same mixture in a diffuser or directly on a light bulb and leave the light on—this will fill the room with a relaxing, stress-reducing fragrance. You can experiment with different combinations of the following essential oils recommended for relieving arthritis pain: nutmeg, lavender, helicrysum, ginger, fir, cedar, and roman chamomile.

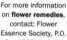

For more information on **flower remedies**, contact: Flower Essence Society, P.O. Box 1769, Nevada City, CA 95959; tel: 800-548-0075 or 916-265-9163; fax: 916-265-6467.

For **dietary recommendations for arthritis**, see Chapter 12: The Arthritis Diet, pp. 250-278.

sion was covering my head, and now it's gone. Best of all, these flower remedies don't have any side effects, like drowsiness, that I got from the anti-depressant medications I used before."

Aromatherapy

Aromatherapy is a unique branch of herbal medicine that utilizes the medicinal properties found in the essential oils of various plants. Through a process of steam distillation or cold-pressing, the volatile constituents of the plant's oil (its essence) are extracted from its flowers, leaves, branches, or roots. The immediate and often profound effect that essential oils have on the central nervous system also makes aromatherapy an excellent method for stress management.[36] The term *aromatherapy* was coined in 1937 by the French chemist Rene-Maurice Gattefosse, who observed the healing effect of lavender oil on burns.

Essential oils have a number of pharmacological properties—antibacterial, antiviral, antispasmodic, as diuretics (promoting production and excretion of urine), and as vasodilators (widening blood vessels). They are able to energize or pacify, detoxify, and help digestion. The oils' therapeutic properties also make them effective for treating infection, interacting with the various branches of the nervous system, modifying immune response, and harmonizing moods and emotions. Aromatic molecules that interact with the nasal cavity give off signals that travel to the limbic system, the emotional switchboard of the brain.[37] There they create impressions associated with previous experiences and emotions. The limbic system is directly connected to those parts of the brain that control heart rate, blood pressure, breathing, memory, stress levels, and hormone balance.

John Steele, Ph.D., of Sherman Oaks, California, and Robert Tisserand, of London, England, leading researchers in the field of aromatherapy, have studied the effects on brain-wave patterns when essential oils are inhaled or smelled. Their findings show that oils such as orange, jasmine, and rose have a tranquilizing effect and work by altering the brain waves into a rhythm that produces calmness and a sense of well-being.[38] Essential oils like citronella and *Eucalyptus citriodora* can be diffused in the air or rubbed on the wrists, solar plexus, and temples for quick and effective relaxation. Lavender oil added to the bath or sprayed on the bed sheets reduces tension and enhances relaxation.[39] Roman chamomile (*Anthemis nobilis*) is also recommended to calm an upset mind or body. A drop rubbed on the solar plexus can bring rapid relief of mental or physical stress.

How to Use Aromatherapy

How to Use Aromatherapy—Aromatherapy uses essential oils to affect the body in several ways. The benefits of essential oils can be obtained through inhalation, external application, or ingestion.

■ Through a diffusor: Diffusors disperse microparticles of the essential oil into the air. They can be used to achieve beneficial results in respiratory conditions, or to simply change the air with the mood-lifting or calming qualities of the fragrance.

■ External application: Oils are readily absorbed through the skin. Convenient applications are baths, massages, hot and cold compresses, or a simple topical application of diluted oils.[40] Essential oils in a hot bath can stimulate the skin, induce relaxation, and energize the body. In massage, the oils can be worked into the skin and, depending on the oil and the massage technique, can either calm or stimulate an individual. When used in compresses, essential oils soothe minor aches and pains, reduce swelling, and treat sprains.

■ Floral waters: These can be sprayed into the air or sprayed on skin that is too sensitive to the touch.

■ Internal application: For certain conditions (such as organ dysfunction), it can be advantageous to take oils internally. It is essential to receive proper medical guidance for internal use of oils.

For information about **aromatherapy oils,** contact: PhytoMedicine Company, 6701 Sunset Drive, Suite 100, Miami, FL 33143; tel: 305-662-6396; fax: 305-667-5619.

CAUTION

In their pure state, certain oils, such as clove and cinnamon, can cause irritation or skin burns. These oils require careful and expert application. It is recommended that they be diluted with a less irritating essential oil before being applied to the skin. Essential oils can cause toxic reactions if ingested. Consult a physician before taking any oils internally.

For information on **nutrients and herbs to support the adrenal glands and reduce stress,** see Chapter 13: Supplements for Arthritis, pp. 280-313.

12 The Arthritis Diet

DIETARY PRACTICES have a major impact on arthritis. In fact, if you eat the typical American diet, it could be making your arthritis worse. Among the offenders are saturated fats (which occur in cooking oils and fried foods), white flour and sugar, red meat, chemical additives, yeast, and milk and dairy products. These foods can increase inflammation, invoke allergies, and interfere with hormone production, cellular integrity, and the function and mobility of the joints.

Changing the way you eat will change the way you feel. The right foods can keep you free of stiff joints, swelling, and fatigue while also promoting longevity and overall health. If you adhere to only one therapy from this book, choose to eat right by eliminating problematic foods and increasing your daily intake of vegetables, fruits, and whole grains. In this chapter, we explain which foods are "arthritis-friendly" and which foods should be avoided. We also look at the different types of dietary fats and their effect on inflammation. Finally, we provide recipes tailored to specific types of arthritis to give you easy—and delicious—ways to incorporate these dietary changes and relieve your arthritis symptoms.

In This Chapter

- The Arthritis Diet
- The Fats Connection to Arthritis
- Success Story: Diet and Detoxification Defeat Gout
- Arthritis Recipes

The Arthritis Diet

What we call the "Arthritis Diet" is primarily a vegetarian, whole foods diet consisting of fruits and vegetables, raw seeds and nuts and their butters, fermented bean products, fish, and grains—all considered "arthritis-friendly" foods. (See

"Friendly and Unfriendly Arthritis Foods," pp. 254-256). These foods are high in dietary fiber, which helps move food and wastes through the digestive tract before they have a chance to form toxic substances. Many degenerative illnesses, including arthritis, are related to a diet low in fiber.

Whole (unprocessed) foods are rich in the nutrients needed to fight destructive free radicals, promote skin and tissue health, repair bones, muscles, and tendons, and promote regularity. In addition, being more nutrient-dense, whole foods are more filling and decrease the likelihood of overeating and subsequent weight gain; losing weight and reducing the stress on weight-bearing joints are crucial steps to recovering from arthritis. Whole foods also put less overall stress on the body, because they are more easily digested and contain fewer toxic substances than processed foods.

Dietary fats are an important consideration for anyone with arthritis. The wrong kind of fats can increase inflammation in joints, while the "good" fats will help keep inflammation in check. As a percentage of calories, most vegetables contain less than 10% fat and most grains contain 16%-20% fat. By comparison, whole milk and cheeses contain 74% fat (even low-fat milk contains 38% fat on a percentage-of-calories basis). Most animal foods contain large quantities of fat, mostly saturated fats, which raise levels of inflammatory compounds in the body and increase arthritic symptoms. Commercially produced, corn-fed meat and dairy products

Changing the way you eat will change the way you feel. The right foods can keep you free of stiff joints, swelling, and fatigue while also promoting longevity and overall health.

For more on **types of fat and their effect on arthritis**, see this chapter, pp. 253-264.

and shellfish are also high in arachidonic acid (SEE QUICK DEFINITION), which is converted by the body into powerful pro-inflammatory compounds. Whole foods, however, are typically high in healthy fats, including the essential fatty acids, which research has proven help decrease inflammation and improve the health of people with rheumatoid arthritis, psoriatic arthritis, and osteoarthritis.

Arthritis sufferers commonly have a high level of acidity (a urine pH—SEE QUICK DEFINITION—that is lower than 6.3), which increases the potential for developing inflammatory conditions. Acidity can be decreased by reducing your intake of acid-forming foods and increasing intake of alkaline-forming foods in the diet. The most acid-forming foods are sugar, alcohol, vinegar, coffee, meat, and dairy

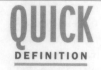

products. Foods known to increase the alkalinity of the body include all vegetables (except tomatoes), aloe vera, and green foods, such as chlorella, barley grass, wheat grass, chlorophyll, parsley, and alfalfa. As a general rule of thumb, the greener the vegetable, the more it will help increase alkalinity in the body.

Tips to Ease the Shift to Healthier Foods

1. Begin by changing one meal a day to healthful eating. This makes shopping and cooking more manageable while you adjust to the new lifestyle. Maintain this for about a month until you tackle the next meal. Within three months, your habits will be transformed.

2. Stop buying snack foods such as sodas, chips, and cookies. Substitute trail mix, popcorn, and herb teas as an interim step.

3. Cook large quantities of main dish recipes so there will be leftovers for lunch or the next day's dinner. Avoid freezing foods as this process may kill important nutrients.

4. Do not insist that children or other family members eat your diet. Simply serve an increasing number of healthful choices with each meal. This, combined with weaning them from sugar and refined flour products, will produce a hunger for good food.

5. When dining at other people's homes, eat lightly, focus on what you can have, and pass up the allergenic foods. Avoid debates about diet. Soon your improved health may prompt a great deal of positive interest in your diet.

6. Choose restaurants where there are healthful choices. Ask if the chef will modify a dish (skip the cream sauce, for example) to make it fit your new diet. If that is not possible, you can eat beforehand at home and just sip a beverage while enjoying the social contact. Be positive, keep the focus off your diet, and, above all, do not be self-righteous.

The Arthritis Diet Daily Menu Plan

General Tips: Avoid simple sugars; eat daily amounts of onions or garlic; five or more servings of fruits and vegetables; 4 oz of blueberries or blackberries; 3 oz of soy products; and drink green tea instead of coffee.[1]

Breakfast: 8 oz of filtered water with freshly squeezed lemon juice.

One piece of fresh fruit such as pineapple, pear, papaya, or apple.

Protein shake: in a blender, mix the recommended amount of protein drink powder (Naturade Vegetable Protein Powder is a good choice and is available in most health food stores), ¼ cup to ½ cup organic or frozen berries, and 1 tbsp flaxseed oil.

Lunch: Green Goodness Salad with Herb Dressing (see recipe below).

One to two medium bowls of steamed vegetables, such as squash (butternut, summer, or spaghetti), kale, collard greens, beets, broccoli, and carrots or one sheet of nori seaweed (available in Asian grocery stores and natural food stores) filled with sliced avocado, shredded carrots, diced cucumbers, and sprouts, drizzled with herb dressing (see recipe below).

If you are not pursuing a detoxification program, you may eat a small portion of free-range chicken, beef, or game. Buffalo, ostrich, venison, and emu are meats particularly high in omega-3 essential fatty acids.

Snack: Fresh fruit or vegetables and nuts and seeds, such as almonds or sesame seeds. Soak seeds in filtered water to increase protein content and ease digestion.

Dinner: One or more of the main dish recipes (see below) for your type of arthritis.

Acid-Forming Foods

Alcohol, cocoa, coffee, and caffeinated teas; vinegar; meat and other animal proteins; sugar and all products that contain sugar; some fruit (especially cranberry, plums and prunes); many fats and oils; some nuts and seeds (cashew, peanut, pecan, filbert, and Brazil nut); cheese; white flour and baked products, pasta, wheat, corn, and oats; and many beans and legumes.

Alkaline-Forming Foods

Fresh vegetables except tomatoes; avocados and most fruit; some nuts and seeds (particularly almond, chestnut, coconut, flax, pumpkin, sesame, and sunflower seeds); herbal teas (dandelion, ginseng); and soy products.

The Fats Connection to Arthritis

The kinds of fats that make up your diet directly affect the severity of inflammation and other arthritic symptoms. There are "good" and "bad" dietary fats, and if your diet contains too many of the bad fats, it may be making your arthritis worse or helping to create it in the first

Friendly and Unfriendly Arthritis Foods

Nuts and Seeds

Include
Limited amounts of natural raw nuts, particularly walnuts, almonds, and pecans; raw nut butters; seeds such as chia, sesame, pumpkin, and flax.

Avoid
Roasted or salted nuts and seeds; nuts with a high omega-6 oil content, such as cashews, brazil, pine nuts, and peanuts.

Oils

Include
Expeller-pressed, unsaturated oils such as flaxseed, sesame, walnut, soy, and soy lecithin spread, cod liver, and hempseed. These oils should never be heated.

Avoid
Butter, oils containing hydrogenated fats, trans-fatty acids, or saturated oils such as shortening, margarine, and cottonseed.

Fish

Include
Cold-water fish (trout, cod, salmon, halibut, bluefish, sardine, and smelts). Wild fish are better than farm raised.

Avoid
All shell fish.

Vegetables

Include
Raw or steamed organic vegetables such as artichokes, asparagus, beets and beet greens, broccoli, Brussels sprouts, cabbage, carrots, celery, chives, corn, cucumbers, endive, green and wax beans, green peas, kale, lima beans, lentils, onions, yams, watercress, lettuce, arugula, radish, parsley, cilantro.

Sprouts such as mung, lentil, alfalfa, radish, soy, and wheat grass.

Wild greens such as burdock, dandelion leaves, chickweed, yellowdock root, wild allums, purslane, lambs quarter, pigweed, and sorrel.

Avoid
Nightshade vegetables including eggplant, bell peppers, potatoes, and tomatoes.

Spices and Seasonings

Include

Chives, garlic, parsley, laurel, marjoram, sage, thyme, savory, kelp, and other vegetable or herb seasonings; Bragg's Liquid Aminos, Celtic Sea Salt; lemon juice and silken tofu salad dressings (if not allergic).

Avoid

Pepper and refined table salt; products that contain yeast such as soy and tamari sauce; vinegar, mustard, or mayonnaise; chemical additives such as monosodium glutamate (MSG).

Grains ✓

Include

Organic breads (yeast-, gluten-, and preservative-free) made of whole grains including millet, quinoa, rye, or buckwheat.

Rice made of millet, wild or brown rice; egg-free noodles and macaroni made from buckwheat, rice, quinoa, soy, or vegetable flours.

Cereals made from millet, oatmeal, brown and wild rice, buckwheat groats, barley, quinoa, amaranth, and teff.

Avoid

Bleached grain products such as white bread and rice, blended breads, processed cereals that are puffed or flaked.

Fruits ✓

Include

Fresh organic fruits such as apples, apricots, berries, cherries, currants, guavas, grapefruit, lemon, mangos, melons, nectarines, oranges, papaya, peaches, pineapple, pears, plums, persimmons, tangerines; use citrus fruits sparingly.

Avoid

All dried fruits.

Meat ✓

Include

Small amounts of wild game, free-range beef, organic chicken, except when undergoing a supervised fast or detoxification program.

Avoid

Non-organic meat products.

Friendly and Unfriendly Arthritis Foods (*cont.*)

Beverages

Include

Filtered water, using certified water filter.

Herb teas containing mint, spearmint, licorice root, eucalyptus, dandelion leaves and roots, red clover, pero, roma, caffix, postum, or ginger.

Fresh, unsweetened juices of organic lemon, orange pear, pineapple, prune, beets, carrots, cucumber, celery, garlic, onion, radish, red cabbage, and turnip; dilute all juices by 75% with filtered water. If you have candidiasis, avoid all fruit juices and other foods containing naturally occurring sugars.

Milk substitutes such as soy, almond or tahini milk. Use nut milk sparingly and dilute with water.

Avoid

Alcohol, cocoa, coffee (regular and decaffeinated), all dairy products, soft drinks, all juice concentrates, canned or frozen apple, orange, berry, cherry, grape, and grapefruit juices.

Eggs and Cheese

Include

Soy, rice, or almond cheese.

Avoid

All dairy, goat, or sheep cheeses, and eggs.

Desserts and Sweeteners

Include

Desserts containing fresh fruits, natural fruit gelatin, or whole tapioca sweetened with moderate amounts of sorghum, raw honey, maple syrup, or stevia (a natural sugar alternative).

Avoid

Foods containing white sugar, yeast, bleached flour, dairy products; canned fruits, ice cream, custards, and candy. Avoid all sugar, except fresh fruit and stevia, if you have tested positive for *Candida* or *Klebsiella* or have hypoglycemic diabetes.

place (see "A Quick Guide to Fats," pp. 258–259). The inflammatory process can become uncontrollable when certain dietary factors skew the delicate balance of inflammation-mediating substances. Prostaglandins, complex fatty acids that can either cause or decrease inflammation, are composed of different fatty acids. The type of prostaglandins (anti- or pro-inflammatory) manufactured by the body depend upon the fats in your diet, as well as the presence of certain nutrients (vitamins C, B3, and B6, magnesium, and zinc).

Prostaglandins that cause inflammation are formed when the diet is high in animal fats, which contain high amounts of arachidonic acid. Arachidonic acid is a long-chain polyunsaturated omega-6 fatty acid, found primarily in animal foods such as meat, poultry, and dairy products. When the diet is abundant in arachidonic acids, they are stored in cell membranes. An enzyme transforms these stored acids into prostaglandins and leukotrienes that instigate inflammation. If there is an overabundance of arachidonic acid or "bad" fats, more pro-inflammatory agents will be produced by the body.

Merely eliminating the inappropriate fats from the diet can produce immediate benefits for arthritis sufferers. Doctors at the Karolinksa Institute in Stockholm, Sweden, found that when 14 rheumatoid arthritis patients fasted for seven days, their joint pain and inflammation decreased. The researchers explained that the cessation of fat intake reduced leukotriene formation and favorably altered fatty-acid composition, thereby reducing inflammation.[2] Researchers at the National Hospital in Oslo, Norway, reported that both fasting and long-term vegetarian diets can reduce arthritic symptoms. "Dietary treatment can reduce the disease activity in some patients with rheumatoid arthritis," they concluded.[3]

Increase Your Intake of the "Good" Fats

Essential fatty acids (EFAs), which are derived only from the diet and not manufactured in the body, help control inflammation and maintain the integrity of cell membranes. EFAs are the building-blocks of prostaglandins, hormone-like substances that either encourage inflammation (prostaglandins of the 2 and 4 series) or discourage inflammation (prostaglandins of the 1 and 3 series). In healthy individuals, the body maintains these prostaglandins in a strict ratio to ensure adequate immune function and to limit inflammatory responses.

The two principle types of essential fatty acids are omega-3 and omega-6. Deficiencies in EFAs, particularly the omega-3s, are quite

A Quick Guide to Fats

Fat or oil (lipid is the biochemical term) is one of the six basic food groups. Fats and oils are made of building-blocks called fatty acids. Structurally, a fatty acid is a chain of carbon atoms with a certain quantity of hydrogen atoms attached. The more hydrogen atoms attached to the carbon atoms, the more "saturated" the fat. Fats come in three natural forms (saturated, monounsaturated, and polyunsaturated) and one man-made form (called hydrogenated or trans fats).

Saturated Fats—A fatty acid that has its full quota of hydrogen atoms is a saturated fatty acid. Saturated fats are solid at room temperature and are primarily found in animal foods and tropical oils such as coconut and palm oil. The body produces saturated fats from sugar. That's one reason why 'low fat' foods do not decrease body fat—their high sugar content is converted into stored fat in the body. Although high fat intake from animal sources has been associated with heart disease, some amount of saturated fat in the diet is necessary to help the body's cells remain healthy and resistant to disease.

Unsaturated Fats—These tend to be liquid at room temperature. Most vegetable oils (coconut and palm oil are exceptions) are unsaturated. Unsaturated means some of the carbon molecules are not filled with hydrogen.

■ Monounsaturated Fats: When a fatty acid lacks only two hydrogen atoms, it is a monounsaturated fatty acid. Monounsaturated fats are consid-

ered healthier than polyunsaturated fats because of their ability to lower blood levels of "bad" cholesterol and maintain or raise levels of "good" cholesterol. Canola oil and olive oil are naturally high in monounsaturated fats. Olive oil is the best oil for cooking, because it does not break down easily into singlet oxygen molecules (free radicals) like most fats and oils do when they are heated. Olive oil is probably the most widely used oil, both for cooking and raw on salads, on a worldwide basis.

■ Polyunsaturated Fats: A fatty acid lacking four or more hydrogen atoms is a polyunsaturated fatty acid. They can be found in both healthy and unhealthy fats and oils. Oils high in polyunsaturated fats include flaxseed and canola oils, as well as pumpkin seeds, purslane, hemp oil, walnuts, and soybeans, which contain omega-3 and omega-6 essential fatty acids.

Hydrogenated and Trans Fats—These terms refer to a synthetic process in which natural oils are broken down into a semi-solid fat by adding a hydrogen atom to an unsaturated fat molecule. This process is widely used to prolong the shelf-life of commercial baked goods, packaged foods, most salad oils and dressings, margarines, and cooking oils such as corn and safflower. The molecules that make up these fats, called trans-fatty acids, are known to interfere with the healthy functioning of our bodies due to their unusual molecular shape.

Essential Fatty Acids (EFAs)—Unsaturated fats required in the diet are called essential fatty acids.

Omega-3 and omega-6 oils are the two principle types of essential fatty acids. A balance of these oils in the diet is necessary for good health. Fish oils, such as salmon, cod, trout, and mackerel, are rich in omega-3 oils. Linoleic acid, the main omega-6 oil, is found in vegetable oils, including safflower, corn, peanut, sunflower, soybean, and sesame. In arthritis and other inflammatory conditions, the most important concern is to increase the intake of omega-3 oils and to decrease the intake of "bad" oils. Once in the body, omega-3 and omega-6 are converted to prostaglandins, hormone-like, complex fatty acids that affect smooth muscle function, inflammatory processes, and constriction and dilation of blood vessels.

common in America because of modern food-processing techniques. Humans evolved on a diet that contained small but roughly equal amounts of omega-3s and omega-6s. When the food supply began to change about one hundred years ago to more processed foods, the amount of omega-3 in many commercial products declined. At the same time, the domestic livestock industry began to use feed grain, which happens to be rich in omega-6 fatty acids and low in omega-3s. Because of these changes, the American diet now has 20 to 25 times more omega-6s than omega-3s, rather than the ideal 1:2 ratio. When there is a deficiency of EFAs in the body, anti-inflammatory prostaglandins (1 and 3 series) tend to decline and individuals tend to develop food sensitivities (allergies) as well as increased inflammation, which can lead to joint destruction and other symptoms of arthritis.

For the arthritis sufferer, it is advisable to avoid foods high in omega-6 fatty acids (such as most vegetable oils, including safflower, corn, peanut, and sesame) because they are converted by enzymes in the body into pro-inflammatory prostaglandins as well as arachidonic acid and leukotrienes (which both cause inflammation). Instead, boost your dietary intake of omega-3 fatty acids (which are anti-inflammatory) by eating more green, leafy vegetables; hemp seed, soy, and walnut oils; pumpkin seeds, sesame seeds, walnuts, and almonds; and the wild plants chia, cattail, and purslane.

The primary omega-3 fatty acid is alpha-linolenic acid (ALA), which is abundant in flaxseed oil. Three tablespoons of unheated flaxseed oil can be put on salads, steamed vegetables, or other foods. Purchase oils that are "expeller-pressed," not just "cold-pressed." Check the expiration date and adhere to it; flaxseed oil can rapidly turn rancid and should be stored in the refrigerator. Organic, whole flaxseeds can also be used to add a nutty flavor to cereals, vegetables, or casseroles; place a few tablespoons in a coffee grinder to release the

Assess Your Fatty-Acid Intake

The first step in looking at dietary fats is to assess your intake of essential fatty acids. We generally rely on two approaches. First, we have the patient complete a "diet diary," detailing their typical food choices over a 1-2 week period, enabling us to evaluate the levels of good and bad fats they are receiving through their regular diet. We then perform a darkfield microscopic analysis of their blood, which will show physiological changes of a poor diet. For example, through darkfield examination, poor red blood cell membrane formation reflects a fatty-acid deficiency, usually of omega-3s.

Second, we may use the Red Blood Cell Membrane Fatty Acid Analysis. This test, developed at the Johns Hopkins Kennedy-Krieger Institute, in Baltimore, Maryland, determines the composition of the fatty acids in the patient's body, which can be used to structure their diet to increase levels of deficient fatty acids and decrease levels of detrimental ones. Usually, it takes six months of supplementation—a bolstered nutrient regimen—before we see a change in the fatty acid composition of a patient's cell membranes. Then there is commonly a remarkable correlation between a change in fatty-acid status—an increase in anti-inflammatories—and the abatement of the joint pain and swelling associated with arthritis.

For information about **Red Blood Cell Membrane Fatty Acid Analysis**, contact: MetaMetrix Medical Laboratory, 5000 Peachtree Industrial Blvd., Suite 110, Norcross, GA 30071; tel: 800-221-4640 or 770-446-5483; fax: 770-441-2237. Body Bio Centre, Five Osprey Drive, Suite 9, Millville, NJ 08332; tel: 888-320-8338 or 609-825-8338; fax: 609-825-2143.

seeds' oils. Purslane (*Portulaca oleracea*), often considered a weed, is actually a nutritious vegetable high in omega-3 fatty acids. Less than one cup supplies a full day's supply of ALA. Purslane also contains vitamin E, a potent antioxidant that is necessary for the formation of the anti-inflammatory prostaglandins, as well as vitamins A and C.

Other types of omega-3 fatty acids include eicosapentaenoic acid (EPA) and docosahexaenoic acid (DHA), which are chemically closer to becoming prostaglandins than ALA. Food sources high in EPA/DHA include salmon, bluefish, bass, trout, organ meats, and brown and red algae. High cooking temperatures can destroy the EFA content in certain foods and oils, so baking or grilling fish is a preferable cooking method to frying. For arthritis, we recommend supplementing with all three forms of omega-3s (ALA, EPA, and DHA).

Fish Consumption Can Benefit Arthritis, But Be Cautious—Increased use of fish, both as a whole food and as fish oil supplements, is a sound beginning in reversing arthritis. Research shows that fish oils can

Finding Healthy Oils

All vegetable oils contain levels of unsaturated and saturated fats. Generally, those with a higher percentage of unsaturated fats and a lower percentage of saturated fats are more healthful.[4]

Oil	Monounsaturated	Polyunsaturated	Saturated
Olive	72%	9%	14%
Flax	72%	19%	9%
Pumpkin seed	57%	34%	9%
Hempseed	80%	12%	8%
Safflower	12%	75%	9%
Canola	62%	32%	6%
Peanut	48%	32%	17%
Corn	24%	59%	13%
Soybean	23%	59%	14%
Sunflower	20%	66%	10%
Sesame seed	40%	40%	18%

block the activity of arachidonic acid, which otherwise produces inflammation. Rheumatologists at the Royal Adelaide Hospital in South Australia found that rheumatoid arthritis patients who took fish oil supplements (18 g daily) for 12 weeks had a 30% reduction in leukotrienes (pro-inflammatory agents).[5] In another study, 49 rheumatoid arthritis patients took either fish oil (DHA) or olive oil in varying dosages for 24 weeks. Both fish and olive oils reduced the number of tender and swollen joints; a high dose of fish oil proved most effective.[6]

But while fish, especially salmon and other cold-water fatty fish, have high levels of beneficial EFAs, there are a few problems associated with eating fish. Increasingly, the salmon reaching the North American market are farm-raised rather than caught from rivers and streams. Commercially produced or "farmed" fish have a less desirable fatty-acid profile than wild fish; specifically, researchers have found that farmed fish are lower in omega-3s.[7] Seafood and fish products are becoming increasingly less healthy. According to research conducted by Vincent Buyck, Ph.D., of the College of Complementary Medicine and Sciences, in Washington, D.C., as water temperatures rise, some microorganisms mutate into forms that can cause disease. When these microorganisms are ingested by seafood or fish, and subsequently by humans, they present a threat to human health.[8]

Eating fish that is boiled or baked is preferable to eating it fried. Foods that are fried have a high level of polychlorinated phenols, a toxic by-product caused by heating oils to frying temperatures. These phenols increase inflammation and worsen arthritis symptoms.[9]

Dietary Recommendations—The following recommendations can help you increase the level of "good" fats in your diet:

- Eat foods rich in the three types of omega-3 fatty acids: alpha-linolenic acid (ALA)—the oils flaxseed (58%), chia seed (30%), poppy seed (15%), pumpkin seed (15%), canola (7%), walnut (5%), and soy (9%), purslane and cattail, and dark green leafy vegetables (50%);[10] eicosapentaenoic acid (EPA)—cold-water fish, salmon, mackerel, halibut, and Chinese snake oil; docosahexaenoic acid (DHA)—cold-water fish and Neuromins™, a commercial supplement containing vegetable sources of DHA.

For information about **Neuromins™**, contact: Martek Biosciences, 6480 Dobbin Road, Columbia, MD 21045; tel: 888-880-2229 or 410-740-0081; fax: 410-740-2985; website: www.martekbio.com.

- Obtain an adequate supply of niacin, vitamins B6 and E, zinc, and magnesium to enhance fatty-acid metabolism. Beans, especially lima, soy, great northern, kidney, and navy, poultry, and fish contain these important nutrients as well as omega-3 fatty acids. Be sure to check for food allergies first.

- Reduce carbohydrate intake and avoid all refined sugars, processed foods, margarine, hydrogenated oils, and gluten-containing foods such as wheat, oats, and barley.

- For better mineral density, increase consumption of raw nuts and seeds, seaweeds, fish, tempeh, tofu, and legumes.

- Incorporate certain spices and herbs into the diet, such as fresh mint leaves, thyme oil, and ginger; these foods contain substances that will help stabilize fats in the cell membranes.

- Avoid all fats and oils containing very-long-chain fatty acids, such as mustard, peanut butter, peanut oil, and canola oil.

Avoid the "Bad" Fats

Hydrogenated fats and trans-fatty acids can directly contribute to inflammation and the destruction of joint tissues. We recommend avoiding foods that contain these fats, which are, unfortunately, a common ingredient in most refined foods. Read the labels of packaged foods before you buy to determine if they contain hydrogenated fats. In the list of ingredients, you will see them described as either "hydrogenated" or "partially hydrogenated" oils. The "Nutrition Facts" label will also provide you with amounts of saturated and unsaturated fats.

The membrane of every cell is a thin envelope of fats that encases and protects the internal biochemical components. Within this fatty envelope are thousands of proteins that facilitate communication and transport—acting like a gate—across the cell membrane. The ability of the cell wall to change shape, so that life sustaining nutrients can be absorbed and wastes expelled, is dependent upon fatty acids.[11] Normal fatty acids have a "rounded" shape and help to form a strong yet flexible membrane surface. But trans-fatty acids have a "straight" shape that forms a weak, brittle cell wall that cannot efficiently transport nutrients and wastes. A weak cell wall can break or become distorted, leaving it vulnerable to attack by free radicals and other processes that break down cell membranes, which leads to cell destruction.[12] When this process of cell destruction occurs in joint tissues, it causes pain, inflammation, and the degenerative process leading to arthritis.

> ## Common Foods That May Contain "Bad" Fats
>
> - Margarine
> - Diet foods
> - Mayonnaise
> - Crackers and chips
> - Cookies, cakes and cake mixes, pastries, and doughnuts
> - Candy
> - Packaged breads
> - Canned, creamed soups and gravy
> - Breakfast cereals and frozen waffles
> - Microwave popcorn
> - Frozen entrees, French fries, fish sticks, and chicken nuggets

It is estimated that as a nation we consume over 600 million pounds of trans-fatty acids a year, mostly in the form of frying fats and margarine. Studies have connected an abnormal fatty-acid pattern with the beginning of arthritic symptoms. Researchers at the University of Verona in Italy studied the fatty-acid composition of 25 patients with psoriatic arthritis and found "significant direct correlations" between levels of fatty acids, specific red blood cell factors, incidence of morning stiffness, and the duration of illness.[13]

Arthritis and Olestra™, The "Fake" Fat—The new "fake" fats, Olestra being the most well-known, pass through the digestive tract without being absorbed. When Olestra is in the digestive tract, it mixes with

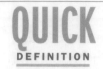
and absorbs fat-soluble vitamins (A, D, E, and K), carotenoids (coenzyme Q10, lycopene, and lutein) and other essential nutrients and antioxidants. These are nutrients in which arthritis sufferers tend to be deficient.[14] Olestra, along with these absorbed nutrients, pass right through the digestive tract and are eventually excreted from the system. As a result, fake fats appear to be potentially detrimental to those with arthritis.

Success Story: Diet and Detoxification Defeat Gout

Ramsey, 56, came to us complaining of fatigue, fever, and severe pain in the big toe of his left foot. The pain in his toe had begun suddenly and without warning two days earlier. A blood test revealed high levels of uric acid (a waste product of the urine cycle) and a darkfield (SEE QUICK DEFINITION) microscopic examination of his blood showed elevated numbers of sharp crystalline structures and his white blood cells were overactive (indicative of an inflammatory response). Ramsey was diagnosed with an acute attack of gout.

Ramsey had just returned from a two-week vacation. During his trip, he had indulged in rich foods, including large quantities of steaks and other meats, rich desserts, and alcoholic beverages. We often see attacks of gout preceded by a dietary change such as Ramsey's vacation indulgences. The body, overwhelmed by these rich and strange foods, is unable to process the uric acid as it normally would. Sodium urate crystals then build up in the joints or skin leading to inflammation.

We immediately recommended dietary changes for Ramsey, both to reduce his exposure to foods that would aggravate his gout and to help his body detoxify. He was to avoid meats, alcohol, coffee, sugar, bread, and wheat. We recommended a soup made from the following organic ingredients: cabbage, onion, garlic, carrots, zucchini (yellow and green), Jerusalem artichokes, and kale. To this, he was to add Bragg's Liquid Aminos, an amino acid supplement to provide a source of protein. Ramsey could eat as much of this soup as he wanted. However, he was to have no other solid food.

We also recommended black cherry juice, which is specifically helpful for gout due to its high bioflavonoid content and its ability to block the enzyme xanthine oxidase (which increases uric acid in the body). Ramsey was to drink six to eight 4-ounce glasses throughout the day. He was also to drink a vegetable juice made from carrots, ½ beet, a two-inch ginger slice, cucumber, zucchini, and one tablespoon of turmeric powder; two to three 8-ounce glasses daily. In addition, we recommended a detoxification tea made from burdock, dandelion, prickly ash, milk thistle, yellow dock, and red clover (½ teaspoon of each brewed in 48 ounces of water); six 8-ounce cups of tea (hot or cold) per day.

Ramsey was to stay on this mostly liquid diet for five days. We also recommended folic acid (10 mg daily) and quercetin (300 mg, three times daily), both of which help control the buildup of uric acid, along with homeopathic remedies for liver and kidney support during the detoxification process. Another support therapy we included was hydrotherapy—Ramsey soaked his foot in warm, salted water two to three times per day. Ramsey also prepared an herbal poultice containing a mixture of one white potato (grated), one teaspoon of turmeric powder, and ½ cucumber (grated). He covered his toe with this mixture and wrapped it in gauze (changing the dressing 2-3 times per day).

After three days on this protocol, Ramsey called to say that his toe was completely better and, in addition, he felt more energetic and clear-headed. When we re-tested his blood after one week, his uric acid levels had returned to normal. As an extra benefit from the cleansing diet, Ramsey's cholesterol levels had dropped and he'd also lost five pounds.

Arthritis Recipes

The recipes below are divided into two major categories, recipes most appropriate for rheumatoid arthritis and those for osteoarthritis, but these recipes can be used by anyone regardless of arthritis type. They are also quite healthy, whether or not you have arthritis. We suggest that you keep a food diary, recording what you eat each day and any changes in your arthritis symptoms (including joint stiffness, swelling, tenderness, and fatigue). If symptoms worsen, use your food diary to locate potential problem foods; experiment the next day with those particular foods to identify the triggering agent, then eliminate it from your diet. A food diary can thus help you determine which foods are most beneficial for reducing your arthritis symptoms.

Chef Harris offers personal and phone consultations on diet. For **Chef Elleth Amenl Harris**, contact: Nature's Feast Catering, 37 Geraldine Circle, Trumbull, CT 06611; tel: 203-261-6256. For a **mail-order source of organic foods**, contact: Walnut Acres Organic Farms, Walnut Acres Road, Penns Creek, PA 17862; tel: 800-433-3998 or 570-837-0601.

In general, the recipes in this chapter eliminate foods that aggravate or escalate arthritis symptoms, particularly the common culprits such as eggs, dairy, wheat, or fried foods. Our chef, Elieth Ameni Harris, has developed and written these recipes specifically for arthritis sufferers so that they can begin to eat healthfully without sacrificing flavor. Most ingredients are available in local supermarkets, health food stores, or farmers markets. All produce should be purchased just prior to use to ensure freshness and should be organic and non-irradiated. If certain vegetables or herbs are difficult to find in your area, consider planting a small outdoor garden and raising your own.

Rheumatoid Arthritis Recipes

Main Dishes

Island Pumpkin Soup with Herb Dumplings

4 cups steamed pumpkin, butternut, or buttercup squash
8 cups vegetable stock
2 cups tofu cream (1 cup silken tofu and 1 cup soy milk; puree in food processor 3-4 minutes)
1 cup onion, chopped
²/₃ cup chopped celery
½ cup leeks, sliced thin
3 tbsp vegetable oil
1 tsp cumin powder
½ tsp nutmeg
1 cinnamon stick
2 tbsp parsley, chopped
4 cloves garlic, minced
1½ tsp sea salt
½ cup Bragg's Liquid Aminos (contains soy)
4 tbsp unbleached (non-wheat) flour slurried in ½ cup water

In a large soup pot, sauté onions, celery, and leeks in the vegetable oil over medium heat for seven minutes. Add vegetable stock, squash, and cinnamon stick; simmer for 15 minutes. Next, add the tofu cream and whisk together with a hand whisk. Season with cumin, nutmeg, garlic, and parsley, while continuing to cook for an additional ten minutes. Meanwhile, make herb dumplings and add teaspoonfuls of the dumpling mixture to the simmering soup. Cook for an additional ten minutes before serving.

Herb Dumplings for Soup—
2½ cups spelt flour
½ tsp baking powder
1 tbsp extra virgin olive oil
1 cup soy milk
¼ cup Irish moss solution*
1 tsp lite gray Celtic sea salt (sea salt may be substituted)
2 tbsp chopped chives
2 tsp fresh thyme, chopped
In a medium-sized mixing bowl, combine the baking powder and unbleached spelt flour. Then add the remaining ingredients and mix until homogenous. Make teaspoon-size dumplings for the soup.

*Irish moss solution: Dissolve Irish moss (available at health food stores) in cold water. Simmer over stove, then fold into dry ingredients. Irish moss acts like egg whites in its ability to bind ingredients together.

Hearty Vegetable Stew with Millet Pilaf
The Stew—
2 cups chopped Swiss chard
1½ cups cubed turnip
1½ cups cubed carrot
2½ cups cubed butternut squash
1 cup chopped celery
1 cup chopped onion
½ cup chopped parsley
1½ cups cooked chickpeas
½ cup frozen peas
8 cups vegetable stock
2 bay leaves
1½ tsp cumin
1½ tsp turmeric
⅓ cup Bragg's Liquid Aminos
2 tbsp arrowroot
Salt and pepper to taste
In a large pot, add vegetable stock, carrot, turnips, and bay leaves; cover and cook over medium heat for ten minutes. Add celery, onions, and parsley and simmer for an additional ten minutes. Next, add chickpeas, peas, and chard; cook for five more minutes before seasoning with cumin, turmeric, and Bragg's. Allow stew to simmer for two to three minutes before thickening with the arrowroot (dissolve in ¼ cup cold water). Add salt and pepper to taste.

The Pilaf—
2 cups millet
3 tbsp saffron or sunflower oil
5 cups vegetable stock
½ cup diced carrots
1 cup cauliflower florets
1 cup diced celery
½ cup minced purple onions
¼ cup fresh parsley
1 tsp dried marjoram
1 tsp dried oregano
2 tbsp tamari
Garnish—
½ cup blanched green peas (to blanch, cook for five minutes in boiling water)
½ cup slivered almonds
Toast millet in 1 tbsp vegetable oil over medium heat in heavy pot for 5-7 minutes. Add vegetable stock and a pinch of sea salt. Boil and then simmer for 20-25 minutes. Meanwhile sauté all vegetables in remaining oil for 3-5 minutes. Set aside.

Marinated Tofu (Optional)—
4 tbsp oil
2 tsp lemon juice
1 tbsp honey
¼ cup mirin (unsweetened rice syrup)
½ tsp fresh thyme
2 cloves garlic
1 lb tofu cut into ¼" cubes
Blend first six ingredients. Pour over tofu and let stand at least one hour. Drain marinade and bake tofu at 375° F for 30-35 minutes. Combine millet, vegetables, and tofu (if desired). Garnish with peas and almonds.

Poached Salmon in Creamy Asparagus Sauce
1 lb salmon steak (two steaks)
¾ cup sliced purple onion, sliced ¼" thick
1 cup vegetable bouillon stock
2 tbsp chopped parsley
½ tsp freshly ground black pepper
½ tsp sea salt
1-3" fresh stem of thyme
1 cup chopped asparagus

In a 9" x 12" baking dish, place onion rings on the bottom of dish. Season fish with salt and pepper and place each steak on the bed of onions. Add the stem of thyme, parsley, and vegetable bouillon; sprinkle the asparagus on top of the vegetables and fish steaks. Cover the baking dish and poach in a preheated 375° F oven for 20 minutes. Reserve the steamed asparagus for the creamy asparagus sauce.

Creamy Asparagus Sauce—
1 cup chopped and steamed asparagus
¾ cup creamy soy milk
¾ cup fish and vegetable bouillon stock
2 tbsp mirin (unsweetened rice syrup)
1 tbsp white miso and 3 tbsp water
2 tbsp vegetable oil
2 tbsp oat or barley flour
1 tbsp shallot, minced
¼ tsp celery seeds
¼ tsp white pepper
½ tsp sea salt

In a large saucepan, add the oil and flour while stirring over medium heat for two minutes. Next, add creamy soy milk and fish stock; simmer for eight minutes while stirring. Season sauce with shallot, celery seeds, white pepper, and salt. Cook for an additional five minutes. Remove sauce from heat and stir in mirin and miso paste. Put the chopped asparagus and the creamy sauce into a food processor; puree until smooth. Serve the sauce warm with poached salmon.

Salads

Green Goodness Salad with Herb Dressing
1 bunch romaine lettuce, broken into pieces
1 bunch arugula, chopped
2 bunches watercress, leaves only
1 bunch Swiss chard or spinach
1 medium endive, diced
1 bunch scallion, chopped
4 sheets toasted nori seaweed, cut into strips
½ cup roasted pumpkin seeds
1 pack sunflower sprouts

In a large salad bowl, combine all of the ingredients, except nori and roasted pumpkin seeds. Mix well and set aside. Serve salad with herb dressing; sprinkle seeds and nori strips on top.

Herb Dressing—
½ cup extra virgin olive oil, flaxseed oil, or hemp seed oil
¼ cup lemon juice (may use vinegar if not allergic to yeast)
1 tbsp prepared mustard
1 tsp dried tarragon
2 tsp chopped fresh chives
¼ cup Bragg's Liquid Aminos
Combine all ingredients in a blender except the chives. Stir in chives afterwards.

Quinoa–Black Bean Festival Salad with Cilantro–Lime Vinaigrette
3 cups cooked quinoa
1½ cups cooked black beans
½ cup dried cranberries
1 cup yellow squash, chopped medium size
1 cup zucchini, chopped medium size
1 bunch scallion, chopped
¼ cup finely chopped parsley
Add all of the ingredients into a large mixing bowl and mix well.
Cilantro-Lime Vinaigrette—
Juice of 2 large limes
⅓ cup water
¼ cup Bragg's Liquid Aminos
¼ cup extra virgin olive oil
2 tbsp honey
1 clove garlic, minced
2 tbsp fresh cilantro, chopped
Salt and pepper to taste
In a blender, add all the vinaigrette ingredients and blend for three minutes until homogenous. Drizzle over quinoa–black bean mixture, stir well, and chill before serving.

Exotic Tropical Fruit Salad with Citrus Sauce
Consult with your physician if you have a *Candida* (yeast) or *Klebsiella* infection to determine if this is a good recipe for you.
2 large mangoes, peeled and cubed (1" cubes)
1 large papaya, peeled, seeded, and cubed
3 kiwis, peeled and cut into slices (¼" thick)
1 pint of strawberries, hulled and cut in half
1 star fruit (large), cut into ¼" slices (pineapple may be substituted)
Put all fruit into a large mixing bowl and mix gently until

homogenous. Pour citrus sauce over salad, mix again before chilling in a refrigerator.

Citrus Sauce—
Juice of 2 large oranges (approx. 1 cup)
2 tbsp lemon juice
1 tbsp honey
½ tsp grated nutmeg
In a small mixing bowl, blend all the above ingredients with a hand whisk and serve with fruit salad. Garnish with fresh mint leaves.

Beverages

Inflam-Aid Drink
½ cup fresh black cherry juice (avoid if you have *Candida*)
1 cup fresh organic pineapple juice
1-2 tbsp fresh ginger juice
½ cup spring water
1 cup crushed ice
Combine all ingredients in a blender until well mixed. Yield: two servings. For smoothie, add silken tofu (½ cup) and puree all ingredients in blender for three minutes until smooth.

Dessert

Apple Spice Cake with Cranberry Kanten Glaze
Dry Mixture—
2 cups barley flour or spelt
½ tsp sea salt
1 tsp baking soda
1½ tsp baking powder
1 tsp cinnamon powder
½ tsp allspice
Wet Mixture—
½ cup soy milk
½ cup oil
1 tsp vanilla
1 cup apple juice
1 tsp stevia (a natural concentrated sweetener)
¼ cup honey or maple syrup (decrease amount if you have *Candida*)
2 cups apples, cut into ¼" pieces
¾ cup walnuts

Add the combined dry mixture to the wet mixture. Stir until homogenous. Pour into a lightly oiled 9" cake pan and bake in a preheated oven at 375° F for 30 minutes.

Cranberry Kanten Glaze—
1½ cups cranberries
1½ cups apple juice
1 tbsp and 2 tsp agar-agar
1 tbsp and 2 tsp arrowroot or cornstarch

In a medium sauce pan, add arrowroot and cold apple juice; then simmer. Add agar flakes and cook on medium heat for five minutes. Finally, add cranberries and simmer without stirring for two minutes. Cool to room temperature and spread evenly over cake.

Osteoarthritis Recipes

Main Dishes

Black Bean–Textured Vegetable Protein Soup
4 cups cooked black beans
2 cups TVP (Texturized Soy Vegetable Protein)
12 cups vegetable stock
2 cups chopped green cabbage
1½ cups diced carrots
1½ cups chopped celery
1 large onion, chopped
¼ cup Bragg's Liquid Aminos
4 tbsp miso paste
2 bay leaves (large)
½ tsp cumin powder
4 tbsp chopped parsley
2 tbsp arrowroot powder and ¼ cup cold water
4 cloves garlic, minced
Sea salt and black pepper to taste

In a large soup pot, combine stock, beans, TVP, all vegetables, and bay leaves. Bring to boil at medium high heat, then reduce heat to a simmer and cook for 20 minutes. Meanwhile, slurry miso in about one cup of the vegetable stock (removed from soup pot). Next, add miso solution, parsley, cumin powder, and garlic. Continue cooking for an additional 5-7 minutes, stirring occasionally. Dissolve arrowroot powder in water, then pour the mixture into soup pot while mixing. Allow to simmer for five minutes before seasoning with Bragg's and salt.

Rice, Lentil, and Vegetable Salad

2 cups cooked long-grain brown rice
1 cup cooked lentils (do not overcook)
½ cup finely chopped purple cabbage
½ cup diced carrots
½ cup diced zucchini or cucumber
¼ cup chopped parsley
¼ cup chopped scallion
2 tbsp Bragg's Liquid Aminos
6 tbsp extra virgin olive oil
2 tbsp lemon juice
½ tsp marjoram (dried)
¼ tsp oregano (dried)
Add sea salt and freshly ground black pepper to taste
1 tbsp honey (optional)

In a large bowl, combine the first seven ingredients and mix well. Set the bowl aside, then in a smaller bowl, whisk together the Bragg's, oil, lemon juice, honey, and herbs. Drizzle the dressing over the rice, lentil, and vegetable mixture while stirring. Chill in the refrigerator for at least one hour. Yield: 3-4 servings.

Stuffed Green and Purple Cabbage with Shiitake Mushroom–Red Onion Sauce

1 large green cabbage, cored and steamed 20 minutes
1 large purple cabbage, cored and steamed 20 minutes
4 cups cooked wild and long-grain brown rice blend (¼ cup wild, ¾ cup brown rice)
2 cups chickpeas, cooked and mashed
1 cup diced carrots
1 cup steamed peas
½ cup minced shallots
½ cup chopped parsley
1 tbsp cilantro, chopped
½ tsp cumin powder
1 tsp minced ginger
4 tbsp Bragg's Liquid Aminos
4 tbsp sesame oil
½ tsp sea salt
¼ tsp black pepper powder
1½ cups chopped shiitake mushrooms

In a large saucepan, sauté the peas, carrots, mushrooms, shallots, and ginger in the oil for five minutes over medium high heat. Add the mashed chickpeas, parsley, cilantro, cumin, and Bragg's Liquid Aminos and continue cooking for an additional three minutes while stirring. Season the mixture with salt and pepper before removing from heat and adding the wild rice blend. Mix well and set aside to cool.

Meanwhile, remove the stems of the cabbages by coring them with a paring knife. Next, steam the whole cabbages for 10-15 minutes or until the leaves are pliable but still firm to the touch. Allow the cabbages to cool so that the leaves can be handled. While the cabbages are cooling, prepare the mushroom–red onion sauce. To stuff the cabbages, first remove the leaves. Place one leaf in the palm of one hand, fill one end of the leaf (the end where the mid-rib of leaf is thickest) with 3-4 heaping tablespoons of rice-bean-vegetable mixture. Tightly and slowly wrap the filling with the leaf to form a "log." Holding one end of the log in your palm, stuff the cabbage leaves into one end. Turn the filled log over and stuff the opposite end. Place stuffed cabbages in a 12" x 18" baking dish, cover with mushroom–red onion sauce. Bake covered in a preheated 350° F oven for 30 minutes.

Shiitake Mushroom–Red Onion Sauce—
2 cups sliced mushrooms (patients with yeast allergies should omit mushrooms)
1 cup coarsely chopped red onion
2 tbsp vegetable oil
2 cups vegetable stock
4 tbsp Bragg's Liquid Aminos
2 tbsp white miso paste
2 tbsp mirin
1 tbsp arrowroot and 2 tbsp cold water
Salt and pepper to taste

In a medium-size saucepan, sauté mushroom and red onion in oil for 3-5 minutes. Dissolve the miso into the vegetable stock and simmer for five minutes over medium heat. Next, combine the water, Bragg's, and mirin. Slurry the arrowroot in the mixture. Add the slurry into the vegetable-miso mixture while stirring and allow to cook for an additional three minutes. Season with salt and pepper. Drizzle sauce over stuffed cabbages.

Saffron Rice and Peas
1 tsp saffron
1½ cups pigeon peas (soak overnight and cook until pea yields to firm pressure, about 30 minutes); black-eyed peas can be substituted
2 cups brown basmati rice

3½ cups water
1 cup lite coconut milk
1 bunch scallions, crushed
4 stalks thyme
1 tsp sea salt
2 Scotch bonnet peppers (optional)
2 cloves garlic, crushed
In a medium-size pot, add the partly cooked beans, rice, water, and garlic; bring to a boil over medium heat. Add coconut milk, scallion, thyme, saffron, and salt; continue to simmer at medium low heat, with cover on, for 25-30 minutes. Carefully remove peppers without breaking the skin. Also remove scallions and thyme stalks. Mix the rice combination so that the peas are thoroughly blended. Serve hot. Yield: 5 6 servings.

Vegetable Bryani

2 cups cooked basmati rice (brown)*
1 cup frozen mixed vegetables, steamed and drained
½ cup whole cashews (substitute other nuts if you have *Candida*)
¼ cup raisins
½ tsp saffron threads plus 2 tbsp soaking water
1 tbsp chopped cilantro
4 tbsp chopped green onion
3 tbsp vegetable oil
Salt and pepper to taste
In a large saucepan, add cilantro and green onion to oil; sauté for five minutes. Add saffron threads (which have been soaked for 10-15 minutes) to rice and mix well. Next, stir in the rice, mixed vegetables, raisins, and cashews along with the sautéed cilantro and onions. Cook for an additional ten minutes over medium heat, stirring until mixture is heated through.
*To cook rice: 1½ cups basmati rice with 3 cups water and ½ tsp sea salt.

Curried Cauliflower and Bean Stew

½ cup yellow split peas, washed
½ cup red lentils, washed
¼ cup barley
1½ cups chickpeas, soaked overnight and cooked
4 cups vegetable stock
1 large cauliflower, broken into florets

¾ cups coarsely chopped onions
¾ cups coarsely chopped celery
4 tbsp canola or cold-pressed olive oil
2 tsp ground cumin seeds
1½ tbsp coriander powder
1 tbsp turmeric powder
2 tbsp fresh ginger, minced
1 lb fresh spinach, stems removed, washed, and coarsely chopped
2 tsp sea salt
½ tsp black pepper
In a medium saucepan, add vegetable stock, yellow peas, red lentils, and barley. Simmer over medium heat for 25 minutes, until beans and grains are cooked. Meanwhile, in a large skillet, put oil, onions, celery, and cauliflower florets, and sauté over medium high heat for ten minutes, stirring. Add the spices and continue cooking for five minutes. Next, stir in spinach and chickpeas, along with cooked peas, lentils, and barley mixture. Simmer for 3-5 minutes and season with salt and pepper. Can be served with Vegetable Bryani.

Scrambled Tofu
1 tsp dried basil
1 lb soft tofu (mashed)
1 tsp turmeric
2 cloves of garlic, minced
3 tbsp onion, chopped fine
3 tbsp chopped parsley
1 tsp sea salt
¼ tsp black pepper
2 tbsp oat flour
2 tbsp cold-pressed olive oil
In a medium-size bowl, mash tofu, add turmeric, salt, pepper, and oat flour. Add onions, parsley, and garlic with oil into a skillet; sauté for three minutes on medium heat. Next, add tofu mixture and cook for 5-7 minutes. Garnish with parsley and radish flowers.

Beverages

Dr. Zampieron's Zingiber Zing
1" slice of fresh, organic ginger root
1 organic green Granny Smith apple
1 piece of organic pineapple

1-2 drops of stevia extract
Seltzer or sparkling water
Juice all fruits and add seltzer to desired taste. Add stevia if more sweetness is desired. Add more ginger for more of a flavor "bite."[15]

Very Berry Banana Shake
1 cup blueberries
1 cup strawberries
1 large, very ripe banana
1½ cups plain soy milk
3 tbsp raw honey
1 cup ice cubes (optional)
¼ tsp ground nutmeg

Combine all ingredients in a blender and blend until smooth. Precaution: Not to be consumed if you have *Candida*.

Green Mobility Juice
¼ cup organic green cabbage juice
¼ cup organic broccoli juice
½ cup organic carrot juice
½ cup organic Granny Smith apple juice
¼ cup organic spinach juice
2 tbsp organic parsley juice
2 tbsp fresh organic ginger juice

Juice each vegetable in a quality juicer. Add ½ tsp vitamin C powder to the mixture. Drink juice right away. If juice is too concentrated, dilute by half with filtered water.

Dessert

Pineapple-Cherry Crisp
Filling—
3 cups crushed pineapple
1 cup fresh or frozen cherries
¾ cup pineapple juice
1 tsp vanilla extract
½ tsp lemon rind
1 tbsp agar-agar flakes
1 tsp arrowroot
Top and Bottom Crust—

Juice for Gout Attacks

Here is an excellent juice combination for gout:

1 dandelion (roots, leaves, and flowers)
1 burdock root
½" yellow dock root
1 bunch parsley
1 bunch cilantro
1 bunch water cress
2 carrots

3 cups of your favorite granola, coarsely chopped
½ cup safflower or canola oil
¾ cup succanat or maple sugar (reduce amount if you have *Candida*)
½ cup whole wheat (avoid if allergic to wheat) or oat flour
1 tbsp ground cinnamon
½ tsp sea salt

In a large saucepan, simmer together the pineapple, cherries, vanilla extract, rind, and agar flakes on a medium low heat for five minutes while stirring. Meanwhile, slurry the arrowroot in cold pineapple juice and pour them into the simmering fruit mixture. Allow to cook for an additional five minutes, mixing well. Set aside to cool. Next, combine all of the ingredients for the crust in a large bowl. Spread half of the crust mixture evenly in a 9" x 12" baking dish; add fruit filling over the bottom crust. Top the fruit layer with last half of the crust mixture. Bake in a preheated 375° F oven for 35-40 minutes. Allow to cool to room temperature before cutting into 3" x 3" inch squares. This makes a healthy and delicious snack or dessert. Yield: 12 servings.

Use chopped apples (Rome, Cortland, or Granny Smith), apple juice, and dried cranberries as an alternative to pineapple and cherries.

If cartilage breaks down as a result of

inadequate nutrition, then other bodily functions dependent

on similar nutrients, such as the immune system,

suffer as well. We urge all arthritis sufferers to adopt an

"arthritis-friendly" diet and pursue a

supplement program tailored to the person's specific

nutritional deficiencies.

13 Supplements for Arthritis

FOOD AS MEDICINE is an old but forgotten (at least by conventional medicine) concept that is critical to health and wellness in general and to arthritis patients in particular. Deficiencies of important nutrients have immediate and direct consequences on joint function and cartilage structure. For example, low levels of antioxidant vitamins (such as C and E) increase the potential for free radicals to attack and destroy sensitive joint tissues. Deficiencies in amino acids (the building-blocks of proteins), vitamin C, iron, selenium, and manganese contribute to the breakdown of cartilage, leading to arthritic changes in the joints, loss of mobility, and bone deterioration. If cartilage breaks down as a result of inadequate nutrition, then other bodily functions dependent on similar nutrients, such as the immune system, suffer as well. We urge all arthritis sufferers to adopt an "arthritis-friendly" diet and pursue a supplement program tailored to the person's specific nutritional deficiencies.

In This Chapter

- Vitamins
- Minerals
- Cartilage Builders
- Herbs
- Amino Acids
- Antioxidants
- Bioflavonoids
- Enzymes
- Homeopathic Remedies

Although a program of nutritional supplementation should be individualized, we discuss in this chapter the most common nutrient deficiencies associated with arthritis, along with recommendations for preventative and therapeutic dosages. We also give advice on how to obtain these nutrients through both food choices and as supplements. We know that the rows of nutritional supplements on grocery-store shelves can be confusing and intimidating and you may have heard claims and counter-claims about "arthritis cures" such as MSM, glucosamine sulfate, and chondroitin, among others. In this chapter, we will explain the real story behind these substances and how they can help treat your arthritis when combined with a multi-faceted nutritional program.

Vitamins

The vitamins most therapeutic for arthritis are ones with active antioxidant properties, such as vitamins C and E; those involved in bone structure and joint mobility, such as vitamins A and K; and those typically deficient in arthritis patients that improve symptoms after supplementation, such as vitamins B3 and B5.

Vitamin A and the Carotene Complexes—Vitamin A (retinol) is needed for the growth and repair of body tissues; it creates smooth and supple skin, protects all mucous membranes, and establishes stronger immune function.[1] Cortisone drugs, frequently prescribed for rheumatoid arthritis, decrease the amount of vitamin A available in the body. The body obtains vitamin A from food sources or manufactures it through the conversion of carotenes (alpha, beta, gamma).

> Food as medicine is an old but forgotten (at least by conventional medicine) concept that is critical to arthritis patients. Deficiencies of important nutrients have direct consequences on joint function and cartilage structure.

Because high levels of vitamin A can be toxic, it is usually safer to boost your intake of carotenes, which will be converted by the body into sufficient amounts of vitamin A. Carotenes also have many therapeutic effects on the reproductive and immune systems, protect cells from free-radical damage, and are anti-carcinogens.[2]

Food sources of vitamin A: fish oil, such as cod liver oil. RDA: 5,000 IU; therapeutic dose: 10,000-20,000 IU. Precautions: Very high levels of vitamin A can cause headaches and irritability and can be toxic; high levels should be avoided during pregnancy.[3] Food sources of carotenes: all yellow and green vegetables, including carrots, beet greens, spinach, and broccoli.[4] Supplements: most broad-spectrum multivitamins contain beta carotene and other carotenoids, including lycopene and lutein. RDA: none; therapeutic dose: 100,000-300,000 IU.

Vitamin B3 (Niacin)—Vitamin B3 maintains the integrity of the mucosal lining of the intestines, plays a role in nervous system function, and improves circulation. Low levels of B3 can cause muscle

See *The Supplement Shopper* (Future Medicine Publishing, 1999; ISBN 1-887299-17-3); to order, call 800-333-HEAL.

weakness, fatigue, skin sores, irritability, and depression. Eating a diet high in refined sugar as well as prolonged use of antibiotics will deplete B3 reserves in the body. Research by William Kaufman, M.D., and Abram Hoffer, M.D., in the 1950s demonstrated that niacinamide (the synthetic version of niacin) helped control and reverse symptoms of arthritis, including impaired joint mobility and joint pain.[5]

Food sources: meat, chicken, fish, peanuts, brewer's yeast, and wheat germ. Supplements: niacin is the natural form of vitamin B3 available in supplement form. When taken in dosages of over 100 milligrams, niacin can cause a very distinctive flushing, tingling, and redness that begins in the lower part of the body and moves up to the face, hands, and head; this sensation typically subsides after 15-20 minutes and causes no harm.[6] Niacinamide causes no flushing and is the niacin of choice in many modern supplements.[7] RDA: 15-20 mg; therapeutic dose: 50 mg. Precautions: Liver enzymes may be affected when utilizing high levels of B3 or niacinamide. Use of inositol hexoniacinate has shown no toxicity and may be the best choice for this supplement.

Vitamin B5 (Pantothenic acid)—Vitamin B5 is involved in the production of adrenal hormones and red blood cells and also helps metabolize fat and carbohydrates. Levels of vitamin B5 are typically low in patients with rheumatoid arthritis[8] and can be used therapeutically to help decrease pain and increase joint mobility.[9]

Food sources: liver, meat, chicken, whole grains, and legumes; eating a variety of foods can ensure adequate levels of vitamin B5. RDA: none; therapeutic dose: 10 mg to 2,000 mg.

Vitamin B6 (Pyridoxine)—Vitamin B6 helps form prostaglandins (pro- and anti-inflammatory agents) and red blood cells[10] and is also involved in the function of the nervous and immune systems.[11] We use vitamin B6 to alleviate pain associated with arthritis, as well as depression and carpal tunnel syndrome. Deficiencies of vitamin B6 can cause depression, skin eruptions, and even convulsions in children.[12] Deficiencies occur as a result of eating a diet high in fats and low in fruits and vegetables. In up to 25% of the population, a deficiency in vitamin B6 is due to excess protein, dyes that are used in food (especially FD&C yellow #5), and the conventional drug penicillamine, frequently prescribed for arthritis patients;[13] these substances prevent the absorption of B6 into the body's cells.

Food sources: whole grains, legumes, nuts and seeds. Supplements: there are two forms of B6, pyridoxine hydrochloride and pyridoxal-5-phosphate (the most active form). For efficient absorption of pyridoxal by the body, sufficient levels of riboflavin and magnesium should be present.[14] RDA: 2 mg; therapeutic dose: 50 mg. Precautions: High levels of pyridoxine can cause toxic side effects.[15]

Vitamin C—Both an antioxidant and anti-inflammatory, vitamin C helps repair and maintain healthy connective tissues. It is essential for collagen production and the maintenance of joint lining,[16] helps tissue repair, and reduces the bruising and swelling often associated with arthritis.[17]

Food sources: most fruits and vegetables, especially oranges, grapefruit, kiwis, lemons, avocado, and parsley. Supplements: the most cost-effective form of vitamin C is ascorbic acid, which is extracted from rosehips or acerola. There is also a new form of vitamin C called ester-C, which is purported to stay in the body longer, thereby increasing absorption.[18] RDA: 60 mg; therapeutic dose: 500-5,000 mg (to bowel tolerance).

Vitamin D—Vitamin D is a fat-soluble nutrient, considered to be both a vitamin and a hormone. It controls the absorption of calcium and phosphorus used in bone formation.[19] The major diseases caused by vitamin D deficiency, rickets and osteomalacia, are now relatively rare in the United States, but new evidence has found that mild deficiencies of vitamin D cause aches and pains in the hips and other joints, which are often found in arthritis.[20] A deficiency of vitamin D has been linked to increased likelihood of hip fractures and osteoporosis-related bone problems. Researchers at the Brigham and Women's Hospital in Boston, Massachusetts, studied 30 women with acute hip fractures and found that 50% of them were deficient in vitamin D.[21]

Vitamin D can be synthesized in the body through sunlight exposure. About 20 minutes a day of sunlight is necessary, although older people and those with very dark skin may need an hour. The sun can hit any part of the body but has to contact the skin directly; it is not effective through clothing, glass windows, or a sunscreen. People with sun sensitivity are advised to cover areas that are very sensitive with a sunscreen but allow the sun to hit areas that are less sensitive. People who are house-bound due to arthritis should attempt to be outside 20 minutes a day or at least a few hours a week to generate enough vitamin D for healthy bone repair.

Food sources: cod liver oil, fatty fish such as salmon and mackerel, butter, and egg yolks. Supplements: D2 ergocalciferol is synthetically derived; D3 (cholecalciferol) is the natural form from fish oils. RDA: 400 IU; therapeutic dose: 400 IU. Precautions: Vitamin D can be toxic if taken in high amounts—over 1,000 IU per day of vitamin D on an ongoing basis could cause malaise, drowsiness, extreme thirst, nausea, and calcification of soft tissues.

Vitamin E—Vitamin E protects cell membranes from oxidative damage and acts as an anti-inflammatory, blocking the activity of an enzyme that provokes inflammation. It also maintains the elastic quality in cells, which, in turn, increases elasticity in muscles. Levels of vitamin E are typically low in those with rheumatoid arthritis. Several studies indicate that there is a decrease in pain and joint swelling reported by people given vitamin E. Many patients also reported that they were able to reduce their doses of nonsteroidal, anti-inflammatory drugs (NSAIDs) while taking vitamin E.[22]

Food sources: cold-pressed oils such as sunflower and safflower, almonds, hazelnuts, and wheat germ. Supplements: vitamin E is actually a group of compounds called tocopherols. When purchasing supplements of vitamin E, avoid products that contain vitamin E in the DL-alpha tocopherol acetate form—this means that it is a petroleum-based synthetic form of the vitamin. The natural form of vitamin E will be designated with the letter "D". Research has shown that the natural form of vitamin E has better antioxidant protective properties and recent research indicates that mixed tocopherols may, in fact, be the best. Avoid taking iron supplements at the same time of day as vitamin E supplements as they mutually prevent absorption. Drink filtered water (no chlorinated water) and avoid polyunsaturated fats, since these may destroy vitamin E. RDA: 30 IU; therapeutic dose: up to 3,000 IU per day has shown no negative effects.

Vitamin K—Vitamin K is important for bone health because it is needed in the process of bone repair. Deficiencies have been found in people with osteoporosis and ankylosing spondylitis (a form of arthritis

---

A Quick Guide to Nutrients for Building Healthy Joints

Vitamins:

Vitamins A, B3 (niacin and niacinamide), C, D, E, and K

Minerals:

Calcium, Magnesium, Manganese, Copper, Zinc, and Boron

Cartilage Builders:

Glucosamine Sulfate and Chondroitin Sulfate

---

that affects the spine). Vitamin K can help the healing process in broken bones and for joint support in osteoarthritis.

Food sources: green leafy vegetables (high in chlorophyll, a source of vitamin K), parsley, cabbage, and broccoli. Supplements: there are three main kinds of vitamin K: K1 is the natural form from plants; K2 is produced from intestinal bacteria; and K3 is synthetically produced. RDA: 50 mcg; therapeutic dose: 20-40 mg per day, with meals.

Folic Acid—Folic acid has been shown in research studies to be more effective than the drug allopurinol, a commonly prescribed conventional drug, in inhibiting the enzyme xanthine oxidase (which controls the buildup of uric acid), thereby decreasing tissue destruction in gout. For this purpose, folic acid must be used in a therapeutic dose (10-40 mg per day). Precautions: Although no side effects have been noted, these doses may interfere with some epilepsy drugs and might mask a vitamin B deficiency; consult with a health-care practitioner before using high doses.

Minerals

In order to maintain health, concentrations of minerals in the body must be in specific ratios. Minerals are essential cofactors for enzyme reactions, aid in the uptake of vitamins, and are structural components of the skeleton. Some minerals cannot be manufactured by the body and must be obtained from the diet or nutritional supplements.

Boron—Boron helps maintain bone and joint function and activates the metabolism of vitamin D. Low levels of boron in the soil—and thus in foods grown in that soil—have been linked in many countries to increased osteoarthritis levels.[23] Boron supplementation helps to reduce the excretion of calcium and magnesium, important minerals in bone structure and muscle function.[24] Studies in Germany have found that boron can improve joint pain in osteoarthritis as well as decrease bone loss.[25]

Food sources: boron can be found in most fruits and vegetables, if organically grown (chemicals and artificial fertilizers tend to deplete boron levels). Supplements: boron is commonly found in many multivitamin/multimineral supplements, usually as either sodium borate or sodium tetra borate decahydrate. RDA: none; therapeutic dose: 5-10 mg. Precautions: Over 500 mg per day may cause nausea, vomiting, and diarrhea.

Copper—Copper, along with vitamin C and other nutrients, is important in the synthesis of collagen and elastin, the components of cartilage that provide support and structure. A copper deficiency can lead to joint degeneration, a general feeling of weakness, immune dysfunction, and skin fragility (easily bruised or torn). The body's absorption of copper may sometimes be blocked by a diet high in refined foods or from taking high levels of vitamin C, zinc,[26] and iron.

Food sources: beans, lentils, shellfish (especially oysters), liver, nuts, and green leafy vegetables. Supplements: there are various forms of supplemental copper, such as copper sulfate, copper gluconate, copper picolinate, and others. RDA: 2 mg; therapeutic dose: 2-5 mg. Precautions: Copper toxicity is seen more often than is copper deficiency. Use only after copper levels are measured through hair or urine analysis.

Calcium—Calcium, the most abundant mineral in the body, has gained recognition in the media for its role in health and disease. The main function of calcium (along with phosphorus) is in forming a matrix that hardens bones and teeth. Calcium is also involved in muscle contraction, nerve function, and heartbeat regulation. It moderates the acid-alkaline balance and the way nutrients cross the cell membrane.[27] Calcium absorption into the cells can be compromised by whole grains and cereals, spinach, and by tannins in tea, a diet high in protein, commercial soda, and refined sugar, and antacids that contain aluminum.[28] Although found in dairy products, this form of calcium is not easily absorbed, especially by arthritis sufferers who typically have deficiencies of stomach acid.[29]

Food sources: broccoli, cabbage, almonds, hazelnuts, oats, lentils, beans, figs, currants and raisins, Brussels sprouts, cauliflower, kelp, and green leafy vegetables, especially kale. Kale is very high in an easily absorbed form of calcium.[30] Supplements: bone meal, dolomite, and oyster shell calcium have been found to have the highest levels of lead contamination and should not be used as a supplement.[31] Calcium citrate and calcium gluconate have a much better absorption level.[32] One of the best forms of absorbable calcium is microcrystalline hydroxyapatite. RDA: 1,200 mg; therapeutic dose: 1,000 mg to 1,500 mg. Precautions: Excessive intake of calcium oxalate may cause the formation of kidney stones, but this risk can be decreased by using the calcium citrate and calcium gluconate forms. High calcium intake can interfere with iron absorption, cause chronic constipation, and may also increase blood pressure, if taken along with NSAIDs.[33] If heavy metal toxicity is present (often seen in arthritis), increasing calcium intake may make arthritis symptoms worse; check for heavy metals through hair or urine analysis.

Iodine—Iodine is involved in the development and function of the thyroid gland, which is responsible for producing thyroid hormones important for energy production, mental processes, and speech. Iodine also is important in the condition of the skin, nails, hair, and teeth, and the synthesis of cholesterol. Deficiencies in iodine can cause thyroid dysfunction, which can lead to degenerative illnesses including muscle weakness and arthritis. Food sources: seaweed, kelp, and fish. In the United States, table salt is iodized, which provides sufficient levels of iodine. People using sea salt as a replacement for table salt should consider supplementing with kelp, a vegetable rich in elemental iodine (the most therapeutic form).[34] Certain foods, called goitrogens, prevent iodine absorption. These include soybeans, turnips, cabbage, and pine nuts, especially if eaten raw.[35] Supplements: supplements often contain inorganic iodine such as sodium iodide and potassium iodide. These kinds are not as beneficial as elemental iodine, found in iodine caseinate.[36] RDA: 150 mg; therapeutic dose: 150 mg. Precautions: Iodine, at very high doses, can cause acne and have a reverse effect on the thyroid gland and actually lower thyroid function.[37]

Iron—Eighty percent of people with rheumatoid arthritis have deficiencies of iron in their blood, which can cause anemia. Prolonged use of NSAIDs or commercial antacids, low levels of folic acid, or menstrual difficulties contribute to iron-deficiency anemia. An iron deficiency can also decrease hydrochloric acid in the stomach, impairing digestion and contributing to further nutritional deficiencies. Food sources: red meat, organ meat, shellfish, and egg yolk. Liver contains heme iron that is very well absorbed by humans. Non-heme iron is found in vegetable foods such as oats, millet, parsley, kelp, brewer's yeast, and yellowdock root.[38] Supplements: the form of iron (heme) found in desiccated liver or liquid liver extract supplements is most easily absorbed and has fewer side effects. Of the non-heme forms of iron, ferrous fumerate and ferrous succinate are recommended. RDA: 10-15 mg; therapeutic dose: 10-15 mg. Precautions: Ferrous sulfate, commonly used in conventional supplements, can cause the production of free radicals and should not be used. Elevated levels of iron in the blood are associated with an increased risk for heart attacks and other cardiovascular problems, as well as joint problems and lowered immunity.[39] Overdose in infants can be serious or even fatal, so be sure that your iron supplements are out of the reach of children.

Manganese—Manganese has many functions in the body, including normal growth and metabolism. It helps to activate enzymes, is used for normal bone development, and acts as an anti-inflammatory.[40] Rheumatoid arthritis sufferers are usually significantly deficient in manganese and supplementation is recommended.

Food sources: nuts, egg yolk, dried fruits, whole grains, and green leafy vegetables. Supplements: forms that are not readily absorbed include manganese sulfate and manganese chloride—manganese picolinate and manganese gluconate are better absorbed. RDA: none; therapeutic dose: 150 mg.

Magnesium—Magnesium is second only to potassium as the most concentrated mineral within the cells. Magnesium helps form bones, relax muscle spasms, and decrease the pain involved in arthritis. It activates cellular enzymes and plays a large role in nerve and muscle function as well as helping to regulate the acid-alkaline balance.[41] Magnesium deficiency can cause anxiety, muscle tremors, confusion, irritability, and pain. Processed food or foods cooked at high temperatures can be depleted of their magnesium content.

Food sources: tofu, nuts and seeds, and green leafy vegetables, especially kale, seaweed, and chlorophyll. Supplements: magnesium is absorbed well when taken as an oral supplement and will increase the measurable levels inside red and white blood cells.[42] Epsom salts (magnesium sulfate), an old-fashioned remedy, is an excellent addition to a bath, but has a strong laxative effect if taken as an oral supplement. We recommend using magnesium glycinate, fumerate, or citrate, which are usually better absorbed with less of a laxative effect.[43] RDA: 400 mg; therapeutic dose: 500-1,000 mg. Precautions: Very high doses of magnesium may be dangerous if kidney disease is present.

Selenium—The importance of selenium, which is often deficient in people with inflammatory diseases (such as arthritis), is its activity as an antioxidant and anti-inflammatory. Selenium works in conjunction with vitamin E in cell membranes to fight free radicals.[44] Selenium can also protect against the absorption of heavy metals such as aluminum, mercury, and lead.[45]

Food sources: the small amount of selenium needed by the body is often hard to obtain through the diet because foods are now grown in mineral-poor soils.[46] If grown in fertile soil, grains are a good source of selenium, as are liver, meat, and fish. Supplements: avoid multimineral supplements that contain sodium selenite, an organic salt that is not well absorbed. Organic selenium from yeast or the chelated mineral (seleno-methionine) are better sources. RDA: 26 mcg; therapeutic dose: 200-1,000 mcg per day. Precautions: Selenium toxicity is possible but rare, as only very small amounts are needed by the body. An overdose can cause hair loss, nail malformations, weakness, and slowed mental function.[47]

Zinc—Zinc is found in bones, nails, and skin, among other body organs. It helps synthesize protein, repairs wounds and fractures, and supports immune function. A zinc deficiency (often indicated by white spots on the fingernails) can cause painful knee and hip joints, especially in young men; this condition can often be misdiagnosed as arthritis.[48] In both adults and children suffering from arthritis, zinc levels have been found to be low.[49]

Food sources: whole grains, nuts, seeds, oysters, shellfish, and pumpkin seeds. Supplements: zinc sulfate, found in many multivitamin/multimineral preparations, is not easily absorbed by the body. Other, more readily absorbed forms of zinc are zinc picolinate, zinc citrate, and zinc monomethionine. RDA: 15 mg; therapeutic dose: 50 mg. Precautions: Toxicity of zinc is rarely reported, however, prolonged use of over 150 mg a day can cause anemia.

Cartilage-Building Supplements

Healthy joints are made up of pliable cartilage that absorbs shock and ensures smooth motion. New cartilage cells are constantly replacing old dead cells worn out from use. But when the cycle of cell production is altered or when enzymes that "eat" dead cartilage become overly aggressive or the patient is chronically dehydrated, cartilage loses its vital water content and begins to dry out. This leads to the degradation of joint tissue in osteoarthritis and also in advanced forms of rheumatoid arthritis. This physiologic imbalance allows more and more cartilage to be broken down, while not enough healthy new tissue is built up. Cartilage-building supplements provide the raw materials to rebuild damaged cartilage and stop the unnecessary destruction of healthy cells.

Glucosamine Sulfate—Glucosamine is a building-block of proteoglycans, the cells within cartilage that absorb water and make cartilage

When the cycle of cell production is altered or when enzymes that "eat" dead cartilage become overly aggressive, cartilage loses its vital water content and begins to dry out. Cartilage-building supplements provide the raw materials to rebuild damaged cartilage and stop the unnecessary destruction of healthy cells.

resilient to shock. Glucosamine's presence in the joint tissues also stimulates the production of GAGs (glycosaminoglycans), a complex sugar in cartilage and the lubricating substance inside joints; it also decreases the activity of the enzymes that break down cartilage cells. As people age, it is suspected that their level of glucosamine drops off, resulting in less joint repair activity. When levels of glucosamine are increased (typically through supplements), eroded cartilage is restored and normal joint maintenance resumes. Glucosamine should be used in all types of arthritis.

In a study in Milan, Italy, 80 patients with severe osteoarthritis were given a 30-day course of glucosamine sulfate (1.5 g daily). The treated patients experienced a reduction in pain, tenderness, and over-all symptoms. Examination of cartilage samples from the patients treated with glucosamine sulfate shared many structural aspects of healthy cartilage. The researchers concluded that glucosamine sulfate rebuilt damaged cartilage, thereby reducing pain and other symptoms.[50] Glucosamine is also an effective pain reliever. In studies in Germany and Italy, ibuprofen (the main ingredient of Advil, Motrin, and Nuprin) was compared to glucosamine in patients with osteoarthritis of the knee. Patients experienced pain relief one month after starting on oral glucosamine sulfate—a slower response than with ibuprofen—but they also experienced greater pain relief and fewer gastrointestinal side effects than they did with ibuprofen.[51]

Oral glucosamine supplements are made from the exoskeletons of shellfish, called chitin. There are several forms of glucosamine available, but glucosamine sulfate appears to be the form that shows the maximum absorption when taken orally.[52] The therapeutic dosage of glucosamine sulfate that is necessary for an individual can vary, but we typically recommend starting with 500 mg, three times a day, on an empty stomach. Precautions: There is no known toxicity, even with long-term use, but some people occasionally experience gastrointestinal upset, which can be alleviated by taking it with food.

Chondroitin Sulfate—Chondroitin sulfate is another important ingredient in proteoglycans (which fill in the space between collagen cells and hold water in the joints for shock absorption). Proteoglycans are shaped like bottle brushes with a stem composed of proteins and radiating sugar chains that look like the brush's bristles. Located in the long sugar chains are glycosaminoglycans (GAGs) of which chondroitin sulfate is the most critical. Chondroitin seems to protect joints from breaking down and can speed the recovery of injured bones.[53]

Chondroitin is enjoying widespread popularity for the treatment of arthritis, however, there is much debate about the body's ability to assimilate and use chondroitin orally (see "A Note About Chondroitin Sulfate"). The injectable forms of chondroitin, however, have proven to be effective therapies for arthritis.[54] Thousands of patients in Europe, South America, and other countries, have been successfully treated with various forms of injectable chondroitin, but chondroitin-based injections are not widely available in the United States. However, the Access to Medical Freedom Act, approved in several states in the U.S., allows patients and their holistic doctors to use this treatment if the patient signs a waiver indicating their knowledge that it is not approved by the U.S. Food and Drug Administration. Due to the proven efficacy of these treatments on thousands of patients in Europe and the lack of side effects, chondroitin-based injections may be worth trying.

We recommend three injectable chondroitin products that have been clinically tested (outside the U.S.) with beneficial results, including pain and inflammation reduction, improvement in joint mobility, and, in some cases, cessation of joint deterioration. Arteparon® contains glycosaminoglycan polysulphate, which is extracted from bovine trachea and lung; a typical course of treatment is 10-15 injections at a rate of two per week. Rumalon® is usually given in 25 injections at a rate of

A Note About Chondroitin Sulfate

Much media attention over the last few years has extolled the virtues of chondroitin sulfate as a supplement for the treatment of arthritis. Many products in health food stores contain a combination of chondroitin sulfate and glucosamine sulfate. However, chondroitin sulfate is a complex sugar or polysaccharide, while glucosamine is a disaccharide (containing only two sugars). This makes chondroitin a much larger molecule—200 times larger than glucosamine—and thus very difficult to absorb intact through the intestines. So, taking chondroitin sulfate orally has not been shown to be as efficacious as oral supplements of glucosamine sulfate (and other forms of glucosamine) for rebuilding and supporting cartilage in arthritis sufferers.

For more information on **Sulconar**, contact: BUH Health Foundation, Avenue De La Paz, Numero 16420, Tijuana 22370, Mexico; tel: 011-526-624-0939.

2-3 per week. Sulconar® is made from cartilage, bone marrow, and liver enzyme, among other substances; the usual course of treatment involves ten injections, one daily for ten days. There is also an injectable prescription available in the U.S. called Syn-Visc®, a form of hyaluronic acid that is injected by a physician directly into a painful joint, which can help relieve pain for up to one year after injection. In our clinical experience, we have seen some remarkable results using this therapy. One patient with osteoarthritis, Luke, who'd had much of the cartilage in his right knee removed through surgery, was able to live pain-free and resume normal activities with the use of Syn-Visc.

Cetyl Myristoleate—The existence of this rare anti-arthritis substance was stumbled upon in 1962 by Harry W. Diehl, Ph.D., a researcher for the National Institutes of Arthritis, Metabolism, and Digestive Diseases. Assigned to inject an arthritis-inducing agent into laboratory mice for the purposes of testing a new synthetic drug, Dr. Diehl found that the mice were strangely resistant to developing arthritis symptoms. Dr. Diehl eventually identified in the mice an oil called cetyl myristoleate responsible for preventing arthritis.

Cetyl myristoleate occurs in only a few animal species—Swiss albino mice, sperm whales, and the male beaver. To make this useful substance available to the public, Dr. Diehl found that a mixture of myristoleic acid (from fish oils and cow's milk butter) and cetyl alcohol, a molecule found in coconut and palm oils, rendered the same chemical substance found in the mice. Cetyl myristoleate appears to have three modes of therapeutic action that are helpful for both osteoarthritis and rheumatoid arthritis: it acts as a lubricant for the smooth motion of joints and muscles, modulates immune system function, and has anti-inflammatory effects.[55]

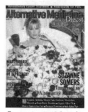

Typical recommended dose: Cetyl myristoleate is usually given orally for a one-month period at a dose of 10 g to 15 g. It is also available as a topical cream that can be rubbed into sore and painful joint areas. Because cetyl myristoleate is a fatty substance, we advise taking it in conjunction with 100 mg of lipase, an enzyme that helps digest fat.[56]

For more on **cetyl myristoleate**, see "Quick-Acting Natural Arthritis Relief," *Alternative Medicine Digest* 20 (October/November 1997), pp. 90-94; www.alternativemedicine.com

Sulfur Compounds—Sulfur-containing compounds are used by the body to regenerate cartilage cells, maintain cellular functions, and produce the amino acid glutathione, which is used by the liver to process toxins. Food sources rich in sulfur include garlic, onions, Brussels sprouts, and cabbage. Supplementation with sulfur-containing compounds has proven to be effective in reducing inflammation, relieving pain, and rebuilding cartilage for arthritis suffers.

■ S-adenosylmethionine (SAMe) is a natural substance produced by the human body when the amino acid methionine combines with adenosine triphosphate (ATP), an energy source present in muscle cells.[57] SAMe is a methyl-donor, meaning that it gives its sulfur molecules to important cellular activity such as rebuilding cell membranes, removing toxins and wastes, and producing mood-elevating brain chemicals (dopamine and serotonin). If the body is deficient in vitamin B12, folic acid, or methionine, production of SAMe may decrease. Research has also found that levels of SAMe drop off as people age or in patients with osteoarthritis, muscle pain, liver disease, and depression. SAMe was first used to treat depression in the 1970s, but has recently been found to ease joint and muscle pain and may contribute to cartilage regeneration. In one double-blind study, SAMe reduced pain in osteoarthritis patients as effectively as the drug ibuprofen, and produced fewer side effects.[58] Similar studies have found that SAMe is an anti-inflammatory and pain reliever in arthritis of the hip and knee.[59] Dose: 400 mg, four times a day. Precautions: Certain side effects have been found with the use of SAMe, such as nausea and gastrointestinal disturbances, although this usually clears if it is taken with a meal.

■ Dimethylsulfoxide (DMSO) is also a source of sulfur (derived from wood pulp, garlic oil, or as a by-product of petroleum) and thought to be a free-radical scavenger with anti-inflammatory properties. DMSO acts as a "carrier substance" increasing the absorption rate of other substances. There are several forms of DMSO available through prescription or over-the-counter: intravenous solutions, intramuscular injections, oral capsules, and topical lotions and ointments. Precautions: DMSO has shown great promise as a pain-relief therapy, but its side effects include occasional nausea, a strong sulfur smell on the skin and the breath, and skin irritation.

■ Methylsulfonylmethane (MSM) is a sister compound of DMSO derived from food sources. MSM is also naturally produced in the body, but levels decrease with age, in degenerative illnesses such as arthritis, and in people with poor dietary habits. Supplementing with MSM can reduce inflammation and scar tissue, relieve pain, increase blood flow for improved exchange of nutrients, reduce muscle spasms, promote peristalsis, increase cell-wall flexibility, and reduce allergic

Arthritis Help From the Sea

The green-lipped mussel, an edible shellfish native to New Zealand, is high in a unique kind of fatty acid known to reduce inflammation. ETA (eicosatetraenoic acid) is a previously unidentified type of omega-3 fatty acid with more biological activity than other omega-3s. Green-lipped mussels also contain amino acids, trace minerals, and GAGs (glycosaminoglycans, a component of cartilage). Dose: a typical recommended dose is 500 mg, three times per day with food. Precautions: Side effects are rare and mild, but include temporary aggravation of joint pain and tenderness, stomach discomfort, gas, nausea, and fluid retention.[62] People with known shellfish allergies should not use green-lipped mussel.

For more on **green-lipped mussel extract**, see "New Zealand's Green-Lipped Mussel for Arthritis Relief," *Alternative Medicine Digest* 21 (December 1997/January 1998), pp. 74-77; www.alternative-medicine.com

Sea cucumber (beche-de-mer) is a small marine animal related to the starfish traditionally used as an ingredient in Japanese and Chinese soups and stews.[63] Health benefits of sea cucumber include the relief of symptoms of rheumatoid arthritis, osteoarthritis, and ankylosing spondylitis.[64] Sea cucumbers also contain GAGs and chondroitins, which are important components of cartilage tissue.[65] Dose: a typical recommended dose is 500 mg, twice a day. Precautions: People with seafood or shellfish allergies should not take sea cucumber.

reactions.[60] Of special relevance in rheumatoid arthritis, MSM can help normalize the immune system and reduce the autoimmune response. MSM is a source of biologically active sulfur, which has an extensive role in the body. It is a component of amino acids, the building-blocks of proteins, which, in turn, build cell walls, tissues, cartilage, bones, muscles, and organs. MSM does not have the unpleasant side effects associated with DMSO.[61] MSM is available without a prescription in powder form, capsules, eye drops, and topical creams. Dose: typical recommended dosage levels range from 500 mg to 1,000 mg per day; under a doctor's supervision, therapeutic amounts may be prescribed.

Herbs

Bitter Melon (*Mormordica charantia*)—Bitter melon, also called cerese root, is helpful for psoriasis and psoriatic arthritis because it acts to slow the rapid cellular proliferation that causes the scaly skin buildup so common with psoriatic conditions.

Boswellia serrata (Salai Guggul or Indian Olibanum)—*Boswellia serrata*, also known as boswella, has been used for centuries by Ayurvedic (SEE QUICK DEFINITION) physicians for arthritic conditions. Its chemical component, boswellic acid, has powerful anti-inflammatory and analgesic activity.[66] Several studies have found that boswellic acid inhibits inflammation-causing agents, prevents interference with GAG (glycosaminoglycan) synthesis, and improves blood and lymphatic circulation to the joints.[67] Clinical studies on humans have also revealed the potent anti-rheumatic activity of this phytomedicine. In one study, boswellic acids given to patients with rheumatoid arthritis for six months caused a dramatic reduction in the levels of C-reactive protein, an indicator of the amount of inflammation in the body.

A standardized extract containing 60% boswellic acid is the most effective preparation. Dose: 400 mg, three times daily. Precautions: Boswella contains high levels of gum resins, which can strain the kidneys when used for an extended period; supplement with boswella only for a six-week period, then discontinue use for one week before resuming treatment.[68]

Chinese Thoroughwax (*Bupleurum radix*)—Bupleurum

is an herb that modern scientific investigation has validated for its use as an anti-inflammatory. The active components, saikosaponins, significantly increased blood levels of ACTH (adrenocorticotropic hormone, a pituitary hormone that causes the adrenal glands to secrete cortisol) and cortisone (a hormone that reduces pain) 30-60 minutes after treatment.[69] Bupleurum also benefits the adrenal glands and protects this organ from the damaging effects of pharmaceutical drugs such as corticosteroids.

Cayenne Pepper (*Capsicum anuum*)—Cayenne pepper

contains capsaicin, a chemical component involved in pain relief. When applied topically, capsaicin enhances circulation to painful areas to help distribute nutrients, oxygen, and healing hormones to the afflicted area and remove waste products. Capsaicin also depletes body reserves of substance P (SEE QUICK DEFINITION), believed to be responsible for intensifying and prolonging muscle and joint inflammation and pain.[70]

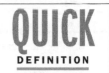

DEFINITION

Ayurveda is the traditional medicine of India, based on many centuries of empirical use. Its name means "end of the Vedas" (which were India's sacred scripts), implying that a holistic medicine may be founded on spiritual principles. Ayurveda describes three metabolic, constitutional, and body types (doshas), in association with the basic elements of Nature in combination. These are *vata* (air and ether, rooted in intestines), *pitta* (fire and water/stomach), and *kapha* (water and earth/lungs). Ayurvedic physicians use these categories (which also have psychological aspects) as the basis for prescribing individualized formulas of herbs, diet, massage, breathing, meditation, exercise and yoga postures, and detoxification techniques.

Substance P is several amino acids bonded together normally present in minute amounts in the nervous system and intestines. Typically involved in the pain response, substance P expands and contracts smooth muscles in the intestines and other tissues and muscles. Substance P also suppresses serotonin, a precursor to melatonin the hormone that regulates sleep/wake cycles.

Cinnamon (*Cinnamon cassiae*)—In Chinese medicine, cinnamon is one of the most widely used warming herbs for promoting circulation in joints and limbs. It is also helpful for indigestion, gas, and diarrhea. Hot topical application of cinnamon tea or cinnamon oil helps to improve circulation and ease the pain of fibromyalgia and arthritis.

Feverfew (*Tanacetum parthenium*)—Frequently used to treat migraine headaches, feverfew can be more effective at controlling inflammation than aspirin or NSAIDs (nonsteroidal, anti-inflammatory drugs).[71] It blocks the production of inflammatory chemicals and slows the migration of certain white blood cells to the inflamed area, thus modulating inflammation and pain. A double-blind study from England determined that feverfew was effective in reducing the pain of migraine headaches and was also useful for rheumatoid arthritis.[72] We recommend using the product BotanoDyne, which contains standardized whole plant feverfew extract at 0.75% parthenolide (one of feverfew's active ingredients).

For more about BotanoDyne, contact: Nature's Answer, 320 Oser Avenue, Hauppauge, NY 11788; tel: 800-439-2324 or 516-231-7492; fax: 516-231-8391; website: www. naturesanswer.com.

Ginger (*Zingiber officinale*)—Sitting on the produce shelf of most American grocery stores is one of nature's most cost-effective and powerful medicines—ginger root. Ginger is an expectorant, anti-tussive (cough suppressant), gastrointestinal stimulant, anti-nausea, circulatory tonic, antioxidant, and anti-inflammatory. It is also used in Chinese medicine to increase the movement of *qi* (life force), blood, and lymph. Ginger's high concentration of proteolytic enzymes (which break down proteins) is responsible for its ability to subdue pain and inflammation. Proteolytic enzymes block several inflammatory substances, including pro-inflammatory prostaglandins and leukotrienes.[73] In one study, arthritis patients (many of them with mixed rheumatoid arthritis, osteoarthritis, and fibromyalgia) were given supplements of ginger over two-and-a-half years. In 89% of rheumatoid arthritis patients and 88% of osteoarthritis patients, ginger brought about relief from pain and swelling.[74] In another study, patients with rheumatoid arthritis consumed 5-50 grams of fresh ginger per day. All patients reported that they had dramatic relief of pain, swelling, inflammation, and morning stiffness as well as increased joint mobility. Ginger also helps soothe the gastrointestinal system, so it can be of special assistance to those suffering from irritable bowel, leaky gut syndrome, gastritis, or nausea.[75] The more ginger consumed, the better the effects.[76]

Jamaican Dogwood (*Piscidia erythrima* and *Piscidia piscipula*)—Jamaican

dogwood, a member of the pea family, is one of the most powerful herbal medicines for pain. Typically used as an anti-spasmodic, it can ease painful cramping in both smooth and skeletal muscles.[77] The Jamaican dogwood grows in Jamaica, the Bahamas, Mexico, southern Texas, and Florida; pieces of the roots or outer bark are used to extract its active components.[78] We mix equal parts of Jamaican dogwood with kava-kava, white willow bark, ginger, turmeric, *Boswellia*, and other botanicals for a potent remedy. This combination is available commercially in BotanoDyne from Nature's Answer.

Kava-Kava (*Piper methysticum*)—We have successfully used kava-kava in

botanical mixtures designed to ease pain, anxiety, and depression. Kava-kava functions as one of the least toxic yet most powerful herbal skeletal muscle relaxants and has been used traditionally by Hawaiians for rheumatism and the treatment of arthritis. Chemicals contained in kava, known as pyrones, are responsible for the plant's relaxing properties. Kava-kava seems to function as a spinal, rather than a cerebral, sedative. In one study, kava-kava reduced pain in a manner unlike that of opiates, NSAIDs, or other pain relievers, as it did not bind to any of the normal pain-relieving receptors in the body. In addition, as yet undetermined chemicals in kava are postulated to be responsible for its analgesic effects.[79]

For relief of arthritis pain and fibromyalgia, a typical dose of 100-150 mg of kava-kava (depending on body weight) may be taken three times per day. For insomnia, a dose of 200-300 mg of kava-kava is recommended, taken prior to bedtime. When used properly, kava does not cause over-sedation, nor does it affect reaction time, like alcohol. Instead, kava improves sociability, reduces anxiety, eases depression, and enhances alertness.[80] Precautions: There is concern about long-term use of kava-kava and its effect on the liver; we do not recommend taking this herb for extended periods of time. Kava causes drowsiness in some individuals—use kava for the first time in the evening, while not operating heavy machinery or driving.

EDITOR'S NOTE
Drs. Zampieron and Kamhi have co-authored a book entitled *The Natural Medicine Chest* (M. Evans, 1999), which contains additional information on many of the supplements discussed in this chapter.

Licorice Root (*Glycyrrhiza glabra*)—Licorice root, used to fla-

vor candies and liqueurs, is also one of the most thoroughly studied phytomedicines.[81] A common ingredient in Chinese medicinal formulas, licorice has significant antiviral and antibacterial activity.[82] It stimulates interferon (a cytokine with antiviral activity) and enhances the body's production of cortisone (a natural painkiller).[83]

Lignum vitae (*Guiacum officinale* and *Guiacum sanctum*)—Lignum vitae is a tree native to South Florida, the Caribbean, and South America. The gum of this tree, guaia-gum, contains therapeutic resins and oils used as a pain reliever for arthritis, rheumatism, and gout.[84] An alcohol extract that dissolves the gummy resin is the preferred medicinal application. Clinical trials are under way at the Naturopathic Medical Center of Middlebury, Connecticut, to evaluate Lignum vitae and sarsaparilla extracts to treat Lyme disease, which can cause debilitation of the nervous system and severe arthritis.[85]

Oregon Grape Root—Oregon grape root contains high levels of hydrastine and berberine, two alkaloids which have been shown to inhibit the formulation of polyamines in the gut. Polyamines are bowel toxins that are abnormally high in individuals with psoriasis and psoriatic arthritis. They can also increase leaky gut, a factor in most cases of arthritis. Particularly helpful for psoriasis and psoriatic arthritis.[86]

Turmeric (*Curcuma longa*)—Turmeric, the bright yellow spice used in Indian cooking, is a powerful anti-inflammatory, liver protector, and antioxidant.[87] Its anti-inflammatory properties are credited to the chemical component curcumin. Curcumin was found to be better at reducing acute inflammation than cortisone and phenylbutazone, two commonly prescribed pharmaceutical drugs.[88] Turmeric is a key component of Botanodyne, an herbal combination from Nature's Answer.

White Willow Bark (*Salix alba*) and Black Willow Bark (*Salix nigra*)—These herbs have been used traditionally to reduce inflammation, fever, and pain. The active chemical components of willow are the herbal equivalents of synthetic aspirin, without the gastrointestinal side effects of most aspirin products. Of the many species of willow, white willow contains the highest amount of salicin (the active component). The effectiveness of white willow bark may be reduced if dysbiosis (imbalance in the gastrointestinal microflora) exists. It is advised to use standardized extracts (at 15% salicin) of white willow bark instead of the whole herb. Taking supplements of *acidophilus* may improve the absorption and effectiveness of white willow.

Wintergreen Oil (*Oleum Gaultheria procumbens*)—Purified wintergreen oil contains high levels of methylsalycilate, an aspirin-like compound that blocks prostaglandins and helps to stop pain and inflammation, and has been used for arthralgia (nerve pain in the joints). The application of wintergreen oil to joints or other afflicted areas can help relieve pain.

Amino Acids

Amino acids are the building-blocks of proteins. There are over 22 amino acids linked in various combinations to form 1,600 basic proteins necessary for body structure and the formation of antibodies, hormones, enzymes, organs, and cell membranes. Some amino acids are manufactured in the body while others (the essential amino acids) must be obtained from dietary sources.

When buying amino acids look for USP pharmaceutical grade, L-crystalline, free-form amino acids. The designation USP means that the product meets the standard of purity set by the United States Pharmacopeia. The term *free-form* refers to the highest level of purity of the amino acid. The L refers to one of the two forms of most amino acids, designated D- and L (for example, D-lysine or L-lysine). The L-form amino acids are proper for human biochemistry, as proteins in the human body are made from this form. The exception is phenylalanine, an amino acid which consists of a combination of the D- and L- forms (thus its full name, DL-phenylalanine).

Below, we discuss the amino acids that are typically deficient in arthritis sufferers and may be able to improve symptoms. We do not, however, recommend taking individual amino acid supplements for indefinite periods, because this can create an imbalance of other amino acids and may contribute to the development of other health conditions.

Cysteine—Cysteine is a sulfur-containing amino acid typically found in the protein complexes of hair, fingernails, and toenails. It acts as an antioxidant, shields the liver from toxic heavy metals, and helps prevent infections by augmenting the actions of vitamin C. Food sources: poultry, yogurt, oats, egg yolk, red peppers, broccoli, Brussels sprouts, and wheat germ. Typical therapeutic dose: 1,000 mg a day in the form of N-acetyl-cysteine (NAC).

Glutamine—Glutamine is an essential amino acid that plays an important role in maintaining the integrity of the intestinal wall and can be very helpful in reversing a permeable (leaky) gastrointestinal lining.[89] It is used in the synthesis of an important nutrient known as N-acetyl-D-glu-

Chinese Herbal Formulas

Traditional Chinese medicine (TCM), practiced for over 5,000 years, is complex and often difficult for Westerners to understand. One important concept in Chinese medicine is the free-flowing motion of *qi* (SEE QUICK DEFINITION) and blood through channels, or meridians, in the body. A Chinese medicine physician considers the flow of *qi* in a patient through close examination of the patient's pulse, tongue, body odor, voice tone and strength, and general demeanor, among other elements. Underlying imbalances and disharmony in the body are described in terminology analogous to the natural world (heat, cold, dryness, or dampness). The concept of balance, or the interrelationship of organs, is central to TCM. Disease arises when obstructions occur to impede the flow of *qi* and thus disturb the regulation of related organs and body systems. The primary symptoms of arthritis, according to TCM, are related to obstructions in the liver meridian, which governs the joints, tendons, sinews, ligaments, and muscles, and oversees their proper function.

According to Kim Vanderlinden, N.D., D.T.C.M., a naturopathic physician and doctor of traditional Chinese medicine who practices in Vancouver, B.C., Canada, Chinese herbs are classified by energetic functions (distinguished as cold, cool, warm, or hot) and the organs that their energies affect (lung, kidney, or liver). Similarly, the diseases that affect the human body are classified accordingly—by excess or deficient energy and organ imbalances. Inflammatory conditions are classified as an excess of hot and, after considering other factors, a cooling herb might be prescribed to balance the excess quality. Joint pain is characterized by wind or dampness and therapeutic herbs may dispel wind or damp. The following Chinese herbs are used, usually in combination with other herbs, to treat many aspects of a person's individual arthritic symptoms:

- Angelica Family (*Dong Quai, Du Huo, Chuan Xiong, Gao Ben, Qiang Huo, Fang Feng*)—These herbs are traditionally used to alleviate pain and to improve blood circulation. They work by dispelling wind and eliminating blockages to circulation. Angelica herbs also relax smooth muscle cells and have been used to treat arthritis, uterine cramps, trauma, and headaches.[90]

- Bai Shao and Chi Shao (White and Red Peony)—A cousin of the ornamental peony found

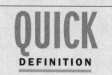

QUICK
DEFINITION

Qi (pronounced CHEE) is a Chinese word variously translated to mean "vital energy," "essence of life," and "living force." In Chinese medicine, the proper flow of *qi* along energy channels (meridians) within the body is crucial to a person's health and vitality. There are many types of *qi*, classified according to source, location, and function (such as activation, warming, defense, transformation, and containment). Within the body, *qi* and blood are closely linked, as each is considered to flow along with the other. *Qi* may be stagnant (non-moving), deficient (partially absent), or excessive (inappropriately abundant) in a given organ system. *Qi* has two essential qualities: yang (active, fiery, moving, bright, energizing) and yin (passive, watery, stationary, dark, calming).

in North American gardens, these medicinal peonies are frequently used to treat arthritis. They have an affinity for the liver and spleen meridians and invigorate blood. Both peonies are often mixed with other Chinese herbs, such as cinnamon, bupleurum, *dong quai*, licorice, and Chinese lovage, for broad-spectrum arthritis formulas.

■ Camphor (*Cinnamonium camphora*)—Camphor is used in traditional Chinese medicinal balms and salves for the treatment of myalgia (muscle pain) and joint pain. Camphor is used topically to break up stagnate blood, warm the meridians, conduct *qi*, and dispel wind and damp. It has a warming, anesthetic effect on the skin that eventually feels like a cool sensation and is often mixed with menthol to expel wind and heat from the body. These essential oils are available in plasters, an adhesive patch saturated with medicine that is applied to the affected area of the body for extended periods.

■ Clematis (*Radix clematis*)—A common ingredient in Chinese medicinal formulas, clematis expels damp wind and moves *qi*. An effective pain reliever, clematis is used to treat calcium deposits in the joints and calcium spurs in the synovial region of the joint, especially in gouty arthritis.

■ Niu Xi or Ox Knee (*Achyranthus bidentala*)—Closely resembling a segmented joint, this herb was used traditionally to strengthen the ligaments, tendons, and sinews, because of its tonic effect on both the liver and the kidneys. It is especially useful in treating swollen and painful knee joints and enhances the circulation of blood and

qi. Research on this plant shows that it can dramatically relieve pain, particularly when it is combined with ligusticum, aconiti, peony, ginseng, and licorice.[91]

■ Sheng Di Huang (*Rehmannia glutinosa*)—Rehmannia promotes muscle growth, lowers blood sugar, and nourishes yin and is used to treat damaged tendons and sprained joints.[92] In one clinical study with 12 subjects, all showed a marked decrease in joint pain and swelling, an increase in function, and a decrease in temperature. After two to seven weeks, there was a decrease in the biologic inflammatory markers in the blood indicating that inflammation had decreased. Follow-up within 3-6 months showed only one relapse, which was treated successfully with another round of rehmannia.[93] In Chinese medicine, rehmannia is prepared in several different ways (arranged here in descending order of potency): the fresh root, the dried root, and the root cooked and stir-fried in wine. Precautions: Some people can develop edema (water retention) after using rehmannia; patients with high blood pressure should be monitored closely while using this herb.

■ Siberian Ginseng (*Eleutherococcus senticosus*)—An all-purpose herb, Siberian ginseng can enhance the body's production of cortisol, a hormone that reduces pain. Siberian ginseng has a particular affinity for the extremities and removes excess fluid due to swelling. Thanks to its stress-reducing abilities, Siberian ginseng is also helpful for people coping with chronic pain and illness.

continued on next page

Chinese Herbal Formulas (cont.)

■ Xu Duan (*Radix dipsacus*)—Commonly used in formulas for osteoarthritis, *Radix dipsacus* tonifies the liver and kidneys, two of the organs most affected in arthritis. Dipsacus helps strengthen the bones and tendons and prevents damage from wear and tear. It also promotes the circulation of blood and helps "moisten" the joints.

■ Yan Hu Suo (*Corydalis ambigua*)—One of the most powerful Chinese herbs for pain, *Corydalis ambigua*, a member of the poppy family, is virtually unknown in the West.[94] *Corydalis* is also a sedative and is recommended for use at night when arthritis pains are too unbearable to sleep. *Corydalis* is often mixed with Chuan Xiong (*Ligusticum wallichiil*) for body aches and pains, joint inflammation, headaches, toothaches, and stomachaches. Another common mixture includes *Corydalis*, cinnamon, angelica, ligusticum, and lovage root. We recommend the patent medicine Yan Hu Suo Zhi Tong Pian (Corydalis Stop Pain Tablets) or BotanoDyne from Nature's Answer and this herb can also be bought in root form for preparation as a tincture.

For **Kim Vanderlinden, N.D., D.T.C.M.**: West Coast Clinic of Integrated Medicine, 601 W. Broadway, Suite 204, Vancouver, BC, Canada V5Z 4C2; tel: 604-873-0046. For more about **Chinese herbal medicine**, contact: American Association of Oriental Medicine, 433 Front Street, Catasauqua, PA 18032; tel: 610-266-1433; fax: 610-264-2768. To order **patent medicines**, contact: China Herbs, 6333 Wayne Avenue, Philadelphia, PA 19144; tel: 800-221-4372; fax: 215-849-3338. Crane Herb Company, 745 Falmouth Road, Mashpee, MA 02649; tel: 800-227-4118 or 508-539-1700; fax: 508-539-2369; website: www.craneherb.com. For **BotanoDyne**, contact: Nature's Answer, 320 Oser Avenue, Hauppauge, NY 11788; tel: 800-439-2324 or 516-231-7492; fax: 516-231-8391; website: www.naturesanswer.com.

Patent Medicines

The Chinese herbs described above are typically sold in combination remedies with other herbs. Referred to as patent medicines, these remedies are standardized formulas based on recipes that have been used for over 2,000 years. Now available as pills, ointments, or tinctures, patent medicines are easier to take than the traditional tea beverages made from the same ingredients. It is important to find a reliable manufacturer of patent medicines, one who doesn't include ingredients from endangered species, artificial colorings, or sugar coatings. Reputable manufacturers provide a list of ingredients and the symptoms that these ingredients can benefit on the label of their product. Follow the directions carefully and consult with a health-care practitioner before beginning a course of Chinese herbs. Specific patent medicines that are useful in arthritis include Guan Jie Yan Wan (for joint inflammation), Kang Gu Zeng Sheng Pian (for osteoarthritis and ankylosing spondylitis), Hong She Pills (for fibromyalgia and muscle aches), and Shang Shi Zhi Tong Gao (a topical plaster for pain).

cosamine (NAG), which is fundamental in the production of the protective mucus which lines the entire digestive and respiratory tract and the first line of defense against leaky gut syndrome. Glutamine supplementation has also been shown to enhance levels of glutathione, a fighter against free radicals.[95] Food sources: cabbage and okra. Typical therapeutic dose: in patients who have leaky gut syndrome, 3-10 g of glutamine per day, in divided doses between meals, can be very helpful.

Histidine—Histidine is essential for the growth and repair of tissues, maintains the fatty (myelin) sheaths that insulate nerves, and is important in the production of red and white blood cells. During times of stress, histidine is needed more than any of the other amino acids because of its antioxidant and anti-inflammatory properties.[96] In one study, low histidine levels were found in the blood and synovial fluid of patients with rheumatoid arthritis.[97] Patients who were suffering from rheumatoid arthritis received a daily dose of histidine (1 g), which improved their grip strength and ability to walk.[98] Food sources: pork, poultry, cheese, and wheat germ. Typical therapeutic dose: 1-5 g per day.[99] Supplementation should be monitored by measuring histidine levels in the blood and documenting any adverse reactions.

Phenylalanine—Phenylalanine is a building-block of the mood-regulating brain chemicals dopamine and norepinephrine. Typically used for depression, phenylalanine is very effective for arthritis sufferers who are depressed as a result of the pain caused by their illness.[100] Phenylalanine can also be effective for pain associated with rheumatoid arthritis and osteoarthritis due to its analegesic effect.[101] Food sources: meats, especially wild game. Typical therapeutic dose: 3-5 g daily of DL-phenylalanine, between meals on an empty stomach. Precautions: People suffering from phenylketonuria (PKU, a genetic inability to metabolize phenylalanine) should not use supplements or eat foods high in this amino acid.

Antioxidants

An antioxidant is a natural biochemical substance that protects living cells from the damaging effects of free radicals. Free radicals cause oxidation, the same chemical process that causes metal to rust and apples to turn brown. In the body, if left uncontrolled, free radicals cause cell membranes to erode and die, leading to joint dysfunction and other degenerative conditions.

Produced as a by-product of cellular activities, free radicals are typically neutralized and rendered harmless by antioxidants. But when environmental and other toxins (poor diet, pollution, stress, cigarettes) introduce an increased burden of free radicals, the body's reserve of antioxidants is quickly exhausted. Many studies have found that the levels of antioxidants in the blood of people suffering from arthritis are very low and may contribute to the onset and exacerbation of joint destruction and inflammation.

Types of Antioxidants

Amino Acids: cysteine, glutathione, methionine

Bioflavonoids: anthocyanin bioflavonoids (in fruit, especially grapes, cranberries, and bilberries), citrus bioflavonoids (in grapefruit, lemons, and oranges), oligometric proanthocyanidins (OPCs) in pycnogenol (pine bark or grape seed extract)

Carotene: alpha and beta carotene (in red, yellow, and dark green fruits and vegetables), lycopene (in red fruits and vegetables, such as red grapefruit and tomatoes)

Spices: cayenne pepper, garlic, turmeric

Herbs: astragalus, bilberry, ginkgo, green tea, milk thistle, sage

Minerals: copper, manganese, selenium, zinc

Vitamins: A, B1, C, and E, coenzyme Q10, NADH (nicotinamide adenine dinucleotide)

Enzymes: catalase, glutathione peroxidase, superoxide dismutase

Hormones: melatonin

Miscellaneous: lipoic acid

Bioflavonoids

The red of an apple or the many hues of peppers may seem only fanciful adornments, but the chemical pigments responsible for these colors can play an important disease-fighting role in the human body. Known as bioflavonoids, they boost the amount of vitamin C (an antioxidant) inside cells, strengthen capillaries, and fight damaging free radicals. They also have a unique ability to bind and strengthen collagen structures, which are vital for the integrity of connective tissue. Other beneficial effects on collagen include inhibition of enzymes that destroy collagen structures during inflammation and prevention of inflammation-enhancing substances. Health conditions that benefit from bioflavonoids include rheumatoid arthritis, periodontal disease, and other inflammatory problems. Bioflavonoids found in black cherries have been used to reduce uric acid levels and decrease tissue destruction associated with gout.[102] They also exhibit antimicrobial activity, which is helpful for arthritis linked to infections of microorganisms in the intestines.

There are over 4,000 bioflavonoid compounds found in different types of food. The bioflavonoid called anthocyanidin gives the deep red or blue color to blueberries, blackberries, cherries, grapes, and hawthorn berries, and is the most effective of all the bioflavonoid compounds in providing collagen support. Boosting dietary intake of foods containing anthocyanidins is beneficial for arthritis sufferers. Other bioflavonoid compounds include citrus bioflavonoids, catechins, quercetin, hesperidin, and proanthocyanidins. Food sources: fruits such as grapefruit, lemon, oranges, apples, apricots, pears, peaches, tomatoes, cherries, blueberries, cranberries, black currants, red grapes, plums, raspberries, strawberries, hawthorn berries, and other berries; vegetables such as red cabbage, onions, parsley, and rhubarb; herbs such as milk thistle and sage; grape skins, pine bark, red wine, and green tea. Supplements: an excellent bioflavonoid complex supplement is Joint Phyto-Nutrition from Nature's Answer. Typical dose of bioflavonoid complex: 250-500 mg, twice daily.

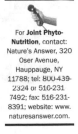

For **Joint Phyto-Nutrition**, contact: Nature's Answer, 320 Oser Avenue, Hauppauge, NY 11788; tel: 800-439-2324 or 516-231-7492; fax: 516-231-8391; website: www.naturesanswer.com.

Green Tea (Camellia sinensis)—Green tea contains the bioflavonoids called catechins, which have anti-inflammatory and antioxidant properties and are helpful in treating rheumatoid arthritis by destroying free radicals that act on synovial membranes.[103] Catechins bind with heavy metals to decrease their harmful potential. Green tea also contains other antioxidants, such as vitamins A (in the form of beta carotene) and C. Other benefits of green tea include a slight stimulating effect from a small amount of caffeine, as well as antimicrobial and cancer-fighting effects. Typical dose: 3-4 cups of organic green tea per day.

Quercetin—A bright yellow pigment, quercetin has outstanding anti-inflammatory properties useful in treating arthritis.[104] Quercetin inhibits uric acid production (beneficial for gout), regulates the release of pro-inflammatory chemicals, and decreases the number of leukotrienes (immune cells that cause inflammation). Quercetin is also useful in helping correct intestinal permeability (leaky gut syndrome) and allergies.[105] Food sources: onions and green tea. Supplements: quercetin works best when combined with the enzyme bromelain.[106] Typical dose: 200-1,000 mg daily.

Pycnogenol—Extracted from grape seeds or pine bark, pycnogenol contains proanthocyanidins, an antioxidant that is 50 times more powerful than vitamins C and E.[107] Proanthocyanidins can also

Essential Fatty Acids for Arthritis Relief

Essential fatty acids (EFAs) are unsaturated fats required in the diet. EFAs are converted into prostaglandins, hormone-like substances that regulate many metabolic functions, particularly inflammatory processes. Prostaglandins can either cause inflammation (pro-inflammatory) or decrease inflammation (anti-inflammatory), depending on which fatty acids are readily available as well as the presence of enzymes and nutrients needed for prostaglandin production. These nutrients include vitamins B3, B6, and C, magnesium, and zinc. There are two types of EFAs, omega-3 and omega-6 oils. More omega-6 is needed by the body than omega-3. However, in the case of arthritis, omega-6 oils can be converted into inflammation-causing agents when levels of arachidonic acid (SEE QUICK DEFINITION) are too high. Therefore, we recommend supplementing with omega-3 oils (from flax, hempseed, wild game, and free-swimming fish) only and avoiding food sources high in omega-6, including the vegetable oils safflower, corn, and peanut.

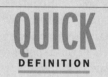

QUICK DEFINITION

Arachidonic acid is a fatty acid found primarily in animal foods such as meat, poultry, and dairy products, and to a lesser extent in fish. When the diet is abundant with arachidonic acids, these are stored in cell membranes; an enzyme transforms these stored acids into chemical messengers called prostaglandins and leukotrienes with instigate inflammation.

For information about the **importance of EFAs in reducing inflammation**, see Chapter 12: The Arthritis Diet, pp. 250-278.

increase the strength of collagen by cross-linking the fibers in the connective tissue matrix.[108] This makes the collagen more resistant to free-radical damage from the arthritic process. Therapeutic dosage: 50-300 mg per day.

Enzymes

Enzymes are an important component of the metabolism of all living organisms. In the body, there are over 3,000 different enzymes, each with a distinct task. Enzymes form new tissue, including bone, cartilage, muscle, and nerve cells. They are important in the normal detoxification processes as well, helping the body get rid of excess toxins and cellular debris (often found in people with degenerative illnesses such as arthritis). Enzymes are also responsible for digestion and the breakdown of foods into nutrients for use in the body. There are three primary enzymes that the body produces to digest foods: amylase digests starch, lipase digests fat, and protease digests proteins.

According to Lita Lee, Ph.D., an enzyme therapist in Lowell, Oregon, many people with arthritis are deficient in the enzyme protease, which digests protein of all kinds, including food proteins and proteins of foreign cells.[109] For this reason, protease is an effective anti-inflammatory that enhances the healing process and controls inflammation. When used to treat conditions involving calcium and bone problems, such as arthritis, osteoporosis, and gout, protease can help decrease inflammation and reduce soreness, swelling, and tenderness.[110]

Enzymes need to be taken on an empty stomach for treating pain and inflammation. To digest food and prevent food allergens and toxins from migrating from the colon to the bloodstream, they should be taken on a full stomach. Protease and other anti-inflammatory enzymes are also available from plant sources and those listed below help reduce inflammation, improve digestion, and fight infections:

Bromelain—Studies have found that bromelain, an enzyme found in pineapples, has anti-inflammatory properties as effective as conventional drugs such as prednisone.[111] According to clinical research, bromelain helps break down fibrin, a substance that accumulates in an inflamed area and blocks off blood and lymph fluid, causing swelling.[112] Bromelain also interferes with the production of prostaglandins (SEE QUICK DEFINITION) and other substances that contribute to inflammation and increases the production of prostaglandins that decrease inflammation. Bromelain can also act along with pancreatic enzymes to help clear the blood of allergens (foreign substances), which can contribute to or trigger inflammation. As a digestive aid, bromelain is usually used in combination with ox bile and hydrochloric acid.[113]

For anti-inflammatory effects, take bromelain on an empty stomach (taken with food, it helps improve digestion).[114] Juicing an organic non-irradiated pineapple along with half of an organic lemon, and a quarter- or half-inch piece of fresh ginger root, is an excellent way to get high amounts of bromelain into your system. But for consistent therapeutic value, supplements containing specific amounts of bromelain should be used. Typical therapeutic dose: 500-2,000 mg, three times daily. Precautions: Bromelain can cause sensitivity in people who are allergic to bee stings, olive tree pollen, or pineapple.[115] Those

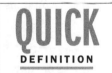

DEFINITION

Prostaglandins are hormone-like, complex fatty acids which affect smooth muscle function, inflammatory processes, and constriction and dilation of blood vessels. Essential fatty acids in the diet (omega-3 and omega-6, found in fish oils) provide the raw material for prostaglandin production; once ingested, these essential fatty acids can be converted to prostaglandins by nearly any cell in the body. Omega-6-derived prostaglandins can have either pro-inflammatory or anti-inflammatory properties, while most prostaglandins converted from omega-3 sources help reduce pain and inflammation. For proper body function, an appropriate balance of both types of prostaglandins must be maintained.

with a history of heart palpitations are advised to limit the dose of bromelain to 460 mg per day.[116]

Papaya—A tropical fruit, papaya contains the digestive enzyme papain, which has the power of digesting 300 times its own volume in protein. The skin of the fruit, especially when it is still green, has been used to treat ulcers and infectious wounds.[117] As with all digestive enzymes, papain helps to break down circulating immune complexes, which aggravate arthritis and inflammation. Papain is included in many digestive enzyme combinations, often along with bromelain and hydrochloric acid. Therapeutic dose: 250-500 mg daily.

Homeopathic Remedies

Homeopathic medicine, established in Germany in the 18th century, is based on three principles: like cures like (Law of Similars); the more a remedy is diluted, the greater its potency (Law of Infinitesimal Dose); and an illness is specific to the individual (a holistic medical model). According to homeopathy's founder, Dr. Samuel Hahnemann, disease can be permanently and rapidly reversed by using a medicine that is capable of producing (in the human system) the most similar and complete symptoms of the disease in a healthy person. Each homeopathic medicine is "proven" or tested in healthy people and their symptoms recorded. When treating ill patients, a homeopathic practitioner matches the patient's symptoms with a remedy that produced similar symptoms in a healthy person. Treating "like with like" works effectively to reverse disease because the homeopathic remedy works on an energetic level (having been diluted to the point that no chemical components remain).

Dr. Hahnemann found that the more a substance was diluted and shaken, the higher its potency. Homeopathic remedies are prepared in a series of dilution steps using water and succussing (vigorous shaking). Potency levels are designated with "X" and "C". The "X" means that the homeopathic remedy has been serially diluted on a 1:10 scale (one part substance to nine parts water) and the "C" means the remedy has been diluted on a 1:100 scale (one part substance to 99 parts water). A number value is placed before the scale designator to identify how many dilutions the remedy has undergone. A remedy designated "6X" has undergone six dilutions at one part substance to nine parts water; a remedy that is designated "12X" has undergone 12 dilutions and is stronger than the 6X remedy. Common potencies available over-the-counter are 6X, 12X, 30X, 6C, 12C, and 30C.

Hydrochloric Acid for Improving Digestion

Many people with arthritis are deficient in digestive factors (hydrochloric acid and pancreatic enzymes) needed to adequately break down food so that cells can absorb important nutrients. When digestion is incomplete or inadequate, food molecules can be inappropriately absorbed into the bloodstream, contributing to the onset of arthritis and other diseases.[118]

Inside the stomach, a very low pH (acid level) is needed to break down food. To maintain the optimal pH (around 2, which is very acidic), the stomach secretes hydrochloric acid (HCl). With age, HCl levels tend to decline, leading to impaired digestion. Research has shown that insufficient hydrochloric acid is common in people suffering from rheumatoid arthritis.[119]

In order to determine HCl levels, physicians use the Heidelberg Gastric Analysis. After a 12-hour fast, the patient swallows a Heidelberg capsule, a device about the size of a vitamin that has a pH meter and radio transmitter inside. Once the capsule is swallowed the patient drinks a solution of bicarbonate of soda, which stimulates the stomach to secrete hydrochloric acid. The capsule measures and transmits the changing pH levels to a receiver placed over the patient's stomach, indicating whether or not they are producing adequate HCl. The capsule can easily pass through the gastrointestinal tract for excretion.

A combination of physical symptoms can also indicate low levels of hydrochloric acid or a deficiency in digestive and pancreatic enzymes. If you answer "yes" to at least three of the questions below, your body may not be producing enough digestive enzymes for optimal digestion.

After eating, do you suffer from:

_____ gas?

_____ bloating?

_____ abdominal discomfort?

_____ undigested food in stool?

The correct dose of HCl supplementation can often be determined by independent experimentation. Typically, start with 600 mg of hydrochloric acid for a medium-size meal; if a warm sensation occurs in the stomach, then decrease the amount of hydrochloric acid for the following meals of the same size.

For more about the **Heidelberg Gastric Analysis**, contact: Heidelberg International, Inc., 933 Beasley Street, Blairsville, GA 30512; tel: 706-745-9698; fax: 706-781-6229.

Classical homeopathic remedies are prescribed for a patient based on each person's unique and distinguishing symptoms. This individualized prescription considers not only the physical symptoms but also the mental and emotional states as well. This is vastly different from conventional medicine, which will generally give one medicine to every patient for a specific disease condition. In homeopathy, any number of homeopathic remedies could be prescribed for that condition, but a specific remedy can be identified after reviewing the person's individual symptoms.

Building the Totality of Symptoms

The main symptom profile includes physical complaints, the effect of motion and temperature on pain, food cravings, and personality or emotional disposition. In homeopathy, the subjective quality of how a pain "feels" is extremely useful in identifying a remedy. When pursuing homeopathic treatment, pay attention to your pain and try to match it to the following categories:

- Sharp: stabbing, cutting, stitching, piercing, pricking. splinter-like, stinging
- Shooting: radiates from one location to another
- Stiff: constricted or contracted
- Pressing: squeezing, compressing, crushing, pinching
- Changeable: wandering in any direction or is hard to locate
- Burning: cold or hot needles
- Lame: dislocated, broken, sprained, or paralytic area
- Other types of pain: throbbing or pulsating, digging, twisting, drawing, pulling

Frequency and duration of symptoms are also important. Do they occur regularly at a particular time or in correlation with the weather? Do they come on strongly and persist for only a short time? In musculoskeletal diseases, physical signs are also part of the patient profile. The affected areas may be swollen and discolored (red, white, pale, waxy, or bruised), or hot or cold to the touch. Protrusions or bone deformities may be visible, especially on finger joints, as arthritis progresses. It is unusual for many Americans to consider that their emotional disposition factors into their physical ailments, but in homeopathy, these qualities are as important as the location and duration of pain. Homeopaths look for the following emotional patterns: restlessness, irritability, quick to overreact, or cries easily. A strong desire for rest or remaining still, a constant need for motion or activity, desire to be outdoors, or fear of crowds help construct the personality profile.

For **Ann Seipt, N.D.**: 3003 North Central, Suite 103-117, Phoenix, AZ 85012; tel: 602-274-1340; fax: 602-604-9655. For **referrals to practicing homeopaths in your area**, contact: National Center for Homeopathy, 801 North Fairfax, Suite 306, Alexandria, VA 22314; tel: 703-548-7790.

Common Homeopathic Remedies for Arthritis

There are many remedies that can be effective in treating arthritis, depending upon the type of arthritis, location of pain, affinity for warmth or cold, and emotional state. Below, Ann Seipt, N.D., a homeopathic practitioner in Phoenix, Arizona, describes the most commonly prescribed remedies based on their symptom profile. If a remedy is well-suited for your condition, you will experience immediate improvements or, in some cases, a healing crisis (a brief worsening of symptoms followed by improvement). If symptoms persist, however, it indicates an incorrect potency, dosage, or remedy, or perhaps deeper underlying problems. As with all medicinal substances, one should be cautious in self-prescribing homeopathic remedies and seek professional medical advice before beginning a homeopathic course of treatment.

Remedies for Inflammation

Apis mellifica (Apis): Symptoms of acute arthritis that comes on rapidly; wandering joint pain that feels stiff and sore to any pressure; burning and stinging pains; stiffness and lameness in the shoulder blades; edema (swelling) in affected parts; sensation of joints being stretched tightly; red or shiny white coloration in affected parts; pain and swelling worsen when the temperature is warm and improve from application of cold water.

Bryonia alba (Byronia or Bry.): Symptoms of pale, tense, and swollen joints that come on slowly, continuous, or remittent; stitching and tearing pains that are aggravated by motion and relieved after rest; desire to remain still and quiet; extremely irritable disposition; white-coated tongue; dry mouth and lips; no thirst or great thirst; frequent constipation.

Dulcamara (Dulc.): Symptoms of rheumatism during sudden changes of weather from hot and dry to cold and damp; rheumatic complaints alternating with diarrhea; rheumatism may follow the suppression of a skin eruption; "pins and needles" sensation in limbs.

Formica ruffa: Symptoms of intense pain that come and go suddenly; red and swollen joints typically in the right side of the body; swelling decreases when pressure is applied to the joint.

Kali bichromium (Kali bich. or Kali bi.): Symptoms of gouty pains alternating with gastric complaints; rheumatism in spring and summer; pains that occur at the same time every year; pain in small spots that wander within a period of a few days or weeks; pricking pain or stiffness all over; joint symptoms can alternate with diarrhea or nasal discharge.

Rhus toxicodendron (Rhus tox): Symptoms of painful joints, ligaments, tendons, and skin; joints are red, shiny, and swollen; stiffness and lameness of the affected parts; tearing and burning pain as if sprained; tendency to affect the left side of the body; stiffness compels the person to move around but pain worsens from over-exertion; pain relieved by warmth or massage, worsens in damp, cold weather; cravings for cold milk.

Remedies for Degenerative Changes

Causticum (Caust.): Symptoms of stiff and cracking joints, especially knees; contracted muscles and tendons in the fingers and palm of hand; contractions draw the limbs out of shape and cause deformed joints; aching shoulders; paralysis of deltoid muscle (triangular muscle covering the shoulder joint); symptoms decrease in damp weather and worsen in dry, cold weather; aversion to sweet foods and cravings for smoked meats.

Guaiacum: Symptoms of immovable stiffness of contracted parts; rheumatic pain worsens around heat and improves around cold; pain increases with slight motion and the affected part feels hot; nodosities (conspicuous protuberances) on the joints and contracted tendons, hamstrings, and left wrist; craving for apples and aversion to milk.

Ruta graveolens: Symptoms of pain in back or coccyx (lower end of spinal column) as if bruised; pain has an affinity for tendons and bones of the feet causing the patient to walk lightly; all body parts feel bruised, especially the right wrist and both feet; pain worsens around heat; thirst for ice-cold water.

Remedies for Arthritis in Small Joints

Actaea spicata: Symptoms of swelling and severe pain in the joints of the feet, hands, wrists, and ankles; stiffness increases after rest; weakness in the hands; swelling of the small joints during or after walking.

Colchicum: Symptoms of acute arthritis or gout of small joints; a white spot remains on skin after pressed by a finger; sudden onset or increase of tearing or stitching pain especially in the fingers; pain travels from left to right; dark red, swollen joints; enlarged gouty joint nodosities; dark urine with white sediment; may have thick nasal discharge; irritable disposition; sensitive to noise, light, or odors.

Ledum palustre (Ledum or Led.): Symptoms of arthritis starting in the feet and moving upward, especially in small joints; soreness in feet and soles; swelling of body parts that feel cold to the touch; tearing pain in joints, with accompanying weakness; pain changes place quickly with little or no swelling; pain improves with cold water or cold applications; pain worse at night when getting warm in bed; sensitive to wine; later stages will develop arthritic nodosities. This remedy is specific for Lyme disease.

Phosphorus (Phos.): Symptoms of arthritic wrists and finger joints; pains feel as if sprained or cut; pain usually occurs on the left side; back feels as if it is broken; stiffness of knees and the feet; stiffness in the morning; symptoms worsen with cold applications and improve with warm applications; stiffness is prominent, especially in neck, back, and shoulders, or when rising from a sitting position.

Rhododendron: Symptoms of arthritic nodes on smaller joints like the fingers, neck, and heel; pain worsens before a storm or from cold weather, but lessens once a storm begins; pain increases with rest and subsides with motion; sleep better with legs crossed.

Remedies for Arthritis in the Neck and Back

Cimicifuga racemosa (Cimicifuga or Cimic.): Symptoms of fibromyalgia, arthritis, and rheumatism, accompanied by great pain; rheumatism may alternate with depression; wandering pains that feel like an electric shock; frequent pains in the neck that cause stiffness; heat and swelling occurring in affected parts; fibromyalgia worse with menses; menstrual and uterine problems.

Ferrum phosphoricum (Ferrum or Ferr. p.): Symptoms of several joints affected at the same time; stinging and tearing pains that cause constant motion; pain improves from slow motion; face turns red with the least exertion.

Remedies for Arthritis in the Lower Back and Extremities

Berberis vulgaris: Symptoms of shooting, tearing, or burning pains radiating in low back muscles and knees; rapid change of pain within minutes or hours; sticking pain near the kidneys; lameness after walking a short distance; kidney stones or gallstones.

Kali carbonicum (Kali carb. or Kali c.): Symptoms of tearing pain in the small joints; sharp stitching pain in lumbar region that shoots into the buttocks or thighs; back pain; deformed joints; irritable with pain; sensitive to drafts or easily chilled.

Pulsatilla (Puls.): Symptoms of red, hot, and swelling knees and feet; erratic pains that shift rapidly from joint to joint or one-sided pains; drawing, tearing, and shifting pains; pain worsens at twilight or in a warm, stuffy room; craves fresh air and gentle exercise or motion; cries easily.

Lac caninum: Symptoms of rheumatism that migrate and alternate from one side to the other or from one site to another.

Ranunculus bulbosa: Symptoms of pain in nerves and muscles in the back, upper arms, and between ribs; pains tend to occur on the left side; pain worsens in a cold and damp place or when the temperature changes from warm to cold; pain worsens with motion; may be associated with herpes zoster (shingles); sensitive to wine.

14

Exercises and Physical Therapies

WHILE DAILY EXERCISE and physical activity are important components of any healthy lifestyle, they are an absolute necessity for people who suffer from arthritis. Regular exercise improves energy levels, provides nourishment for muscles and connective tissues, and maintains a healthy weight. By keeping muscles toned and fit, they can then adequately support joints, reduce pain and stiffness, and halt the progression of the disease.

The best exercise program for arthritis should target flexibility, strength, circulation of blood and lymph fluid, and relaxation. We recommend working with a qualified health-care practitioner or physical therapist to develop a daily routine to suit your specific type of arthritis and physical limitations. Start off slowly with home or office stretches, then add aerobic exercises. Isometric (resistance training) and aquatic exercises build muscle and increase flexibility without placing excess strain on joints. *Tai chi*, yoga, and other meditative exercises achieve the same goals as well as relaxing an anxious mind. Daily exercise should be further augmented by massage, acupressure, or other physical therapies that promote relaxation and improve the circula-

Exercises

- Stretches for Home and Work
- Exercises for Specific Parts of the Body
- Isometric Exercises
- Aquatic Exercise
- *Tai chi*
- *Qigong*
- Yoga

Physical Therapies

- Hydrotherapy
- Bodywork
- Energy Medicine

tion of blood and lymphatic fluid. You may want to incorporate therapeutic baths and other water treatments into your daily routine as well. Water has a therapeutic effect and can be used to improve circulation, detoxify the body of toxins, and initiate healing of internal organs. In this chapter, we discuss some of the most widely available physical therapies so that you and your health-care professional can determine which ones would be most beneficial.

Exercises

People with arthritis should ease into an exercise program and never try to do too much too quickly. Gentle stretches are an excellent way to gain flexibility and begin exercising joints and muscles. Other exercise therapies, including isometric and aquatic exercises, *tai chi*, *qigong*, and yoga, provide an effective workout without putting excessive strain on the body. They are also effective for relieving stress and focusing the mind.

Stretches for Home and Work
This program is designed to help reduce muscle tension and stress in the neck, shoulders, and back, with stretching routines to be done at work and at home.[1] It should be undertaken in conjunction with a sound exercise and nutrition program. See pages 316-318 for instructions and illustrations for this program.

Isometric Exercises
In arthritis, muscles stay abnormally contracted for long periods, causing a buildup of waste products in the muscle tissues and even a shortening of the muscle. This can starve portions of the cartilage (or discs in spinal arthritis), leading to degeneration and osteoarthritis. The goal of isometric exercises is to relax the muscle so that it will stretch to its normal length and move more freely, eliminating wastes and feeding cartilage more efficiently. An isometric exercise applies resistance (or force) to a contracted (stiffened) muscle in order to improve motion and flexibility. The basic premise is that a muscle is easier to stretch after it has been contracted for at least 10-15 seconds. In an isometric contraction, the muscle is opposed by an immovable force (a wall, for example); after holding the contraction, the muscle is relaxed and will then stretch with more ease.

CAUTION
You should feel tightness but never pain while doing these exercises. If you experience any pain, stop and check with your doctor.

Daily Office Routine

If you spend eight hours or more sitting at a desk or standing behind a counter, your joints and muscles are not receiving the proper amount of motion necessary for healthy flexibility. Be sure to take a break from your normal working position to walk around and stretch your muscles, which helps circulate nutrients to muscles and other tissues, or take a walk during your lunch break to reduce stress and avoid afternoon weariness. The stretches described below can be done at your desk throughout the day without interrupting your work schedule. Take a ten minute break to do these exercises and repeat the entire routine two to three times a day. Work into each stretch slowly and hold it steady for 15-30 seconds; do two to three repetitions of each position. Try to avoid a bouncing motion as this causes stress on your joints and remember to take deep, relaxing breaths during each stretch.

If exercise causes pain that persists for more than one hour, you are over-exercising, which can cause stress to the joints and cartilage and subsequent damage or deterioration. Aerobic exercises such as jogging are not recommended for patients with arthritis in the knees, hips, or ankles. The frequency, duration, and kind of any exercise program should depend upon the individual's weight, age, sex, the health of the cartilage, and many other factors. Consult with a health-care practitioner to design a program that will suit your individual profile.

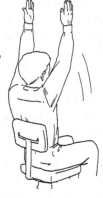

1 With arms straight at sides, raise them forward and upward over head, stretch, hold.

2 With hands clasped behind neck (dotted position), pull elbows together and hold. Bring elbows back out to side, hold.

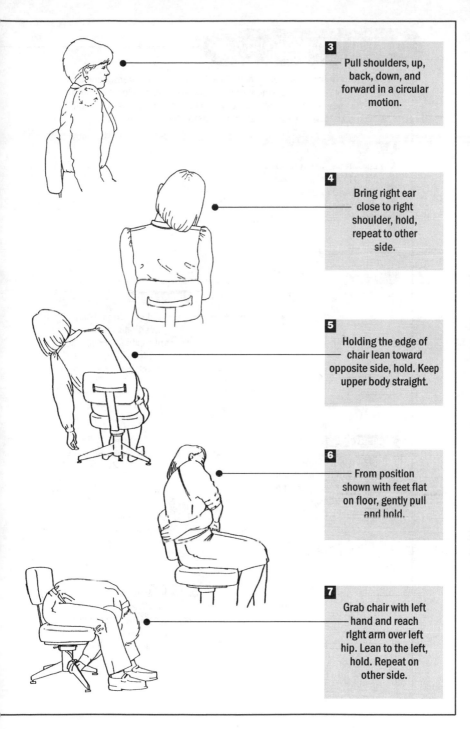

3 Pull shoulders, up, back, down, and forward in a circular motion.

4 Bring right ear close to right shoulder, hold, repeat to other side.

5 Holding the edge of chair lean toward opposite side, hold. Keep upper body straight.

6 From position shown with feet flat on floor, gently pull and hold.

7 Grab chair with left hand and reach right arm over left hip. Lean to the left, hold. Repeat on other side.

Daily Home Routine

The stretches described below can be done in the morning after waking or before going to bed at night. Do the entire routine and repeat particular stretches if that area of the body is tight or sore. Before beginning the routine, warm up your muscles with a brisk walk or a soak in a warm tub for 10-20 minutes.

Back

Lay flat on the floor. Pull knee to chest and raise the head to the knee. When stretch is felt, hold.

Upper Body

Sit in a chair. From position shown with arms extended twist the body and head until stretch is felt and hold.

Hamstrings

From position shown, using a belt or towel pull gently until stretch is felt and hold.

Shoulders

Put elbow behind the head. Gently pull elbow toward the center of back until stretch is felt hold.

Exercises for specific parts of the body

These exercises target the head, neck, shoulders, and back. For many people, stress and tension tend to build up in these areas, causing muscle contractions and pain. Do these exercises two to three times per day to stretch contracted muscles and strengthen weakened joints. When doing these stretches, concentrate on breathing to provide a deeper, more relaxed stretch.

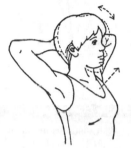

Base of head and neck

A. With chest up, tuck chin down and in, as if rocking head on neck. Do not bend neck or bob head. Do not hold breath while nodding.

B. Turn head to left and repeat A, then turn head to right and repeat A.

Neck, shoulders, and upper back

This is the starting/ending position. Can be done sitting or standing.

While exhaling, turn head slightly and pull head/neck down in a diagonal direction. Release pressure from hand on head.

When head reaches the end point in B, maintain pressure and rotate head away from arm about 40°. Repeat this rotation motion several times before returning to position A, then repeat. Do to both sides.

Exercises for specific parts of the body

Upper Back Stretch

With chin in, arms straight, raise upper back toward ceiling, inhale. Relax, exhale, and lower spine letting shoulder blades come close to each other.

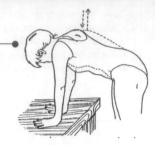

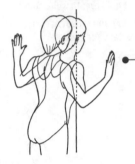

Upper Chest, Shoulders

With hands at prescribed level, lean in toward corner keeping chest up and exhaling.

Shoulder & Middle Back

Interlock fingers and raise arms as high as possible while exhaling. Keep chest up, chin in.

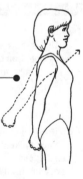

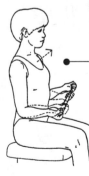

Shoulder Rotation

Holding rubber tubing move hands apart while exhaling and pinching shoulder blades together slightly. Keep elbows bent to 90° and at sides, chest up.

A Simple Isometric Exercise

If you have an elbow that causes pain when straightened, you can do the following isometric exercise:

- Straighten the arm out to the point where it begins to cause discomfort and hold it there.

- Grab the wrist of that hand with your other hand, hold it firmly in place and then continue to attempt to straighten the elbow, applying gentle force in the opposite direction with the arm that is holding it, for a count of ten seconds.

- Release your hold on the wrist. Relax the injured arm and attempt to straighten it further. When you release the opposing force, you will find that it can move more easily.

Doing this several times a day, for about 15 seconds for each stiff joint, should increase mobility of the joint and decrease pain in about a week. If pain persists or increases in intensity after a day or two, stop doing the exercise and consult your health-care practitioner. Flexibility can be further increased by rubbing an analgesic salve on the joint or using a hot pack before stretching. We recommend using BotanoGesic Salve, which contains all natural ingredients, including menthol and capsicum.

For information about **BotanoGesic Salve**, contact: Nature's Answer, 320 Oser Avenue, Hauppauge, NY 11788; tel: 800-439-2324 or 516-231-7492; fax: 516-231-8391.

Aquatic Exercise

Water exercises make the muscles work harder because of the water's increased resistance, but the body's buoyancy diminishes shock and trauma to bones and joints. Swimming is one of the best water exercises and can be used as an aerobic exercise if continued for 20 minutes or more. Try different strokes to exercise different muscles and joints. Using flotation devises like kickboards and water wings can give more support to the body than unassisted swimming. If the lower half of the body needs special attention, walking in water is also highly recommended; the faster you walk, the greater the resistance the muscles encounter and the better the workout. There are also water aerobics classes available at local gyms or health clubs.

Tai Chi

Tai chi is a unique Chinese system of slow, continuous, flowing movements that create a sense of tranquillity, vitality, and calmness. *Tai chi* is perfectly designed for arthritis sufferers, because there is little impact (no bouncing motions). It is gentle and yet effective in stretching muscles, loosening and lubricating the joints, and circulating the blood. Traditional Chinese medicine holds that *tai chi* stimulates and nourishes the body's internal organs by circulating *qi* (SEE QUICK DEFINITION), facilitates emotional and mental well-being, and teaches the mind how to control the body.[2] The art of *tai chi* can be practiced by almost anyone and movements can be modified for those with arthritis.

Qigong

Similar to *tai chi*, *qigong* (also referred to as chi-kung) is an ancient exercise that stimulates and balances the flow of *qi* along acupuncture meridians (energy pathways). *Qigong* cultivates inner strength, calms the mind, and restores the body to its natural state of health. Although less artistic and dynamic than *tai chi*, *qigong* is much easier to learn and can be done by the severely disabled as well as the healthy. *Qigong* practice can range from simple calisthenics-type movements with breath coordination to complex exercises that direct brain-wave frequencies, deep relaxation, and breathing to improve strength and flexibility and reverse damage caused by prior injuries and disease.

Qigong can be especially helpful to arthritis patients because it initiates relaxation, moderates pain and depression, and regulates the immune system, according to Roger Jahnke, O.M.D., director of the Health Action Clinic of Santa Barbara College of Oriental Medicine, in Santa Barbara, California. It also enhances the lymphatic flow, which improves the ability of the body to detoxify and deliver vital, replenishing nutrients to target tissues. *Qigong* can also balance the function of hormone-producing glands, which mediate pain and mood. Dr. Jahnke cites a group of arthritis patients who have been regular participants in *qigong* classes. "After approximately six months, several patients remarked that the stiffness and pain in their hands had diminished and the deformed knuckles characteristic of arthritis had begun to return to normal. The most incredible thing about *qigong* practice is that people actually can feel the operation of the physiological mechanisms of healing in their body. The increase of blood and lymph flow and a shift in neurotransmitters [chemical messengers in the brain] creates a sensation that is clearly perceptible to the individual."[3]

Yoga

Yoga is one of the most ancient systems of self-healing practiced today. Yoga teaches a basic principle of mind/body unity: if the mind is chronically restless and agitated, the health of the body will be compromised. Similarly, if the body is in poor health, mental strength and clarity will be adversely affected. The art of yoga can bring about harmony and oneness of mind, body, and spirit.

Classical yoga is divided into eight branches that give guidance as to the proper diet, hygiene, detoxification regimes, and physical/psychological practices to help the individual integrate their personal, psychological, and spiritual awareness. The most well-known and popular of the yogic branches is Hatha yoga, which teaches certain *asanas* (postures) and breathing techniques to create profound changes in the body and mind. The two types of *asana*, therapeutic and meditative, are designed to improve health and physical well-being and were originally prescribed for those with neck, back, and joint pain. According to Ameni Harris, a nutritionist and yoga teacher trained at the Integral Yoga Ashram in Buckingham, Virginia, yoga can benefit most illnesses if done on a regular basis. One goal of yoga is to harness and stimulate the flow of *prana*, or life energy (similar to *qi* in the Chinese system). The blockage of *prana*, because of improper diet, lifestyle stressors, or imbalance in one's physical, emotional, or spiritual health, can lead to illness. Breathing techniques and duration of holding certain postures remove barriers to the flow of *prana* and can improve oxygen intake by as much as seven times over a normal breath, according to Harris.[1]

"Yoga's profound positive benefits on arthritis stem from its effects on many systems, including the musculoskeletal, lymphatic, endocrine, and immune system,"

For **Ameni Harris'** **yoga and stress management instructional guide or video**, contact: Ameni Harris, 37 Geraldine Circle, Trumbull, CT 06611; tel: 203-261-6256.

For more about **yoga postures**, see *Alternative Medicine: The Definitive Guide* (Future Medicine Publishing, 1995; ISBN 1-887299-33-5); to order, call 800-333-HEAL.

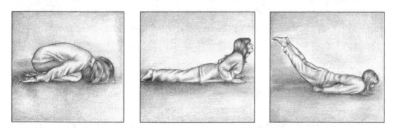

Yoga postures or *asanas*: child's posture, cobra, and locust.

QUICK
DEFINITION

explains Harris. In addition to improving circulation of blood, lymph, and *prana*, yoga corrects imbalances of hormones by regulating chakras (the energy centers that correspond to hormone-producing glands). The lymphatic system (SEE QUICK DEFINITION) doesn't have a pump of its own, instead it depends on movement of the body to transport fluid in and out of tissues. When a person is inactive or motion is imbalanced, the lymphatic fluid can become stagnant and create disease. Through yoga's stretches and postures, lymphatic fluid is pumped throughout the body, removing toxins and waste products from cells and delivering fresh nutrients. The health of all cartilage is dependent on this very process.

"Anyone can do yoga, no matter what age or shape you are in," states Harris. "Even if you are very ill, you can begin with gentle, modified postures, using props, pillows, or the wall to buttress you in weakened areas. Before pursuing a yoga practice, discuss it with a physician and seek out a qualified yoga teacher for proper instruction. Videos are also excellent tools for the beginner, because it is important to see the postures being performed." The safest and most reliable way to use yoga therapeutically is to follow a balanced program of postures to achieve an overall normalizing and health-inducing effect. It is best for the beginner to start with a simple program of basic postures. A structured course can teach the fundamental breathing techniques and postures for exercises later practiced on one's own.

Physical Therapies

A number of physical therapies, including hydrotherapy, bodywork (massage, rolfing, osseous manipulation, oriental body therapies, reflexology), and energy medicine (microcurrent therapy, magnet therapy), can be effective in treating all types of arthritis.

Hydrotherapy

Hydrotherapy is the use of water, ice, steam, and hot and cold temperatures to maintain and restore health. Treatments include full body immersion, steam baths, saunas, and the application of hot and cold compresses. Therapeutically, hot water soothes and relaxes the body, muscles, and connective tissues, according to Douglas Lewis, N.D., chair of the Physical Medicine Department at Bastyr University in Seattle, Washington. Applications of hot water produce a response that stimulates the immune system and causes white blood cells to clean up toxins and assist in eliminating wastes. Organs are affected through the reflex action of the surface nerves located in the skin. Cold water, on the other hand, discourages inflammation by means of vasoconstriction (narrowing the blood vessels) and making the blood vessels less permeable; cold water also tones muscular weakness. When applications of hot and cold water are alternated (known as contrast hydrotherapy), their therapeutic benefits are combined. Contrast therapy stimulates the endocrine system, liver, skin, and lymphatic system. It also improves circulation of fresh blood (containing oxygen, nutrients, and hormones) to the tissues and removal of waste products (such as inflammatory molecules and carbon dioxide).

Naturopathic physicians are trained in hydrotherapy. For **referrals to naturopathic practitioners in your area**, contact: American Association of Naturopathic Physicians, 2366 Eastlake Avenue, Suite 322, Seattle, WA 98102; tel: 206-323-7610.

Clinical Applications of Hydrotherapy—

The following applications of hydrotherapy require supervision by a trained health-care practitioner:

■ Contrast Hydrotherapy: No other therapy can initiate a sense of relaxation, well-being, and relief from spasm and pain as well as whole-body contrast hydrotherapy. The treatment begins with a 10-15 minute session in a whirlpool/Jacuzzi, Finnish sauna, or Russian steam cabinet. After the patient's body has warmed, the practitioner sprays cool water on the patient, starting on the back of the legs and working up the back along the spine, trunk, and head. The cool spray lasts for about 30 seconds. This process is repeated on the front side of the patient for another 30 seconds. The patient immediately returns to the source of heat for three to four minutes. After returning to the heat, they should feel a pleasant tingling sensation, which is caused by the dilation of blood vessels. The application of alternating cold and hot is repeated two more times, ending in a shorter cool application. Contrast applications to arthritic joints and tight muscles are the most effective therapy for increasing blood flow through an area. It aids in removing wastes (which cause pain and inflammation) from joints and connective tissues and helps bring nutrients and oxygen into the area.[5] It also increases the functional activity of the

⚠CAUTION⚠

Low blood pressure upon standing rapidly may occur during hydrotherapy. Patients taking hypertension medication should proceed with caution Although rare, patients have fainted from this therapy. Follow all contrast hydrotherapy by drinking 8 oz of mixed vegetable juice.

For more about **detoxifying fat-stored chemicals and other toxins**, see Chapter 4: General Detoxification, pp. 78-100.

organs; for example, a cool spray of water over the small of the back where the kidneys and adrenal glands are located increases the function of these organs.

■ Hyperthermic Hydrotherapy: Hyperthermia deliberately induces fever in the patient who is unable to mount a natural fever response. Fever is helpful for the body; it is an intelligent response to an internal imbalance or invader and stimulates the immune system by increasing the production of antibodies and white blood cells. Hyperthermia is used in arthritis for detoxification of fat-stored chemicals and drug residues, lymphatic stimulation, or treatment of infections.

The entire hyperthermia procedure takes about 75-90 minutes and includes immersion of the entire body in hot water, followed by a sweating period, and a tepid shower. Before beginning the treatment, the patient should empty his/her bladder. The practitioner records the patient's temperature, pulse, and blood pressure, then the patient is given a cup of tea (peppermint, yarrow, elder, ginger, cayenne, or boneset) and climbs into the whirlpool/Jacuzzi. The temperature of the water should be 104°-106° F and maintained at this level throughout the treatment. The patient is immersed in the water to raise the body temperature; by immersing more body surface area, temperature will increase more rapidly. A wash cloth dipped in ice water should be used as a cold compress for the patient's head and brow; liberal use of the compress is advised (if using a sauna, use a cup of water and periodically pour over the body). Oral temperature and pulse should be taken every 5-10 minutes. Once their temperature reaches 103° F, the patient is helped out of the water and escorted to a bed to begin the second phase of the treatment, the diaphoretic, or sweating, period.

The patient is wrapped in sheets and covered with five to seven layers of wool blankets. Under the blankets, the patient will begin to sweat profusely. We have found that sweating occurs even in people who report a difficult time perspiring. It is important to create a relaxed atmosphere during treatment—soothing or meditative music can be used to induce sleep or a sense of calm. This phase of the treatment usually lasts for an hour, by which time the patient's temperature has dropped to 99° F. A tepid shower will return the body temperature to normal. Vegetable juice or trace-mineral water can be sipped after the shower. The patient should return home and rest, as this treatment can be exhausting.

Using Hydrotherapy at Home—Many of the hydrotherapy techniques used in spas or clinics can be performed in the comfort of your own home, with little equipment or expense.

■ Baths and Showers: A common fixture in every home, bathtubs or showers are the easiest and cheapest form of home hydrotherapy. Baths and showers are soothing, both mentally and physically, help relieve general aches and pains, and can also ease internal congestion and digestive problems. Hot baths and showers stimulate the immune system and induce detoxification through perspiration. Cold baths and showers tone muscles and reduce inflammation. Alternating between cold and hot (contrast hydrotherapy) can also be used to increase circulation of blood and lymphatic fluid. We advise warming the body with a hot shower (at a tolerable temperature) for five minutes and then changing the temperature of the water to warm (for two minutes) and finally to cold (for one to two minutes). Repeat the hot-and-cold cycle three times, always ending with cold water.

■ Whirlpool Baths: We prescribe whirlpool baths for all of our arthritis patients. Whirlpools can rehabilitate injured muscles and joints and alleviate the stresses and strains of everyday life. Although most gyms and clinics have whirlpools, many people with arthritis have found that installing one in

Mineral Baths

Some of the most therapeutic baths come directly from the earth. For instance, seawater contains a similar balance of minerals to that found in human blood. Soaking in the ocean or a bath of dissolved sea salt (Celtic or Dead Sea salts, which are prepared through evaporation of seawater) can help rebalance the body's mineral ratios, which is especially helpful for arthritis sufferers with mineral deficiencies.[6] Because seawater so closely resembles human blood, these minerals can be readily absorbed by the skin in a form that cells can use.

Natural springs are also a source of concentrated minerals such as sodium, calcium, magnesium, and sulfur. Sulfur is especially helpful for rheumatic and arthritic complaints. A vital component of cartilage and synovial fluid, sulfur is typically lower than normal in the joints of many people with arthritis. Bathing in sulfur-rich fluid may initiate cartilage formation and pain relief.

Other therapies include immersion in mineral-rich mud. Originally used in the healing spas of Europe, fango is a combination of mineral-rich clay, anti-inflammatory herbs, and paraffin wax especially useful for arthritis. Fango clay is heated to approximately 116° F and applied as a localized heat pack on problem joints and muscles. The clay molds to the body like a cast and the healing minerals (such as sulfur) and powerful botanicals are absorbed by the skin. Blood flow and metabolic activity increases as capillaries enlarge and pores open, releasing waste products. Other muds, such as Green Argilite Mud, can be used in place of fango.[7]

For information about **body masks and mud preparations**, contact: Gurney's Inn, 290 Old Montauk Highway, Montauk, NY 11954; tel: 800-848-7639 or 516-668-2509; website: www.gurneysweb.com.

Aromatherapy Can Help Arthritis Sufferers

Aromatherapy uses the essential oils of plants for medicinal purposes. Through steam distillation or cold-pressing, the volatile constituents of the plant's oil are extracted from its flowers, leaves, branches, or roots. Essential oils contain beneficial vitamins, minerals, enzymes, and hormones that are easily absorbed into the body's tissues. The benefits of essential oils can be obtained through inhalation or external application. Diffusers are devices that disperse tiny particles of essential oils into the air in any room; inhaling these oils can affect the portion of the brain that controls heart rate, blood pressure, breathing, memory, stress, and hormone balance. Diffused oils are particularly helpful for decreasing muscle tension and increasing relaxation.

For the arthritis sufferer, aromatherapy can reduce inflammation and pain in aching and stiff joints. Aromatherapy can also address other factors involved in arthritis, such as calming and dispelling anxiety and addressing infections or other underlying causes of the disease. The following are particularly helpful for arthritis:

■ Cedarwood: promotes elimination through mucous membranes and acts as an antiseptic and sedative

■ Wintergreen, menthol, and camphor: anti-inflammatory herbs, cooling (apply topically to inflamed joints)

■ Clove, cinnamon, and thyme: anti-inflammatory effects, heating (use with arthritis that is worse in cold, damp weather)

■ Lemon: increases urine flow and acts as an antiseptic

■ Rose: stimulates liver and stomach functions and acts as an antidepressant

■ Tea tree: enhances skin function and can be used as an anti-fungal and antibiotic

Include essential oils in baths, saunas, soaks, and showers to increase the therapeutic value. Essential oils can also be added directly to warm compresses wrapped on a joint to soothe pain. Since the oils are readily absorbed through the skin, direct topical application of oils is extremely beneficial. However, true essential oils can be very strong and may irritate sensitive skin, so usually a few drops of essential oil are diluted in a carrier oil, such as almond or sesame oil.

When purchasing essential oils, watch for labels that state "pure botanical perfume" or "pure fragrance essence." This is a sure indication that the oils are not true "essential" oils, but rather synthetic chemicals have been added. A completely "pure" product is expensive because of the labor and time required to produce it. Up to 1,000 pounds of raw plant material is needed to produce one pound of essential oil, but a little bit of a quality product goes a long way. Chemical components of essential oils are easily altered by exposure to sun or heat; always keep essential oils in dark containers away from damp, moist, or warm places. Essential oils are also sensitive to oxidation when exposed to the air, so keep the bottle tightly sealed. When properly stored, they should remain fresh for one year.

For information on **aromatherapy products**, contact: Amrita Aromatherapy, P.O. Box 2178, Fairfield, IA 52556; tel: 800-410-9651 or 515-472-9136.

their home is affordable and easy. The cost of installing a whirlpool into your home for medical purposes may even be tax deductible, according to Robert Greene, C.P.A., C.M.A., of Staatsburg, New York. To qualify as tax deductible, these expenses must be prescribed in writing by a physician or licensed health-care practitioner "for the mitigation, treatment or prevention of disease or for the purpose of affecting any structure or function of the body." Save receipts and check with your tax advisor to see if your medical expenses qualify.

In a whirlpool or bathtub, you can prepare the following bath for relief of aches and pains: dissolve five or more pounds of Epsom salts or Dead Sea salt or ten drops of lavender essential oil in a bathtub of hot water. Soak for 10-15 minutes and use a cold compress to keep your forehead and head cool. Follow the bath with a cold shower. Perform this soak four times per week if you are in severe pain or twice a week for less debilitating conditions. Epsom salts and Dead Sea salt (prepared by evaporating water from the Dead Sea) are available at grocery or health food stores, drug stores, or through the Internet.

■ Compresses and Packs: These are particularly effective for applying heat or cold to specific parts of the body to relieve muscle spasms, produce local hyperthermia (fever), and help relieve pain.

Hot Packs—Use a commercial hot pack or hot water bottle; if these are not available, use towels that have been soaked in hot water (the water should be hot, but not unbearable). Prepare hot packs to 120° F. Place two or three layers of toweling over the area to be treated, place hot packs on toweling, and cover with an insulating layer of towels. Leave the pack in place for five to 20 minutes; packs may need to be reheated if they cool too much. Follow with a 30-second cold application. Local redness and perspiration will occur indicating circulation of oxygen and nutrients to the area. A number of herbs, oils, and minerals may be used in this procedure for enhanced therapeutic benefits: chamomile (soothes skin, opens pores, eliminates blackheads, aids digestive problems, and promotes sleep), ginger (relaxes sore muscles, improves circulation, and tones the skin), oat straw (relieves sore feet, ingrown toenails, and blisters), and sage (stimulates the sweat glands). Prepare herbs as if preparing a tea or add tinctures or oils directly to a small hot water basin. Soak a towel in the basin, wring out,

CAUTION

Always use the "buddy system" before attempting to enter a hot-water bath or whirlpool for an extended period. Consult with a physician before using a new therapy, especially if you are on prescription medication or have any cardiovascular, thyroid, lung, or diabetic conditions, or are pregnant. Use caution when entering and exiting any potentially slippery area. Get out of a hot bath slowly and carefully; be ready to put your head in a lower position than your body if you feel faint or dizzy. Direct hydrotherapy over the kidneys (if a person has kidney stones) or the liver (if a person has gallstones) can cause the stones to move, creating a medical emergency. Constantly monitor the skin if using cold or hot application for thermal effects.

and apply directly to the skin; cover with an insulating layer. Precautions: Always test a small area of skin for sensitivity to heat or herbs. In general, hot packs wrung from hot tap water are the safest; carefully monitor the skin to avoid burning.

Ice Packs—Helpful in reducing swelling, inflammation, pain, or congestion, ice packs are easy to prepare and inexpensive. Prepare an ice pack by freezing water in waxed paper cups. Once completely frozen, remove from the freezer and peel away a portion of the paper cup. Hold onto the remaining paper cup and rub the exposed portion of the ice over joints, muscles, or painful area. Use for 20 minutes or less and then rest for five minutes before applying ice again; repeat two to three times. Precautions: Applying ice for longer than 20 minutes at a time can cause blood vessels to dilate, creating more inflammation; take frequent breaks so as not to frost the skin.

Heat Compresses—This method starts with a cold compress that is eventually heated by the body. It is recommended for edema, inflammation, and redness occurring in joints or an area of trauma. The compress encourages blood flow and increased metabolic activity in the area. Soak a cotton cloth in ice water and then wring it out, apply it to the area to be treated, cover the cotton cloth with a piece of wool cloth, and wrap plastic around the material and secure in place. Leave the wrap in place for several hours; after the cool sensation wears off, the body will warm the compress. This is an excellent application to leave on overnight or when napping. Variations: A heat compress can also be used after a hot application to remove blood from the treated area.

Bodywork

Hands-on therapies, such as massage, deep tissue manipulation, movement awareness, and energy balancing, are used to improve the structure and functioning of the human body. Bodywork in all its forms helps to reduce pain, soothe injured muscles, stimulate blood and lymphatic circulation, and promote deep relaxation.

Massage—Massage is used for general well-being, stress reduction, resolution of embedded emotions or psychological problems, recovery from sports injuries or muscle soreness, or as an adjunct therapy for medical conditions. According to Thomas Hudak, L.M.T., of Southbury, Connecticut, massage is one of the most important therapies for the treatment of arthritis and fibromyalgia. People with arthritis often experience prolonged muscle tension, which interferes with the elimination of chemical wastes in the muscles and surrounding tissues. Poor circulation in muscle tissues can cause nerve and muscle pain, which may spread to other areas of the body. A nerve that supplies the muscles also supplies the supporting structures of the joint. Pains that seem to emanate from the joints may actually be coming from "trigger points," focal areas where wastes have accumulated in the muscles. Massage helps break up muscular waste deposits and stimulates circulation to troubled regions in the body. Deep pressure on trigger points stretches tissues and loosens shortened muscles to restore muscular balance and proper functioning. Most importantly, certain types of pain can be relieved by massage, as the rhythmic motions sedate the nervous system and promote voluntary muscle relaxation. We recommend that patients with arthritis should pursue a program of massage at least two to three times per week in the early treatment stages, then once a week for several months, with a maintenance schedule of twice a month. Remember, massage therapies should be designed to fit individual profiles, including physical needs and economic limitations.

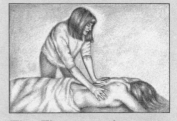

The Therapeutic Effects of Massage

Gertrude Beard, R.N., R.P.T., former associate professor of Physical Therapy at Northwestern University Medical School, summarizes the findings of numerous research studies on the therapeutic effects of massage. Studies indicate that massage helps to:

■ Sedate the nervous system and promote voluntary muscle relaxation

■ Relieve certain types of pain

■ Provide effective treatment of chronic inflammatory conditions by increasing lymphatic circulation

■ Improve circulation through the capillaries, veins, and arteries, and increase blood flow through the muscles

■ Trigger reflex actions in the body to stimulate organs

■ Promote recovery from fatigue

Rolfing—Rolfing, also referred to as "structural integration," is a unique system of soft-tissue manipulation to restore flexibility and improve muscle function and body motion. Developed by biochemist Ida P. Rolf, Ph.D., Rolfing repositions the head, thorax, pelvis, and/or legs so that they are correctly aligned with gravity's force. According to Dr. Rolf, if the body is struggling against gravity to maintain imbalanced postures (standing, walking, or sitting), the muscles become more contracted over time and eventually the fascial tissues (the sheet of connective tissues that envelop muscles, tissues, and organs) begin to break down.[8] This stress causes the fascial tissues to lose their elasticity and become solid, rigid, or sticky, restricting movement of muscles and joints. Eventually osteoarthritis can set in as joints are abnormally compressed and the protective coating between bones deteriorates. Dr. Rolf also observed that physical dysfunction caused the onset of further chronic illness, fatigue, and emotional and psychological problems.

Dr. Rolf reasoned that by manually manipulating and stretching the fascial tissues, she could change the posture and biomechanics of the patient's movement. By applying pressure with the fingers, knuckles, or elbows, the practitioner reorganizes the fascial tissues so that the body's segments regain balance. Educational classes (called Rolfing Movement Education) help the person develop more balanced posture and movement. Our patients with osteoarthritis who had Rolfing sessions experienced improvement in everyday motions. They reported feeling less strain when walking, doing housework, or standing. X rays of their affected joints revealed that erosion of cartilage and bone surrounding the joint had decreased. We have also found that chiropractic adjustments to the spine or other joints remain in alignment longer if the patient completes at least ten sessions of Rolfing treatment. The combination of bodywork, education, and reinforcement of proper posture helps bones to stay in alignment after they are manipulated.

Osseous Manipulation—Osseous manipulation is the repositioning of bones, including the bones of the spinal column, cranium, and other moveable joints. Chiropractors as well as naturopathic or qualified osteopathic physicians are trained and licensed to practice this type of therapy. Chiropractic is concerned with the relationship of the spinal column and the musculoskeletal structures of the body to the nervous system. The nervous system holds the key to the body's incredible potential to heal itself because it controls the functions of all other systems of the body. The spinal column acts as a "switchboard" for the nervous system—when there is interference caused by slight misalignments of the spine (called subluxations), the transmissions of the nervous system can be altered, like an electrical wire which has been impinged. This not only causes localized pain in the spine, but can interfere with neurological information being transmitted to the major organs and cause dysfunction or disease. By adjusting the spine to remove subluxations, normal nerve function can be

For information on **massage**, contact: American Massage Therapy Association, 820 Davis Street, Suite 100, Evanston, IL 60201; tel: 312-761-2682. Thomas Hudak, L.M.T., 190 High Meadow Drive, Southbury, CT 06488; tel: 203-264-0866. For more information about **rolfing**, contact: International Rolf Institute, P.O. Box 1868, Boulder, CO 80306; tel: 303-449-5903.

For more on **chiropractic**, contact: American Chiropractic Association, 1701 Clarendon Blvd., Arlington, VA 22209; tel: 703-276-8800. For **acupressure techniques and referrals**, contact: American Oriental Bodywork Association, 6801 Jericho Turnpike, Syosset, NY 11791; tel: 516-364-5533.

restored. Manipulation can help arthritis (particularly osteoarthritis in the spine) by restoring proper movement and positioning of the joints. Balanced movement prevents "wear and tear" damage to joints, ligaments, and cartilage. Frequent osseous manipulations help decrease the accumulation of scar tissue after injury, thus preventing later osteoarthritic changes in the joints. Chiropractic adjustments, combined with proper nutrition can improve and, in some cases, reverse osteoarthritis.[9]

Oriental Bodywork—The oriental body therapies, such as acupuncture or acupressure, work to balance the flow of *qi* (vital life energy) through energy meridians. These meridians run throughout the body and are associated with different organs—if there is a block in the energy meridian, it will be expressed as health problems in the organs associated with the blocked meridian. Blocked *qi* can be released by applying pressure to specific points along the energy meridians. Acupuncture uses needles, while acupressure (such as shiatsu and *Jin Shin Do*) uses rubbing, kneading, or other types of pressure from the fingers and hands.

Shiatsu means "finger pressure" in Japanese and was originally developed from ancient Chinese acupressure techniques. Shiatsu uses a sequence of firm rhythmic pressure applied to specific points for 3-10 seconds and, like acupuncture, is designed to awaken, calm, and harmonize the meridians. Shiatsu affects not only the acupressure point, but the entire mind and body, making it one of the most effective forms of bodywork for arthritis. *Jin Shin Do* is another Japanese bodywork technique based on the original *Jin Shin Jyutsu* founded by Jiro Murai. Master Murai based his system on moving *qi* through the meridians by

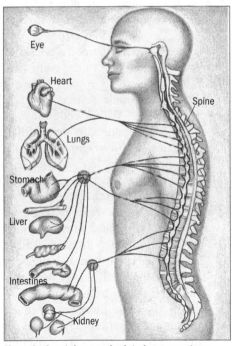

The spinal vertebrae and related organ systems.

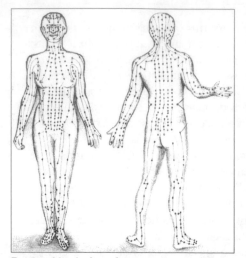

Front and back view of acupuncture meridians.

For more information on **reflexology**, contact: International Institute of Reflexology, P.O. Box 12462, St. Petersburg, FL 33733; tel: 813-343-4811. To learn how to do reflexology, Ellen Kamhi offers an instructional video entitled "The Natural Nurse: How-To Video on Reflexology;" to order, call 800-829-0918.

using certain combinations of acupressure points in a special sequence. Pressure is held for a minute or more until the practitioner can feel the flow of blood and *qi* through the point. Opening and releasing sequences are important to move the *qi* in the proper direction.

Reflexology—Reflexology is the application of pressure to areas of the feet, hands, and earlobes to influence and heal internal organs. Precise pressure releases blockages that inhibit energy flow and cause pain and disease. This pressure is thought to affect internal organs and glands by stimulating reflex points of the body. Typically, practitioners use their thumbs to press on the various zones, or areas of the feet, that correspond to organs or other structural components of the body. For arthritis, reflexology can help to detoxify organs such as the kidneys and liver, as well as stimulate sluggish glands like the thyroid and adrenals.

We use reflexology as an integral part of our physical therapies, as exemplified in the case of Sarah, 53, who came to our office complaining of a "frozen shoulder." She had had difficulty moving her shoulder for the last three years. First, we soaked her feet in warm water and lavender oil for three minutes. After examining the shoulder reflexology points on Sarah's feet, we found that they were quite tender and she felt pain in this area when touched. We applied pressure to each foot for 30 minutes, focusing specifically on her shoulder reflex points. She did not realize the benefit of the treatment until she put on her coat to leave. To her surprise, she easily lifted her arm into the sleeve of the coat—a motion that had been troublesome for years. On Sarah's next visit, she brought her husband, so that they could both learn the basic techniques of reflexology to use on each other. Reflexology is safe and can be used by anyone at home, although treatment by a professional reflexologist is preferable and more effective.

Energy Medicine

Energy medicine uses therapies that employ an energy field (electrical, magnetic, sonic, acoustic) to treat health conditions by detecting and correcting imbalances in the body's own energy fields.

Microcurrent Treatment—Microcurrent treatment devices generate infinitesimally low levels of electrical current in a form that is compatible with the body's own biocurrents occuring in healthy tissues. Used to heal muscle-related back injuries or reduce muscle pain, these almost sub-sensory signals are applied to damaged muscles to recharge the cellular "battery," which in turn leads to healing. Pain relief comes from decreases in swelling and spasms and increases in muscle flexibility. Microcurrent is an application within the larger treatment field

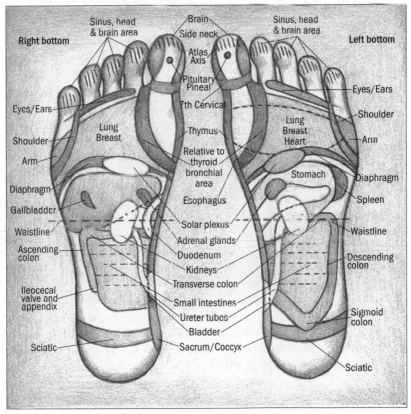

Foot reflexology chart.

Daily Exercise and Physical Medicine Protocol for Arthritis

■ Mornings: Do the daily home routine of stretches. If it fits into your schedule, consider enrolling in a morning yoga or water aerobics class that meets two to three times a week.

■ Afternoons: Do isometric exercises or the daily office routine. Take a brief walk after lunch.

■ Early evenings: If you work, consider taking evening yoga or water aerobics classes.

■ Before bedtime: Use some of the water therapies, such as baths, showers, whirlpool, or sauna. Repeat your morning stretching routine.

■ Weekends: Try to devote more time to stretching, exercise, and meditation. A one-mile walk, *tai chi* and *qigong* classes, and isometric exercise can be distributed throughout the weekend.

■ Two to three times a week, see a licensed professional for massage, reflexology, and chiropractic therapies. Your health-care professional can design a weekly schedule for kinds of therapies and frequencies of treatments.

called electrotherapy, which uses stronger electrical currents for pain reduction. Nearly all U.S. chiropractic offices, physical therapy clinics, and hospital rehabilitation departments employ some form of electrotherapy for pain control, such as ultrasound or the well-known TENS (transcutaneous electrical nerve stimulation) unit.

TENS works by applying a constant electrical stimulation to a painful area of the body. By stimulating certain nerves, TENS reduces the neural transmission of pain and produces large amounts of endorphins (natural opiates that block the transmission of pain messages between the brain and extremities). There are two types of nerve fibers in the arms, legs, and thorax: nerve fibers with a large diameter tend to inhibit pain transmission and prevent pain, while nerve fibers with small diameters tend to facilitate transmission of pain. The application of electrical stimulus to painful areas causes the large-diameter nerves (pain inhibitors) to override the small-diameter nerves (pain transmitters), resulting in reduced sensations of pain.

Magnet Therapy—Magnetic fields exist everywhere: they emanate from the earth, from changes in the weather, and even from the human body. The use of magnetic devices to generate controlled magnetic fields has proven to be an effective diagnostic tool (MRI, magnetic resonance imaging) and therapy for rheumatoid disease, inflammation, cancer, circulatory problems, and other illnesses. Magnetic therapy can influence the flow of varying electrical currents (normally present in all organisms) that govern the nervous system and other biological systems.

A Quick Review of Magnet Basics

All magnets have two poles: positive (or "S" for south, usually marked in red) and negative (or "N" for north, usually marked in green). Negative magnetic energy normalizes and calms systems of the human body, while positive magnetic energy over-stimulates or disrupts the biological system. For this reason, negative poles are most frequently directed towards the body. Do not apply positive magnetic poles directly to the body unless under medical supervision.

The most common types of magnets used in magnetic therapy are ceramic and neodymium (a rare earth chemical). These elements are mixed with iron to increase the magnet's strength or the duration of magnetic charge. The most powerful (and expensive) magnets are neodymium, while ceramic magnets are less expensive but still keep their charge for many years. These types of magnetic materials are incorporated into various types of products available at health food stores or through mail-order catalogs. Ceramic and neodymium magnets are available as plastiform strips that attach to the skin by an elastic adhesive, wrist and back supports, seat pads, and strips worn inside shoes; magnetic blankets and beds are also available for promoting sleep and reducing stress.

The strength of a magnet is measured in gauss units (which measures the intensity of magnetic flux). Every magnetic device has a manufacturer's gauss rating; however, the actual strength of the magnet at the skin surface is often much less than this number. For example, a 4,000-gauss magnet transmits about 1,200 gauss to the patient. Magnets placed in pillow or bed pads will render even lower amounts of field strength at the skin surface, because a magnet's strength quickly decreases with the distance from the subject. The strength of the magnet also depends on its size and thickness. Therapeutic magnets use from 200 gauss to 1,500 gauss (only a fraction of what an MRI machine emits), while a common refrigerator magnet emits 10 gauss.[10]

Controlled use of magnetic fields can benefit arthritis sufferers by increasing blood flow and providing more oxygen to the cells, relieving and even stopping pain, reducing inflammation and fluid retention, inhibiting microorganisms, and dissolving fat and calcium deposits.

For information on **therapeutic magnets**, contact: Philpott Medical Services, 17171 Southeast 29th Street, Choctaw, OK 73020; tel: 405-390-3009. Susan Bucci, tel. 800-285-3430.

■ Reduction of swelling due to inflammation and/or fluid retention: Place magnets directly on the area for about one hour. After you feel a slight reduction in pain, then move the magnets two to three inches toward the torso of the body. Leave magnet at new location for one hour or until you experience further pain reduction. Negative magnetic energy has a pulling effect on fluids, actually drawing it away from the swollen area towards the torso, where excess fluids can be eliminated from the body; removing these excess fluids also reduces pain.

Maintain a Healthy Posture

The way you hold your body when sitting, sleeping, or standing can affect movement of muscles and joints, circulation of blood and lymph fluid, breathing, and use of energy. Poor or imbalanced posture requires a lot of energy to maintain and interferes with circulation. It also contributes to muscle and joint tension, creating the foundation for the development or exacerbation of arthritic changes in the joints. Chiropractic and Rolfing (a therapy for structural alignment) are two of the many therapies used by alternative medicine practitioners to correct poor posture and internal imbalance. You can also follow these guidelines for correcting posture and reducing muscle tension:[11]

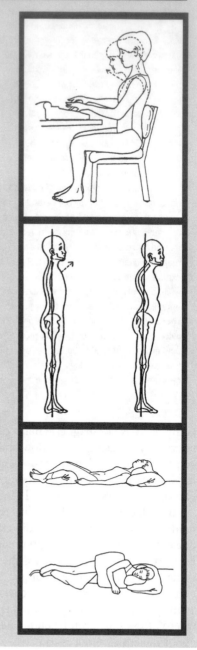

Sitting—When you sit properly, with your spine erect, pelvis centered, and the weight of your upper body supported by your pelvis, your body is actually at rest. Sit towards the front of your chair, feet flat on the floor, parallel and hip-width apart, with knees higher than hips.[12] Sit erect with chest pointing upwards and head and shoulders level. Do not sit with head, neck, and shoulders forward.

Choose a chair with wheels, an unyielding straight back, and an adjustable seat. Do not look down at your work by moving your head, neck, and shoulders forward. Move only your head and keep the rest of the body still. Take deep breaths, soften your gaze, and release the tension in your jaw and mouth. When reading, place a pillow under your arms to remove stress from neck, shoulders, and low back. Reading material should be at eye level.

■ Dissolving calcium deposits: The body attempts to cushion injured joints by placing calcium around the injured area; these deposits can be broken down with the application of negative field magnets, but it requires six weeks to six months of treatment, depending on the magnet strength and severity of the condition. Once the calcium deposits are removed, flexibility returns to the joints and further healing can take place.[13]

Precautions: There are conflicting methods of naming the magnetic poles. To be effective, magnets need to be marked correctly, so be sure to use magnets marked according to the Davis/Rawls system (developed by Dr. Albert Roy Davis in 1936). Avoid touching the sides of thick, therapeutic magnets and never use magnets with holes in the middle. Keep magnets one to two feet away from tape cassettes and computer diskettes. People with cancer or any infection (including *Candida*, viruses, and bacteria) should avoid exposure to bipolar magnets. Do not use magnets on your chest if you have a pacemaker and a pregnant woman should not use magnets on her abdomen. Do not use magnetic beds for longer than 8-10 hours a day. For long-term results, use magnets at night and supplement during the day. It is best to be under the guidance and supervision of a health-care professional.

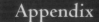

Appendix

Sample Treatment Protocols for Arthritis

The following protocols are meant to serve as general guidelines for each type of arthritis. More specific and detailed information on diet, supplements, exercise, and other topics is provided in the appropriate chapters in this book. Evaluation by a qualified health-care practitioner is always recommended as a first step in the treatment of arthritis. Tests and other diagnostic tools can then be used to design an individual therapeutic program, monitor its effectiveness, and modify it as needed.

Osteoarthritis

Step One: Natural Pain Management

Since pain is a complex interaction of physical, perceptual, cognitive, emotional, environmental, and other factors, a great deal can be done for people with arthritis. In order to wean off or use far less toxic, allopathic, synthetic drugs, it is important to begin to use natural alternative therapies to dampen the amount of pain and inflammation. Often, drugs need to be used simultaneously with natural therapies and supplements in the early stages of treatment, and carefully shifted in favor of the non-toxic approach as time goes on (if possible). This is usually the first step in osteoarthritis treatment. Precautions: Allopathic medication can not and should not be discontinued rapidly without medical supervision.

1. For pain relief, take the following supplements daily:

■ Glucosamine sulfate: 1,500-3,000 mg per day in divided doses on an empty stomach

■ Adrenal Glandular Extract (dosage depends on brand and whether liquid or capsule)

■ Multivitamin/mineral (without iron or copper if pain/inflammation is high)

■ Vitamin E: 1,000-3,000 IU per day in divided doses with meals

■ Vitamin K1 (phytonadione from plant sources): 20-40 mg

■ Selenium: 400-1,000 mcg per day with meals in divided doses

■ EPA/DHA (essential fatty acids): 3,000 mg per day in divided doses (we have had excellent results with Joint Lubrication from Alternative Therapy)

- MSM (methylsulfonylmethane): 250 mg, four times per day
- SAMe (S-adenosylmethionione): 500 mg, three times daily
- DL-phenylalanine: 4-6 grams per day, in divided doses, on an empty stomach
- PCOs or OPCs (proanthocyanidins): 150 mg per day in divided doses with meals
- Lipoic acid: 250 mg per day in divided doses
- Bioflavonoids: Consume several cupfuls per day of blueberries, blackberries, black cherries, acerola cherries, or hawthorne berries. Take a multiple bioflavonoid complex supplement, which may contain the following botanical combinations: grape seed polyphenols, green tea, hawthorn berry, mixed citrus bioflavonoids, acerola cherries, gotu kola (*Centella asiatica*) extracts, amla (Indian gooseberries), and quercetin. Formulas which we have found to be clinically successful include Joint Phyto-Nutrition (Nature's Answer) and Chayawanprash (found in Indian ethnic grocery stores or through Ayush Herbs).
- Glycyrrhiza Glabra Solid Extract (Scientific Botanicals): ¼ tsp, 3-4 times per day, with or without food
- Ananacur (Scientific Botanicals): contains 450 mg bromelain from pineapple (*Anana camosus*) and 300 mg curcumin from *Curcuma longa*; ¼ tsp powder, four times per day on an empty stomach

2. Use a quality oral botanical anti-inflammatory/analgesic formula and a topical botanical analgesic simultaneously. We recommend the following herbs for the oral formula, in one product or a combination of products: *Salix alba* (white willow bark), *Boswellia serrata* (boswella), *Tanacetum parthenium* (feverfew), *Corydalis ambigua*, kava-kava (*Piper methysticum*), *Zingiber officinale* (ginger root), *Angelica spp.* (Du Huo), *Cimicifuga racemosa* (black cohosh), Jamaican dogwood (*Piscidia erythina*), *Uncaria tomentosa* (cat's claw/uña de gato), *Harpagophytum procumbens* (devil's claw), *Guiacum officinale* (Lignum vitae root), *Radix Dipsacus sinensis*, and *Corydalis remota*. Formulas we have had excellent clinical results with include: BotanoDyne (Nature's Answer), PTI (Karuna Labs), and AI Formula (Pure Encapsulations); the Chinese patent formulas Yan Hu Suo Zhi Tong Pian, Du Zhong Hu Gu Wan, Yunnan Feng Shi Leng, and Feng Shi Xiao Tong Wan; and the Ayurvedic formula Boswelya Plus (Ayush Herbs).

Topical botanical formulas, in the form of salve, cream, gel, or liniment, should be massaged into the inflamed joint, muscle, or ligament several (at least four) times daily. These formulas should include combinations of the follow-

For information on **Chayawanprash**, contact: Ayush Herbs, Inc., 2115 112th Avenue NE, Bellevue, WA 98004-2946; tel: 425-637-1400; fax: 425-451-2670; website: www.ayush.com.

ing botanicals: menthol (*Mentha spp.*), camphor (*Cinnamonium camphora*), frankincense, myrrh, boswella, cloves, allspice, aconite, ginger, cinnamon, wintergreen, capsicum, arnica, ruta, and *Dipsacus sinensis*. Formulas which have resulted in clinically significant pain reduction include: the Chinese patent formulas Zheng Gu Shui Liniment, Shang Shi Zhi Tong Gao, Cheong Kun Pain Reliever Oil, and Tiger Balm; and BotanoGesic Salve (Nature's Answer) and Biofreeze (Performance Health). Homeopathic salves that have demonstrated superior clinical results include TRAUMEEL and ZEEL (HEEL/BHI) and ArniFlora (Boericke and Tafel).

3. Follow the Arthritis Diet for three weeks. After your allopathic medicine is discontinued, follow the fasting procedure outlined in this book. Continue to take your natural pain supplements during your fast. Your pain should begin to diminish around the fourth day. Precautions: Some allopathic medicine can cause severe damage to the gastrointestinal system when taken on an empty stomach. Since fasting necessitates the restriction of all solid food, it cannot be accomplished while using NSAIDs, prednisone, and other drugs, which must be taken with food.

4. Use contrast hydrotherapy several times daily to assist in pain relief. Use acupuncture and electrical stimulation (such as TENS) to increase endogenous endorphins.

5. Use mind/body therapies for pain (stress management techniques, meditation, hypnosis, relaxation, guided imagery, biofeedback, cognitive therapy) to achieve an analgesic effect.

6. See a massage therapist, rolf practitioner, Feldenkrais, or Alexander practitioner for postural integration and trigger point evaluation or treatment.

Step Two: Detoxification

Undergo standard tests, especially diagnostic imaging of the joints. See a health-care practitioner to determine digestive capacity, food allergies, intestinal permeability, adrenal and thyroid status, and colonic microflora. Follow therapies discussed in this book to correct imbalances. Use drainage remedies, fasting, and other detoxification procedures to detoxify the body four times per year.

Step Three: Stabilization

1. Consult with a physician trained in physical medicine, manipulation, and restoration of proper biomechan-

For information on **Biofreeze**, contact: Performance Health, Inc., 127 Craighead Street, Suite 105, Pittsburgh, PA 15211; tel: 800-246-3733.

Use the appropriate homeopathic remedies for pain, based on individual signs and symptoms. For more on **selecting homeopathic remedies for pain relief**, see Chapter 13: Supplements for Arthritis, pp. 280-313. For more on **massage and other physical therapies**, see Chapter 14: Exercises and Physical Therapies, pp. 314-339. For **mind/body therapies**, see Chapter 11: Mind/Body Approaches to Arthritis, pp. 226-249.

ics to restore normal range of motion of your joints, attain muscular balance, correct posture or flat feet, correct ergonomic issues at work, strengthen weak muscles, and stretch short muscles.

CAUTION: If you have severe osteoarthritis and have 85% or more cartilage destruction, consult with an orthopedic physician who is knowledgeable on the use of injectable hyaluronic acid preparations (such as SynVisc). We have seen remarkable therapeutic changes in our practice using this approach.

2. Get 45 minutes of exercise four times per week. Especially useful are yoga, *tai chi*, and aquatic exercises. Perform regular stretching and muscle strengthening.

3. Maintain all of the above therapies until you are 90% pain free for one month. When you are no longer in pain, discontinue all herbs for pain and DL-phenylalanine, but continue on all other nutrients. Continue with the physical therapies, but adjust them to your individual needs and schedule.

4. Attain a desirable weight for your height and optimum percentage of body fat, as obesity worsens osteoarthritis.

5. Seek advice from your alternative health-care practitioner to individualize your program as you become increasingly well.

Rheumatoid Arthritis

Step One: Natural Pain Management

Since pain is a complex interaction of physical, perceptual, cognitive, emotional, environmental, and other factors, a great deal can be done for people with arthritis. In order to wean off or use far less toxic, allopathic, synthetic drugs, it is important to begin to use natural alternative therapies to dampen the amount of pain and inflammation. Often, drugs need to be used simultaneously with natural therapies and supplements in the early stages of treatment, and carefully shifted in favor of the nontoxic approach as time goes on (if possible). This is usually the first step in rheumatoid arthritis treatment. Precautions: Allopathic medication can not and should not be discontinued rapidly without medical supervision.

1. For pain relief, take the following supplements daily—

■ Glucosamine sulfate: 1,500-3,000 mg per day in divided doses on an empty stomach

■ Adrenal Glandular Extract (dosage depends on brand and whether liquid or capsule)

■ Multivitamin/mineral (without iron or copper if pain/inflammation is high)

■ Vitamin E: 1,000-3,000 IU per day in divided doses with meals

■ Vitamin K1 (phytonadione from plant sources): 20-40 mg

■ Selenium: 400-1,000 mcg per day with meals in divided doses

- EPA/DHA (essential fatty acids): 3,000 mg per day in divided doses (we have had excellent results with Joint Lubrication from Alternative Therapy)
- MSM (methylsulfonylmethane): 250 mg, four times per day
- DL-phenylalanine: 4-6 grams per day, in divided doses, on an empty stomach
- PCOs or OPCs (proanthocyanidins): 150 mg per day in divided doses with meals
- Lipoic acid: 250 mg per day in divided doses
- Bioflavonoids: Consume several cupfuls per day of blueberries, blackberries, black cherries, acerola cherries, or hawthorne berries. Take a multiple bioflavonoid complex supplement, which may contain the following botanical combinations: grape seed polyphenols, green tea, hawthorn berry, mixed citrus bioflavonoids, acerola cherries, gotu kola (*Centella asiatica*) extracts, amla (Indian gooseberries), and quercetin. Formulas which we have found to be clinically successful include Joint Phyto-Nutrition (Nature's Answer) and Chayawanprash (found in Indian ethnic grocery stores or through Ayush Herbs).
- Glycyrrhiza Glabra Solid Extract (Scientific Botanicals): ¼ tsp, 3-4 times per day, with or without food
- Ananacur (Scientific Botanicals): contains 450 mg bromelain from pineapple (*Anana camosus*) and 300 mg curcumin from *Curcuma longa*; ¼ tsp powder, four times per day on an empty stomach

2. Use a quality oral botanical anti-inflammatory/analgesic formula and a topical botanical analgesic simultaneously. We recommend the following herbs for the oral formula, in one product or a combination of products: *Salix alba* (white willow bark), *Boswellia serrata* (boswella), *Tanacetum parthenium* (feverfew), *Corydalis ambigua*, kava-kava (*Piper methysticum*), *Zingiber officinale* (ginger root), *Angelica spp.* (Du Huo), *Cimicifuga racemosa* (black cohosh), Jamaican dogwood (*Piscidia erythina*), *Uncaria tomentosa* (cat's claw/uña de gato), *Harpagophytum procumbens* (devil's claw), *Guiacum officinale* (Lignum vitae root), *Radix Dipsacus sinensis*, and *Corydalis remota*. Formulas we have had excellent clinical results with include: BotanoDyne (Nature's Answer), PTI (Karuna Labs), and AI Formula (Pure Encapsulations); the Chinese patent formulas Yan Hu Suo Zhi Tong Pian, Du Zhong Hu Gu Wan, Yunnan Feng Shi Leng, and Feng Shi Xiao Tong Wan; and the Ayurvedic formula Boswelya Plus (Ayush Herbs).

Topical botanical formulas, in the form of salve, cream, gel, or liniment, should be massaged into the inflamed joint, muscle, or ligament several (at least four) times daily.

For information on **Chayawanprash**, contact: Ayush Herbs, Inc., 2115 112th Avenue NE, Bellevue, WA 98004-2946; tel: 425-637-1400; fax: 425-451-2670; website: www.ayush.com.

These formulas should include combinations of the following botanicals: menthol (*Mentha spp.*), camphor (*Cinnamonium camphora*), frankincense, myrrh, boswella, cloves, allspice, aconite, ginger, cinnamon, wintergreen, capsicum, arnica, ruta, and *Dipsacus sinensis*. Note: if the rheumatoid process is hot (heat radiating from the joints, high SED rate), avoid hot analgesic herbs (capsicum, ginger) and treat with cooling analgesics (menthol, camphor, wintergreen, eucalyptus, curcumin, *Dipsacus*). If the rheumatoid process is cold, use the warming herbs.

Formulas which have resulted in clinically significant pain reduction include: the Chinese patent formulas Zheng Gu Shui Liniment, Shang Shi Zhi Tong Gao, and Cheong Kun Pain Reliever Oil; and BotanoGesic Salve (Nature's Answer) and Biofreeze (Performance Health). Homeopathic salves that have demonstrated superior clinical results include TRAUMEEL and ZEEL (HEEL/BHI) and ArniFlora (Boericke and Tafel).

3. Follow the Arthritis Diet for three weeks. After your allopathic medicine is discontinued, follow the fasting procedure outlined in this book. Continue to take your natural pain supplements during your fast. Your pain should begin to diminish around the fourth day. Precautions: Some allopathic medicine can cause severe damage to the gastrointestinal system when taken on an empty stomach. Since fasting necessitates the restriction of all solid food, it cannot be accomplished while using NSAIDs, prednisone, and other drugs, which must be taken with food.

4. Use contrast hydrotherapy several times daily to assist in pain relief. Use acupuncture and electrical stimulation (such as TENS) to increase endogenous endorphins.

For information on **Biofreeze**, contact: Performance Health, Inc., 127 Craighead Street, Suite 105, Pittsburgh, PA 15211; tel: 800-246-3733.

5. Use mind/body therapies for pain (stress management techniques, meditation, hypnosis, relaxation, guided imagery, biofeedback, cognitive therapy) to achieve an analgesic effect.

6. See a massage therapist, rolf practitioner, Feldenkrais, or Alexander practitioner for postural integration and trigger point evaluation or treatment.

Step Two: Detoxification

Undergo standard tests, especially diagnostic imaging of the joints. See a health-care practitioner to determine digestive capacity, food allergies, intestinal permeability, adrenal and thyroid status, and colonic microflora. Follow therapies discussed in this book to correct imbalances. Use

Use the appropriate homeopathic remedies for pain, based on individual signs and symptoms. For more on **selecting homeopathic remedies and other supplements for pain relief**, see Chapter 13: Supplements for Arthritis, pp. 280-313.

For **detailed dietary recommendations for arthritis**, see Chapter 12: The Arthritis Diet, pp. 250-278.

drainage remedies, fasting, and other detoxification procedures to detoxify the body four times per year.

1. For dysbiosis and rheumatoid arthritis, a stool analysis will direct the physician to the proper therapies. In general, use PlantiBiotic from Nature's Answer or Biocidin (one pill with each meal; taken only with food). Get 2-3 colonic hydrotherapy treatments per week. For the first eight weeks, use antimicrobial herbs and demulcents in the water. For the last four weeks, use *Lactobacillus* and *Bifidobacteria* cultures as an implant. Repeat stool test to measure results. Repeat intensive therapy if still positive or continue with two treatments per month on a maintenance basis if bowel flora is normalized.

2. For botanical detoxification of all organs: AlteraTonic from Nature's Answer (two pills, three times per day).

3. To treat intestinal permeability: GastroGuard from Nature's Answer (one or two pills, three times per day) or Robert's Formula from Phyto-Pharmica (one or two pills, three times per day). Repeat test and continue on formulas until the tests prove negative.

Step Three: Desensitizing Autoimmunity

1. Have your physician prepare an oral auto-sanguis nosode (take 15 drops, three times per day between meals). Use injectible auto-sanguis therapy from your doctor.

2. Consider urine therapy.

3. Take the following herbs and supplements:
- *Hemidesmus indicus* (MediHerb): one teaspoon, 3-4 times per day
- *Tripterygium wilfordii* (only from a TCM physican): 15-30 ml of the tincture in divided doses
- Lithospermum 15 (a Chinese herbal formula)
- Bovine or chicken cartilage extracts: three grams per day
- MSM (methylsulfonylmethane): 3,000 mg per day in divided doses

4. Use mind/body techniques to help stop the aggressive autoimmune attack. Use counseling and other stress management techniques in the book to become a less stressful person and to deal with emotional issues.

Step Four: Stabilization

1. Consult with a physician trained in physical medicine, manipulation, and restoration of proper biomechanics to restore normal range of motion of your joints, attain muscular balance, correct posture or flat feet, correct ergonomic issues at work, strengthen weak muscles, and stretch short muscles.

2. Get 45 minutes of exercise four times per week. Especially useful arc yoga, *tai chi*, and aquatic exercises. Perform regular stretching and muscle strengthening.

3. Maintain all of the above therapies until you are 90% pain free for one month. When you are no longer in pain, discontinue all herbs for pain and DL-phenylalanine, but continue on all other nutrients. Continue with the physical therapies, but adjust them to your individual needs and schedule.

4. Attain a desirable weight for your height and optimum percentage of body fat.

5. Seek advice from your alternative health-care practitioner to individualize your program as you become increasingly well.

For more on **auto-sanguis therapy**, see Chapter 10: Desensitize the Autoimmune Reaction, pp. 208-224.

Gout

1. Take the following supplements daily:
■ Multivitamin/mineral (low-potency with no more than 100 mg of vitamin C)
■ Folic acid: 10 mg during acute gout attack
■ Omega-3 oils: 3 tbsp
■ Bioflavonoids: 3,000 mg, preferably derived from cherries
■ Quercetin: 300 mg, three times per day

Reduce intake of vitamin C and niacin (vitamin B3) and stop these supplements completely during an acute gout attack, as they increase blood acidity levels and precipitate uric acid crystallization. Continue with low-level supplementation (levels typically found in a high-quality multivitamin) when the acute attack is over. Combine quercetin with bromelain for an increased anti-inflammatory effect.

2. Follow the Arthritis Diet and juice during gout attacks.

3. Eat ½ pound of fresh organic cherries, blueberries, and hawthorn berries daily. These fruits contain flavonoid components that block the enzyme that increases uric acid. No uric acid buildup means no gout attack. Joint Phyto-Nutrition from Nature's Answer contains a potent concentration of flavonoids to support the joints (¼ tsp, four times daily).

4. Avoid eating the following purine-rich foods: liver and other organ meats; sausages and other processed meats; anchovies, crab, and shrimp; all animal products including meats, milk, and eggs; most beans, including soy.

5. Drink 2-3 quarts of filtered (carbon block) water per day to help

keep the urine diluted and flush out uric acid crystals.

6. Stop all alcohol consumption, especially beer. Alcohol increases purine production in the body and makes the blood more acidic. This starts the crystallization process.

7. Lose weight, because obesity is positively correlated with gout. Make a commitment to remaining on the Arthritis Diet and not falling back into unhealthy eating practices, which induce gout in those susceptible to it.

8. Have a health-care physician determine digestive capacity, intestinal permeability, and the health of colon microflora. Follow therapies detailed in this book to correct imbalances in these areas.

9. Use contrast hydrotherapy several times daily to induce a pumping action and flush the afflicted joints with blood and lymphatic fluid, thereby removing uric acid crystals. Continue hydrotherapy indefinitely (once or twice daily) if not in an acute phase of gout.

10. Use a quality oral botanical anti-inflammatory/analgesic formula and a topical botanical analgesic simultaneously. We recommend the following herbs for the oral formula, in one product or a combination of products: *Salix alba* (white willow bark), *Boswellia serrata* (boswella), *Tanacetum parthenium* (feverfew), *Corydalis ambigua*, kava-kava (*Piper methysticum*), *Zingiber officinale* (ginger root), *Angelica spp.* (Du Huo), *Cimicifuga racemosa* (black cohosh), Jamaican dogwood (*Piscidia erythina*), *Uncaria tomentosa* (cat's claw/uña de gato), *Harpagophytum procumbens* (devil's claw), *Guiacum officinale* (Lignum vitae root), *Radix Dipsacus sinensis*, and *Corydalis remota*. Formulas we have had excellent clinical results with include: BotanoDyne (Nature's Answer), PTI (Karuna Labs), and AI Formula (Pure Encapsulations); the Chinese patent formulas Yan Hu Suo Zhi Tong Pian, Du Zhong Hu Gu Wan, Yunnan Feng Shi Leng, and Feng Shi Xiao Tong Wan; and the Ayurvedic formula Boswelya Plus (Ayush Herbs).

Topical botanical formulas, in the form of salve, cream, gel, or liniment, should be massaged into the inflamed joint, muscle, or ligament several (at least four) times daily. These formulas should include combinations of the following botanicals: menthol (*Mentha spp.*), camphor (*Cinnamonium camphora*), frankincense, myrrh, boswella, cloves, allspice, aconite, ginger, cinnamon, wintergreen, capsicum, arnica, ruta, and *Dipsacus sinensis*. Note: if the gout process is hot (heat radiating from the joints, high SED rate), avoid hot analgesic herbs (capsicum, ginger) and treat with cooling analgesics (menthol, camphor, wintergreen, eucalyptus, curcumin, *Dipsacus*). If the process is cold, use the warming herbs.

Formulas which have resulted in clinically significant pain reduction include: the Chinese patent formulas Zheng Gu Shui Liniment, Shang Shi Zhi Tong Gao, and Cheong Kun Pain Reliever Oil; and BotanoGesic Salve (Nature's Answer) and Biofreeze (Performance Health).

11. Cleanse your tissues of toxins and uric acid and help inflammation with AlteraTonic from Nature's Answer (2-3 pills, twice per day between meals).

Ankylosing Spondylitis

Step One: Natural Pain Management

Since pain is a complex interaction of physical, perceptual, cognitive, emotional, environmental, and other factors, a great deal can be done for people with arthritis. In order to wean off or use far less toxic, allopathic, synthetic drugs, it is imperative to begin to use natural alternative therapies to dampen the amount of pain and inflammation. Often, drugs need to be used simultaneously with natural therapies and supplements in the early stages of treatment, and carefully shifted in favor of the nontoxic approach as time goes on (if possible). This is usually the first step in the treatment of ankylosing spondylitis. Precautions: Allopathic medication can not and should not be discontinued rapidly without medical supervision.

1. For pain relief, take the following supplements daily—
■ Glucosamine sulfate: 1,500-3,000 mg per day in divided doses on an empty stomach
■ Adrenal Glandular Extract (dosage depends on brand and whether liquid or capsule)
■ Multivitamin/mineral (without iron or copper if pain/inflammation is high)
■ Vitamin E: 1,000-3,000 IU per day in divided doses with meals
■ Vitamin K1 (phytonadione from plant sources): 20-40 mg
■ Selenium: 400-1,000 mcg per day with meals in divided doses
■ EPA/DHA (essential fatty acids): 3,000 mg per day in divided doses (we have had excellent results with Joint Lubrication from Alternative Therapy)
■ MSM (methylsulfonylmethane): 250 mg, four times per day
■ DL-phenylalanine: 4-6 grams per day, in divided doses, on an empty stomach
■ PCOs or OPCs (proanthocyanidins): 150 mg per day in divided doses with meals
■ Lipoic acid: 250 mg per day in divided doses

■ Bioflavonoids: Consume several cupfuls per day of blueberries, blackberries, black cherries, acerola cherries, or hawthorne berries. Take a multiple bioflavonoid complex supplement, which may contain the following botanical combinations: grape seed polyphenols, green tea, hawthorn berry, mixed citrus bioflavonoids, acerola cherries, gotu kola (*Centella asiatica*) extracts, amla (Indian gooseberries), and quercetin. Formulas which we have found to be clinically successful include Joint Phyto-Nutrition (Nature's Answer) and Chayawanprash (found in Indian ethnic grocery stores or through Ayush Herbs).

■ Glycyrrhiza Glabra Solid Extract (Scientific Botanicals): ¼ tsp, 3-4 times per day, with or without food

■ Ananacur (Scientific Botanicals): contains 450 mg bromelain from pineapple (*Anana camosus*) and 300 mg curcumin from *Curcuma longa*; ¼ tsp powder, four times per day on an empty stomach

2. Use a quality oral botanical anti-inflammatory/analgesic formula and a topical botanical analgesic simultaneously. We recommend the following herbs for the oral formula, in one product or a combination of products: *Salix alba* (white willow bark), *Boswellia serrata* (boswella), *Tanacetum parthenium* (feverfew), *Corydalis ambigua*, kava-kava (*Piper methysticum*), *Zingiber officinale* (ginger root), *Angelica spp.* (Du Huo), *Cimicifuga racemosa* (black cohosh), Jamaican dogwood (*Piscidia erythina*), *Uncaria tomentosa* (cat's claw/uña de gato), *Harpagophytum procumbens* (devil's claw), *Guiacum officinale* (Lignum vitae root), *Radix Dipsacus sinensis*, and *Corydalis remota*. Formulas we have had excellent clinical results with include: BotanoDyne (Nature's Answer), PTI (Karuna Labs), and AI Formula (Pure Encapsulations); the Chinese patent formulas Yan Hu Suo Zhi Tong Pian, Du Zhong Hu Gu Wan, Yunnan Feng Shi Leng, and Feng Shi Xiao Tong Wan; and the Ayurvedic formula Boswelya Plus (Ayush Herbs).

Topical botanical formulas, in the form of salve, cream, gel, or liniment, should be massaged into the inflamed joint, muscle, or ligament several (at least four) times daily. These formulas should include combinations of the following botanicals: menthol (*Mentha spp.*), camphor (*Cinnamonium camphora*), frankincense, myrrh, boswella, cloves, allspice, aconite, ginger, cinnamon, wintergreen, capsicum, arnica, ruta, and *Dipsacus sinensis*. Note: if the ankylosing spondylitis process is hot (heat radiating from the joints, high SED rate), avoid hot analgesic herbs (capsicum, ginger) and treat with cooling analgesics (menthol, camphor, wintergreen, eucalyptus, curcumin, *Dipsacus*). If the process is cold, use the warming herbs.

Formulas which have resulted in clinically significant pain reduction include: the Chinese patent formulas Zheng Gu Shui Liniment,

Shang Shi Zhi Tong Gao, and Cheong Kun Pain Reliever Oil; and BotanoGesic Salve (Nature's Answer) and Biofreeze (Performance Health). Homeopathic salves that have demonstrated superior clinical results include TRAUMEEL and ZEEL (HEEL/BHI) and ArniFlora (Boericke and Tafel).

3. Follow the Arthritis Diet for three weeks. After your allopathic medicine is discontinued, follow the fasting procedure outlined in this book. Continue to take your natural pain supplements during your fast. Your pain should begin to diminish around the fourth day. Precautions: Some allopathic medicine can cause severe damage to the gastrointestinal system when taken on an empty stomach. Since fasting necessitates the restriction of all solid food, it cannot be accomplished while using NSAIDs, prednisone, and other drugs, which must be taken with food.

4. Use contrast hydrotherapy several times daily to assist in pain relief. Use acupuncture and electrical stimulation (such as TENS) to increase endogenous endorphins.

5. Use mind/body therapies for pain (stress management techniques, meditation, hypnosis, relaxation, guided imagery, biofeedback, cognitive therapy) to achieve an analgesic effect.

6. See a massage therapist, rolf practitioner, Feldenkrais, or Alexander practitioner for postural integration and trigger point evaluation or treatment. The focus of physical therapies should be heavily directed at the area typically affected by ankylosing spondylitis—the sacroiliac, lumbar vertebrae, and cervical spine.

Step Two: Detoxification
Undergo standard tests, especially diagnostic imaging of the joints. See a health-care practitioner to determine digestive capacity, food allergies, intestinal permeability, adrenal and thyroid status, and colonic microflora. Follow therapies discussed in this book to correct imbalances. Use drainage remedies, fasting, and other detoxification procedures to detoxify the body four times per year.

1. For dysbiosis and ankylosing spondylitis, a stool analysis will direct the physician to the proper therapies. In general, use PlantiBiotic from Nature's Answer or Biocidin (one pill with each meal; taken only with food). Get 2-3 colonic hydrotherapy treatments per week. For the first eight weeks, use antimicrobial herbs and demulcents in the water. For the last four weeks, use *Lactobacillus* and *Bifidobacteria* cultures as an implant. Repeat stool test

Use the appropriate homeopathic remedies for pain, based on individual signs and symptoms. For more on **selecting homeopathic remedies for pain relief**, see Chapter 13: Supplements for Arthritis, pp. 280-313.

For more information on **TENS and other physical therapies**, see Chapter 14: Exercises and Physical Therapies, pp. 314-339.

to measure results. Repeat intensive therapy if still positive or continue with two treatments per month on a maintenance basis if bowel flora is normalized.

2. For botanical detoxification of all organs: AlteraTonic from Nature's Answer (two pills, three times per day).

3. To treat intestinal permeability: GastroGuard from Nature's Answer (one or two pills, three times per day) or Robert's Formula from Phyto-Pharmica (one or two pills, three times per day). Repeat test and continue on formulas until the tests prove negative.

Step Three: Desensitizing Autoimmunity

1. Have your physician prepare an oral auto-sanguis nosode (take 15 drops, three times per day between meals). Use injectible auto-sanguis therapy from your doctor.

2. Consider urine therapy.

3. Take the following herbs and supplements:

- *Hemidesmus indicus* (MediHerb): one teaspoon, 3-4 times per day
- *Tripterygium wilfordii* (only from a TCM physican): 15-30 ml of the tincture in divided doses
- Lithospermum 15 (a Chinese herbal formula)
- Bovine or chicken cartilage extracts: three grams per day
- MSM (methylsulfonylmethane): 3,000 mg per day in divided doses

4. Use mind/body techniques to help stop the aggressive autoimmune attack. Use counseling and other stress management techniques in the book to become a less stressful person and to deal with emotional issues.

Step Four: Stabilization

1. Consult with a physician trained in physical medicine, manipulation, and restoration of proper biomechanics to restore normal range of motion of your joints, attain muscular balance, correct posture or flat feet, correct ergonomic issues at work, strengthen weak muscles, and stretch short muscles.

2. Get 45 minutes of exercise four times per week. Especially useful are yoga, *tai chi*, and aquatic exercises. Perform regular stretching and muscle strengthening.

3. Maintain all of the above therapies until you are 90% pain free for one month. When you are no longer in pain, discontinue all herbs for pain and DL-phenylalanine, but continue on all other nutrients. Continue with the physical therapies, but adjust them to your individual needs and schedule.

4. Attain a desirable weight for your height and optimum percentage of body fat.

5. Seek advice from your alternative health-care practitioner to individualize your program as you become increasingly well.

Psoriatic Arthritis

1. Take the following supplements daily:
- Multivitamin/mineral supplement
- Vitamin E: 800 IU
- Selenium: 200 mcg
- Zinc: 50 mg
- Omega-3 oils: 3 tbsp
- Flaxseed oil: 1 tbsp, five times a day
- EPA: 10-12 mg
- Glutathione: 200 mg
- Bromelain: 2,000 mg (do not exceed 460 mg per day if you have heart palpitations)

2. Pursue a fasting program consisting of an initial preparation period of juices and "green" drinks, followed by a supervised fast, and ending with a repetition of juices and green drinks.

3. Concentrate your detoxification therapy on colon cleansing and liver support.

4. Have a health-care physician determine digestive capacity, intestinal permeability, and health of colon microflora. Follow therapies detailed in this book to correct imbalances in these areas.

5. Massage sesame oil into your skin prior to a daily shower.

6. Get plenty of sunshine and go swimming in the ocean; traditional medicine and folklore recommend this and our patients have confirmed its effectiveness. However, care must be taken to avoid overexposure in the sun.

7. Use massage therapy, deep tissue work, neuromuscular technique, or other physical therapies to facilitate lymphatic drainage of toxins. Use ultrasound over afflicted joints two to three times per week to provide relief. Use Joint Phyto-Nutrition (from Nature's Answer) to provide optimum nutrition to the joints.

8. Use stress management techniques, such as guided imagery, flotation therapy, biofeedback, visualization, and other mind-body therapies.

9. Eat a well-balanced vegan diet of organic nuts, legumes, grains, fruits, and vegetables.

10. To reduce psoriasis outbreaks, take PlantiBiotic (to cleanse the colon), AlteraTonic (to detoxify the body and support the liver and adrenal glands as well as anti-inflammatory systems), and GastroGuard (to stop leaky gut syndrome). Also, include the herbs *Coleus forskolii* and bitter melon (from Phyto-Pharmica) to help stop the skin lesions from enlarging.

11. Use fresh parsley juice or essential oil of Bergamot and apply to psoriatic lesions before sunbathing to reduce severity of lesions. Care must be taken to avoid excessive exposure, as these remedies may increase photosensitivity. For pain, utilize BotanoDyne (from Nature's Answer) and BotanoGesic salve as needed.

Infectious Arthritis and Lyme Disease

Step One: Natural Pain Management

Since pain is a complex interaction of physical, perceptual, cognitive, emotional, environmental, and other factors, a great deal can be done for people with arthritis. In order to wean off or use far less toxic, allopathic, synthetic drugs, it is important to begin to use natural alternative therapies to dampen the amount of pain and inflammation. Often, drugs need to be used simultaneously with natural therapies and supplements in the early stages of treatment, and carefully shifted in favor of the nontoxic approach as time goes on (if possible). This is usually the first step in infectious arthritis treatment. Precautions: Allopathic medication can not and should not be discontinued rapidly without medical supervision.

1. For pain relief, take the following supplements daily—

■ Glucosamine sulfate: 1,500-3,000 mg per day in divided doses on an empty stomach

■ Adrenal Glandular Extract (dosage depends on brand and whether liquid or capsule)

■ Multivitamin/mineral (without iron or copper if pain/inflammation is high)

■ Vitamin E: 1,000-3,000 IU per day in divided doses with meals

■ Vitamin K1 (phytonadione from plant sources): 20-40 mg

■ Selenium: 400-1,000 mcg per day with meals in divided doses

■ EPA/DHA (essential fatty acids): 3,000 mg per day in divided doses (we have had excellent results with Joint Lubrication from Alternative Therapy)

■ MSM (methylsulfonylmethane): 250 mg, four times per day

■ DL-phenylalanine: 4-6 grams per day, in divided doses, on an empty stomach

■ PCOs or OPCs (proanthocyanidins): 150 mg per day in divided doses with meals

■ Lipoic acid: 250 mg per day in divided doses

■ Bioflavonoids: Consume several cupfuls per day of blueberries, blackberries, black cherries, acerola cherries, or hawthorne berries. Take a multiple bioflavonoid complex supplement, which may contain the following botanical combinations: grape seed polyphenols, green tea, hawthorn berry, mixed citrus bioflavonoids, acerola cherries, gotu kola (*Centella asiatica*) extracts, amla (Indian gooseberries), and quercetin. Formulas which we have found to be clinically successful include Joint Phyto-Nutrition (Nature's Answer) and Chayawanprash (found in Indian ethnic grocery stores or through Ayush Herbs).

■ Glycyrrhiza Glabra Solid Extract (Scientific Botanicals): ¼ tsp, 3-4 times per day, with or without food

■ Ananacur (Scientific Botanicals): contains 450 mg bromelain from pineapple (*Anana camosus*) and 300 mg curcumin from *Curcuma longa*; ¼ tsp powder, four times per day on an empty stomach

2. Use a quality oral botanical anti-inflammatory/analgesic formula and a topical botanical analgesic simultaneously. We recommend the following herbs for the oral formula, in one product or a combination of products: *Salix alba* (white willow bark), *Boswellia serrata* (boswella), *Tanacetum parthenium* (feverfew), *Corydalis ambigua*, kava-kava (*Piper methysticum*), *Zingiber officinale* (ginger root), *Angelica spp.* (Du Huo), *Cimicifuga racemosa* (black cohosh), Jamaican dogwood (*Piscidia erythina*), *Uncaria tomentosa* (cat's claw/uña de gato), *Harpagophytum procumbens* (devil's claw), *Guiacum officinale* (Lignum vitae root), *Radix Dipsacus sinensis*, and *Corydalis remota*. Formulas we have had excellent clinical results with include: BotanoDyne (Nature's Answer), PT1 (Karuna Labs), and AI Formula (Pure Encapsulations); the Chinese patent formulas Yan Hu Suo Zhi Tong Pian, Du Zhong Hu Gu Wan, Yunnan Feng Shi Leng, and Feng Shi Xiao Tong Wan; and the Ayurvedic formula Boswelya Plus (Ayush Herbs).

Topical botanical formulas, in the form of salve, cream, gel, or liniment, should be massaged into the inflamed joint, muscle, or ligament several (at least four) times daily. These formulas should include combinations of the following botanicals: menthol (*Mentha spp.*), camphor (*Cinnamonium camphora*), frankincense, myrrh, boswella, cloves, allspice, aconite, ginger, cinnamon, wintergreen, capsicum, arnica, ruta, and *Dipsacus sinensis*. Note: if the infectious arthritis process is hot (heat radiating from the joints, high SED rate), avoid hot analgesic herbs (capsicum, ginger) and treat with cooling analgesics (menthol,

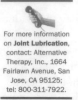

For more information on **Joint Lubrication**, contact: Alternative Therapy, Inc., 1664 Fairlawn Avenue, San Jose, CA 95125; tel: 800-311-7922.

camphor, wintergreen, eucalyptus, curcumin, *Dipsacus*). If the process is cold, use the warming herbs.

Formulas which have resulted in clinically significant pain reduction include: the Chinese patent formulas Zheng Gu Shui Liniment, Shang Shi Zhi Tong Gao, and Cheong Kun Pain Reliever Oil; and BotanoGesic Salve (Nature's Answer) and Biofreeze (Performance Health). Homeopathic salves that have demonstrated superior clinical results include TRAUMEEL and ZEEL (HEEL/BHI) and ArniFlora (Boericke and Tafel).

3. Follow the Arthritis Diet for three weeks. After your allopathic medicine is discontinued, follow the fasting procedure outlined in this book. Continue to take your natural pain supplements during your fast. Your pain should begin to diminish around the fourth day. Precautions: Some allopathic medicine can cause severe damage to the gastrointestinal system when taken on an empty stomach. Since fasting necessitates the restriction of all solid food, it cannot be accomplished while using NSAIDs, prednisone, and other drugs, which must be taken with food.

4. Use contrast hydrotherapy several times daily to assist in pain relief and to restore circulation to the joints. Use acupuncture and electrical stimulation (such as TENS) to increase endogenous endorphins.

5. Use mind/body therapies for pain (stress management techniques, meditation, hypnosis, relaxation, guided imagery, biofeedback, cognitive therapy) to achieve an analgesic effect.

6. See a massage therapist, rolf practitioner, Feldenkrais, or Alexander practitioner for postural integration and trigger point evaluation or treatment.

Step Two: Detoxification

Undergo standard, especially diagnostic imaging of the joints. See a health-care practitioner to determine digestive capacity, food allergies, intestinal permeability, adrenal and thyroid status, and colonic microflora. Follow therapies discussed in this book to correct imbalances. Use drainage remedies, fasting, and other detoxification procedures to detoxify the body four times per year.

1. For dysbiosis and infectious arthritis, a stool analysis will direct the physician to the proper therapies. In general, use PlantiBiotic from Nature's Answer or Biocidin (one pill with each meal; taken only with food). Get 2-3 colonic hydrotherapy treatments per week. For the first eight weeks, use antimicrobial herbs and demulcents in the water. For

the last four weeks, use *Lactobacillus* and *Bifidobacteria* cultures as an implant. Repeat stool test to measure results. Repeat intensive therapy if still positive or continue with two treatments per month on a maintenance basis if bowel flora is normalized.

For information on **Biofreeze**, contact: Performance Health, Inc., 127 Craighead Street, Suite 105, Pittsburgh, PA 15211; tel: 800-246-3733.

2. For botanical detoxification of all organs and to support the liver and anti-inflammatory systems: Altera Tonic from Nature's Answer (two pills, three times per day).

3. To treat intestinal permeability: GastroGuard from Nature's Answer (one or two pills, three times per day) or Robert's Formula from Phyto-Pharmica (one or two pills, three times per day). Repeat test and continue on formulas until the tests prove negative.

Use the appropriate homeopathic remedies for pain, based on individual signs and symptoms. For more information on **selecting homeopathic remedies for pain relief**, see Chapter 13: Supplements for Arthritis, pp. 280-313.

4. Use hyperthermic hydrotherapy: have a naturopathic physician or other practitioner administer hyperthermia treatments three times per week, making sure to raise the body temperature to a minimum of 103° F for one hour. This will kill the spirochetes associated with Lyme disease.

5. Use homeopathic Lyme nosode (available from Professional Health Products): 15 drops, four times per day between meals. Under the supervision of a homeopathic practitioner, take *Ledum* 200C (one dose per day for one week), which often arrests the case immediately and halts the arthralgia.

6. Use equal parts of tincture of sarsaparilla, *Guiacum sanctum*, *Boswellia serrata*, dandelion (*Taraxacum officinale*), goldenseal (*Hydrastis canadensis*), and *Isatis tinctoria* with five drops of thyme oil per ounce of tincture (one teaspoon, 4-5 times daily).

Step Three: Desensitizing Autoimmunity

1. Have your physician prepare an oral auto-sanguis nosode (take 15 drops, three times per day between meals). Use injectible auto-sanguis therapy from your doctor. This acts as a "self-vaccine," not to prevent but to treat the Lyme spirochete.

2. Consider urine therapy.

3. Take the following herbs and supplements:

■ *Hemidesmus indicus* (MediHerb): one teaspoon, 3-4 times per day

■ *Tripterygium wilfordii* (only from a TCM physican): 15-30 ml of the tincture in divided doses

■ Lithospermum 15 (a Chinese herbal formula)

■ Bovine or chicken cartilage extracts: three grams per day

■ MSM (methylsulfonylmethane): 3,000 mg per day in divided doses

4. Use mind/body techniques to help stop the aggressive autoimmune attack. Use counseling and other stress management techniques in the book to become a less stressful person and to deal with emotional issues.

Step Four: Stabilization

1. Consult with a physician trained in physical medicine, manipulation, and restoration of proper biomechanics to restore normal range of motion of your joints, attain muscular balance, correct posture or flat feet, correct ergonomic issues at work, strengthen weak muscles, and stretch short muscles.

For more information on **hydrotherapy**, see Chapter 5: Detoxifying Specific Organs, pp. 102-129. For more on **tests used for diagnosing the underlying causes of arthritis**, see Chapter 3: Diagnosing Arthritis, pp. 52-77.

2. Get 45 minutes of exercise four times per week. Especially useful are yoga, tai chi, and aquatic exercises. Perform regular stretching and muscle strengthening.

3. Maintain all of the above therapies until you are 90% pain free for one month. When you are no longer in pain, discontinue all herbs for pain and DL-phenylalanine, but continue on all other nutrients. Continue with the physical therapies, but adjust them to your individual needs and schedule.

4. Attain a desirable weight for your height and optimum percentage of body fat.

5. Seek advice from your alternative health-care practitioner to individualize your program as you become increasingly well.

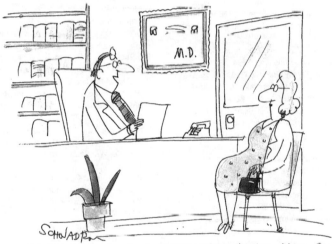

"I'M SENDING YOU TO A SPECIALIST WHO TREATS DRUG SIDE EFFECTS FROM DRUG SIDE EFFECTS."

Endnotes

Chapter 1
Arthritis Can Be Reversed

1 Arthritis Foundation. "Arthritis Fact Sheet." Available from: Arthritis Foundation, 1330 West Peachtree Street, Atlanta, GA 30309; tel: 404-872-7100; fax: 404-872-8694; website: www.arthritis.org. Michael T. Murray, N.D. *Arthritis* (Rocklin, CA: Prima Publishing, 1994), 3.

2 R.P. Grelsamer, M.D., and S. Loevl, eds. *The Columbia Presbyterian Osteoarthritis Handbook* (New York: Macmillan, 1996), xviii.

3 Michael T. Murray, N.D. *Arthritis* (Rocklin, CA: Prima Publishing, 1994), 28.

4 *The PDR Family Guide to Prescription Drugs* 2nd ed. (Montvale, NJ: Medical Economics, 1994), 804-808.

5 P.M. Brooks et al. "NSAIDs and Osteoarthritis–Help or Hindrance?" *Journal of Rheumatology* 9 (1982), 3-5.

6 N.M. Newman et al. "Acetabular Bone Destruction Related to NSAIDs." *The Lancet* (1985), 11-13. L. Soloman. "Drug Induced Arthropathy and Necrosis of the Femoral Head." *Journal of Bone and Joint Surgery* 55B (1973), 246-251.

7 B.F. McAdam et al. "Systemic Biosynthesis of Prostacyclin by Cyclooxygenase (COX)-2: The Human Pharmacology of a Selective Inhibitor of COX-2." *Proceedings of the National Academy of Sciences* 96:1 (1999), 272-277. D.W. Gilroy et al. "Inducible Cyclooxygenase May Have Anti-Inflammatory Properties." *Nature Medicine* 5:6 (June 1999), 698-701.

Chapter 2
What Is Arthritis?

1 R. Weiss. "Geneticists to Arthritics: A Gene's The Rub." *Science News* 138 (1990), 148.

2 David S. Pisetsky, M.D., Ph.D., With Susan Flamholtz Trien. *Duke University Medical Center Book of Arthritis* (New York: Ballantine Books, 1995), 75-76.

3 James Balch, M.D., and Phyllis Balch. *Prescriptions for Nutritional Healing* (Garden City Park, NY: Avery Publishing, 1997), 138.

4 E.L. Rabin. "Mechanical Aspects of Osteoarthritis." *Bulletin of Rheumatic Diseases* 26 (862-865). E.L. Rabin et al. "A Consolidated Concept of Joint Lubrication." *Journal of Bone and Joint Surgery* 54A (1972), 607-616. E.L. Rabin, S.R. Simon, R.M. Rose, I.L. Paul, eds. *Mechanics of Joint Degeneration: Practical Biomechanics for the Orthopedic Surgeon* (New York: John Wiley and Sons, 1979).

5 C.L. Tsai et al. "Estrogen and Osteoarthritis: A Study of Synovial Estradiol and Estriol Receptor Binding in Human Osteoarthritic Knees." *Biochemical and Biophysical Research Communications* 183 (1992), 1287-1291.

6 Michael Murray, N.D., and Joseph Pizzorno, N.D. *The Textbook of Natural Medicine* (Seattle, WA: Bastyr University Press, 1998).

7 I. Machtey and L. Ouaknine. "Tocopherol in Osteoarthritis: A Controlled Pilot Study." *Journal of the American Geriatric Society* 26 (1978), 328-330.

8 G. Krystal, G.M. Morris, and L. Sokoloff. "Stimulation of DNA Synthesis by Ascorbate in Cultures of Articular Chondrocytes." *Arthritis and Rheumatism* 25 (1982), 318-325.

9 W. Kaufman. *The Common Form of Joint Dysfunction: Its Incidence and Treatment* (Brattleboro, VT: E.L. Hildreth, 1949). J.R. DiPalma and W.S. Thayer. "Use of Niacin as a Drug." *Annual Review of Nutrition* 11 (1991), 169-187.

10 R.L. Travers, G.C. Rennie, and R.E. Newnham. "Boron and Arthritis: The Results of a Double-Blind Pilot Study." *Journal of Nutrition in Medicine* 1 (1990), 127-132.

11 J. Kremer et al. "Effects of Manipulation of Dietary Fatty Acids on Clinical Manifestation of Rheumatoid Arthritis." *The Lancet* 1 (1985), 184-187. J.P.

Pelletier and J. Martel-Pelletier. "Role of Synovial Inflammation, Cytokines, and IGF-1 in the Physiopathology of Osteoarthritis." *Review of Rheumatic Education Forum* 61 (1994), 103s-108s.

12 James Balch, M.D., and Phyllis Balch. *Prescriptions for Nutritional Healing* (Garden City Park, NY: Avery Publishing, 1997), 138.

13 R.P. Greisamer, M.D., and S. Loevl, eds. *The Columbia Presbyterian Osteoarthritis Handbook* (New York: Macmillan, 1996), 36.

14 Joseph Candel and David Sudderth. *The Arthritis Solution* (Rocklin, CA: Prima Publishing, 1997), 3.

15 Arthritis Foundation. *Primer on Rheumatic Disease* 8th ed. (Atlanta, GA: Arthritis Foundation, 1983), 39. J.P. Kulka et al. "Early Joint Lesions of Rheumatoid Arthritis." *Archives of Pathology* 59 (1955), 129-150. H.R. Schumacher. "Synovial Membrane and Fluid Morphological Alterations in Early Rheumatoid Arthritis: Microvascular Injury and Virus-Like Particles." *Annals of the New York Academy of Sciences* 256 (1975), 39-64.

16 Joseph Pizzorno, N.D., Michael T. Murray, N.D., and Patrick Donovan, R.N., N.D. "Bowel Toxemia, Permeability and Disease: New Information to Support an Old Concept." *Textbook of Natural Medicine, IV: Bowel Toxemia* (Seattle, WA: Bastyr College Publications, 1985), 2.

17 R.S. Panesh et al. "Delayed Reactions to Food. Food Allergy in Rheumatic Disease." *Annals of Allergy* 56 (1986), 500-503. See also: M.A. Van de Laar and J.K. Ander Korst. "Food Intolerance in Rheumatoid Arthritis: A Double-Blind Controlled Trial of the Clinical Effects of Elimination of Milk Allergens and Azo Dyes." *Annals of Rheumatological Disease* 51 (1992), 298-302. J.A. Hickland. "The Effect of Diet in Rheumatoid Arthritis." *Journal of Clinical Allergy* 10 (1980), 463-467. Gail Darlington, M.D., et al. "Placebo Controlled Blind Study of Dietary Manipulation Therapy in Rheumatoid Arthritis." *The Lancet* i (1986), 236-

238. F. MacCrae et al. "Diet and Arthritis." *Practitioner* 230 (1986), 359-361. H.M. Buchanan et al. "Is Diet Important in Rheumatoid Arthritis?" *British Journal of Rheumatology* 30 (1991), 125-134. Gail Darlington, M.D., et al. "Clinical Review of Dietary Therapy for Rheumatoid Arthritis." *British Journal of Rheumatology* 32 (1993), 507-514.

18 B. Dugas and J.P. Kolb. "Nitric Oxide Production in Human Inflammatory Process." *Research in Immunology* 9:146 (1995), 661-717.

19 Joseph Pizzorno, N.D. *Total Wellness* (Rocklin, CA: Prima Publishing, 1996), 167-168.

20 Richard Leviton. "Rheumatoid Arthritis and Multiple Sclerosis: The Cause May Be In the Blood." *Alternative Medicine Digest* 18 (May/June 1997), 64-68.

21 Hans-Henrich Reckeweg. *Homotoxicology: Illness and Healing Through Anti-Homotoxic Therapy* (Albuquerque, NM: Menaco Publishing, 1980).

22 G.E. Comstock et. al. "Serum Concentrations of Alpha-Tocopherol, Beta Carotene, and Retinol Preceding the Diagnosis of Rheumatoid Arthritis and Systemic Lupus Erythematosus." *Annals of Rheumatic Disease* 56:5 (1997), 323-325.

23 Gail Darlington, M.D., and Linda Gamlin. *Diet and Arthritis* (London, England: Vermilion, 1996), 247.

24 G.V. Ball and L.B. Sorensen. "Pathogenesis of Hyperuricemia in Saturnine Gout." *New England Journal of Medicine* 280 (1969), 1197-1202.

25 Gerald P. Rodnan, M.D., and H. Ralph Schumacher, M.D. *Primer on the Rheumatic Diseases* 8th ed. (Atlanta, GA: The Arthritis Foundation, 1983), 91.

26 Luke Bucci, Ph.D. *Healing Arthritis: The Natural Way* (Arlington, TX: Summit Publishing Group, 1995), 6.

27 M. Proctor et al. "Lowered Cutaneous and Urinary Levels of Polyamines With Clinical Improvement in Treated Psoriasis." *Archives of Dermatology* 115 (1979), 945-949. Editorial. "Polyamines and Psoriasis." *Archives of Dermatology* 115 (1979), 943-944. Editorial.

"Polyamines in Psoriasis." *Journal of Investigative Dermatology* 81 (1983), 385-387. E. Rosenberg et al. "Microbial Factors in Psoriasis." *Archives of Dermatology* 118 (1982), 1434-1444.

28 N.B. Zlatkov et al. "Free Fatty Acids in the Blood Serum of Psoriatics." *Acta Dermato-Venereologica* 64 (1984), 22-25.

29 Editorial. "Leukotrienes and Other Lipoxygenase Products in the Pathogenesis and Therapy of Psoriasis and Other Dermatoses." *Archives of Dermatology* 119 (1983), 541-547.

30 A. Donadini et al. "Plasma Levels of Zinc, Copper and Nickel in Healthy Controls and in Psoriatic Patients." *Acta Vitaminologica et Enzymologica* 1 (1980), 9-16.

31 P.E. Philips. "Seminars in Arthritis and Rheumatism: Infectious Agents in the Pathogenesis of Rheumatoid Arthritis." *Seminars in Arthritis and Rheumatism* 16 (1986), 1-100. See also: M.M. Griffiths. "Arthritis Induced by Bacteria and Viruses." In: B. Henderson, J.C.W. Edwards, and E.R. Pettipher. *Mechanism and Models in Rheumatoid Arthritis* (London, England: Academic Press, 1995), 411-430.

32 Gail Darlington, M.D., and Linda Gamlin. *Diet and Arthritis* (London, England: Vermilion Press, 1996), 109.

33 B.M. Segal et al. "Microbial Products Induce Autoimmune Disease by an IL-12 Dependent Pathway." *Journal of Immunology* 158 (1997), 5087-5090.

34 J.H. Schwab. "Bacterial Cell Wall Induced Arthritis: Models of Chronic Recurrent Polyarthritis and Reactivation of Monoarticular Arthritis." In: B. Henderson, J.C.W. Edwards and E.R. Pettither. *Mechanisms and Models in Rheumatoid Arthritis* (London, England: Academic Press, 1995), 431-446.

35 Gail Darlington, M.D., and Linda Gamlin. *Diet and Arthritis* (London, England: Vermilion Press, 1996), 127.

36 Fred Bayles. "Lyme Disease Not as Rampant as Fear." *USA Today* (August 9, 1999), 3A.

37 Robert Bingham, M.D. *Fighting Back Against Arthritis* (Desert Hot Springs, CA: Desert Arthritis Medical Clinic, 1994), 5-6.

Chapter 3
Diagnosing Arthritis

1 Robert Berkow, M.D. *The Merck Manual* 14th ed. (Rahway, NJ: Merck, 1982), 1177.

2 A.J. Fletcher. *The Merck Manual of Geriatrics* 2nd ed. (White House Station, NJ: Merck, 1995), 933.

3 R. Roubenoff et al. "Abnormal Homocysteine Metabolism in Rheumatoid Arthritis." *Arthritis and Rheumatism* 40:4 (1997), 718-722.

4 W. Emlen et al. "Measurement of Serum Hyaluronic Acid with Rheumatoid Arthritis: Correlation With Disease Activity." *Journal of Rheumatology* 23:6 (1996), 974-978.

5 Robert Berkow, M.D. *The Merck Manual* 14th ed. (Rahway, NJ: Merck, 1982), 1223.

6 U. Wagner et al. "HLA Markers and Prediction of Clinical Course and Outcome in Rheumatoid Arthritis." *Arthritis and Rheumatology* 40:2 (1997), 341-351.

7 M. Hakala et al. "Application of Markers of Collagen Metabolism in Serum and Synovial Fluid for Assessment of Disease Process in Patients with Rheumatoid Arthritis." *Annals of Rheumatic Disease* 54:11 (1995), 886-890.

8 James F. Balch, M.D., and Phyllis A. Balch, C.N.C. *Prescriptions for Nutritional Healing* (Garden City Park, NY: Avery Publishing Group, 1993), 191.

9 Michael T. Murray, M.D. *Arthritis* (Rocklin, CA: Prima Publishing, 1994), 249.

10 H. Mielants et al. "Intestinal Mucosal Permeability in Inflammatory Rheumatic Disease II: Role of Disease." *Journal of Rheumatology* 18:3 (1991), 394-400.

11 Lita Lee, Ph.D. "The 24-Hour Urinalysis According to Loomis." *Earthletter* 4:2 (Summer 1994), 2.

12 Gail Darlington, M.D., and Linda Gamlin. *Diet and Arthritis* (London, England: Vermilion Press, 1996). See also: M.A. Van de Laar et al. "Food Intolerance in Rheumatoid Arthritis II: Clinical and Histological Aspects." *Annals of Rheumatic Disease* 51:3 (1992), 303-306.

13 G.E. Comstock et al. "Serum Concentrations of Alpha Tocopherol, Beta

Carotene, and Retinol Preceding the Diagnosis of Rheumatoid Arthritis and Systemic Lupus Erythmatosus." *Annals of Rheumatic Disease* 56:5 (1997), 323-355.

14 Lawrence Wilson. *Nutritional Balancing and Hair Mineral Analysis* (Scottsdale, AZ: L.D. Wilson Consultants, 1992), 115.

15 Ibid., 44-46.

Chapter 4
General Detoxification

1 William J. Rea, M.D. *Chemical Sensitivity, Vol. 4* (Boca Raton, FL: C.R.C. Lewis, 1997), 2434.

2 William J. Rea, M.D. *Chemical Sensitivity, Vol. 3* (Boca Raton, FL: C.R.C. Lewis, 1996), 1555-1579.

3 William Lee Cowden, M.D., "Is Your Shower Toxic? Some Pollution Solutions." *Alternative Medicine* 29 (April/May 1999), 69.

4 B. Croty "Ulcerative Colitis and Xenobiotic Metabolism." *The Lancet* 343 (1990), 35-38.

5 William Lee Cowden, M.D., "Is Your Shower Toxic? Some Pollution Solutions." *Alternative Medicine* 29 (April/May 1999), 69.

6 W. Melillo. "How Safe is Mercury in Dentistry?" *Washington Post Weekly Journal of Medicine, Science and Society* (September 1991), 4. World Health Organization. *Environmental Health Criteria for Inorganic Mercury* (Geneva, Switzerland: World Health Organization, 1991), 118.

7 William J. Rea, M.D. *Chemical Sensitivity, Vol. 3* (Boca Raton, FL: C.R.C. Lewis, 1996), 1555-1579.

8 *Copper Toxicity Paper 5*. Available from: Eck Institute of Applied Nutrition and Bioenergetics, Ltd., 8650 North 22nd Avenue, Phoenix, AZ 85021; tel: 602-995-1580.

9 D.N. Taylor et al. "Effects of Trichloroethylene in the Exploratory and Locomotor Activity in Rats Exposed During Development." *Science Total Environment* 47 (1985), 415-420. H.N. Arito, T. Suruta, K. Nakagaki, and S. Tanaka. "Partial Insomnia, Hyperactivity and Hyperdipsia Induced by Repeated Administration of Toluene in Rats: Their Relation to Brain Monoamine Metabolism." *Toxicology* 37:1-2 (1985), 99-110.

10 William J. Rea, M.D. *Chemical Sensitivity, Vol. 3* (Boca Raton, FL: C.R.C. Lewis, 1996), 1555-1579.

11 J. Palmblad et al. "Antirheumatic Effects of Fasting." *Rheumatic Disease Clinics of North America 2* (May 1991), 351-352. J. Kjeldsen-Kragh et al. "Controlled Trial of Fasting and One Year Vegetarian Diet in Rheumatoid Arthritis." *The Lancet* 338 (1991), 899-902. J. Kjeldsen-Kragh et al. "Vegetarian Diet After Fasting for Patients with Rheumatoid Arthritis—Status: Two Years After Introduction of the Diet." *Clinical Rheumatology 3* (September 1994), 475-482.

12 R.S. Goodhart and M.E. Shils. *Modern Nutrition in Health and Disease* 6th ed. (Philadelphia: Lea & Febiger, 1980), 738, 983-986, 1086. William J. Rea, M.D. *Chemical Sensitivity* (Boca Raton, FL: CRC Lewis, 1997), 2401.

13 I. Hafstrom et al. "Effects of Fasting on Disease Activity, Neutrophil Function, Fatty Acid Composition, and Leukotriene Biosynthesis in Patients with Rheumatoid Arthritis." *Arthritis and Rheumatology* 5 (May 1988), 585-592.

14 Cherie Calbom, M.D. *The Juice Lady's Juicing for High-Level Wellness and Vibrant Good Looks* (New York: Three Rivers Press, 1999), 7-8.

15 Joseph B. Marion. *The Anti-Aging Manual* (South Woodstock, CT: Information Pioneers, 1996), 195.

16 Ibid., 237.

17 Ronald L. Seibold, M.S., ed. *Cereal Grass: Nature's Greatest Health Gift* (New Canaan, CT: Keats Publishing, 1991), 61.

Chapter 5
Detoxifying Specific Organs

1 Burton Goldberg Group. *Alternative Medicine: The Definitive Guide* (Tiburon, CA: Future Medicine Publishing, 1995), 144.

2 Ralph Golan, M.D. *Optimal Wellness* (New York: Ballantine, 1995), 160.

3 Edmond Bordeaux Szekeley. *Essene Gospel of Peace* (International Biogenic Society, 1937), 16.

4 John Harvey Kellogg, M.D. "Should the Colon Be Sacrificed or May It Be Reformed?" *Journal of the American Medicine Association* 68:26 (1917), 1957-1959.

5 William J. Rea, M.D. *Chemical Sensitivity, Vol. 4* (Boca Raton, FL: CRC Lewis, 1997), 2438.

6 Joseph Pizzorno, N.D. *Total Wellness* (Rocklin, CA: Prima Publishing, 1996), 105.

7 L.K.T. Lam et al. "Isolation and Identification of Kahweol Palmitate and Cafestol Palmitate as Active Constituents of Green Coffee Beans That Enhance Glutathione-S-Transferase Activity in the Mouse." *Cancer Research* 42 (1982), 1193-1198.

8 Howard Straus. "Coffee Corner." *Gerson Healing Newsletter* 11:5 (1996), 9-11.

9 Eugene Zampieron, N.D., A.H.G., and Ellen Kamhi, Ph.D., R.N. *The Natural Medicine Chest* (New York: M. Evans, 1999), 52-54.

10 Michael Tierra. *The Way of Herbs* (Santa Fe, NM: Lotus Press, 1988), 263.

11 J. G. Langer et al. *Indian Journal of Pharmacology* 13 (1982), 98.

12 C. J. Poutinen. *Herbs for Detoxification* (New Canaan, CT: Keats, 1977), 67.

13 M. World et al. "Cyanidanol-3 for Alcoholic Liver Disease: Result of a Six-Month Clinical Trial." *Alcoholism* 19 (1984), 23-29.

14 Eugene Zampieron, N.D., A.H.G. Clinical observations (1986-1998).

15 Arthur C. Guyton. *Basic Human Physiology* (Philadelphia: W.B. Saunders, 1971).

16 John Anderson. "Rebounders: Bounce Your Way to Better Health." *Alternative Medicine Digest* 20 (October/November 1997), 42-46.

17 David L. Hoffmann, B.Sc, M.N.I.M.H. *The Herb User's Guide* (Wellingborough, Northhamptonshire, England: Thorsens, 1987), 141.

18 H.S. Wolf et al. "Detection of Polycyclic Aromatic Hydrocarbons in Skin Oil Obtained From Roofing Workers." *Chemosphere* 11 (1982), 595.

19 D.W. Schnare et al. "Body Burden Reductions of PCBs, PBBs, and Chlorinated Pesticides in Human Subjects." *Ambio* 13 (1984), 5-6.

20 William J. Rea, M.D. *Chemical Sensitivity, Vol. 4* (Boca Raton, FL: CRC Lewis, 1997), 2463.

Chapter 6

Eradicating Bacteria and Yeast

1 Joseph Pizzorno, N.D. *Total Wellness* (Rocklin, CA: Prima Publishing, 1996), 112.

2 Ibid., 112.

3 Ralph Golan, M.D. *Optimal Wellness* (New York: Ballantine Books, 1995), 172.

4 Joseph Pizzorno, N.D. *Total Wellness* (Rocklin, CA: Prima Publishing, 1996).

5 Alan Ebringer, M.D., et al. "Cross Reactivity Between *Klebsiella aerogenes* Species and B27 Lymphocyte Antigens as an Etiological Factor in Ankylosing Spondylitis." In: Jean Dausset and Arne Svejgaard, eds. *HLA and Disease* (Copenhagen: Williams & Wilkins, 1977), 27.

6 Alan Ebringer et al. "Ankylosing Spondylitis HLA-B27 and *Klebsiella* 11: Cross Reactivity Studies with Human Tissue Typing Sera." *British Journal of Experimental Pathology* 61 (1980), 92-96.

7 Alan Ebringer et al. "Ankylosing Spondylitis, *Klebsiella* and HLA-B27." *Rheumatological Rehabilitation* 16 (1977), 190-196. See also: Alan Ebringer et al. "Sequential Studies in Ankylosing Spondylitis: Associated of Klebsiella Pneumonia with Active Disease." *Annals of Rheumatic Disease* 37 (1978), 146-151. Research reported in The Lancet [Vol. 352 (October 3, 1998), 1137-1140] further investigates the link between HLA-B27 and ankylosing spondylitis.

8 Alan Ebringer et al. "Rheumatoid Arthritis and Proteus: A Possible Etiological Association." *Rheumatology International* 9 (1989), 223-228.

9 Alan Ebringer et al., "The Use of a Low-Starch Diet in the Treatment of Patients Suffering from Ankylosing Spondylitis." *Clinical Rheumatology* 15:Suppl. 1 (January 1996), 62-66.

10 Michael T. Murray, N.D. "Chronic Candidiasis: A Natural Approach." *American Journal of Natural Medicine*

4:4 (May 1997), 13.

11. W. Krause, H. Matheis, and K. Wulf. "Fungaemia and Funguria After Oral Administration of *Candida albicans*." *The Lancet* 1:7595 (1969), 598-599.

12 G. Rodman and R. Schumacher, eds. "The Complement System." In: *Primer on the Rheumatic Diseases* 8th ed. (Atlanta, GA: Arthritis Foundation, 1983), 20-21.

13 William G. Crook, M.D. *The Yeast Connection Handbook* (Jackson, TN: Professional Books, 1997), 47-48.

14 Simon Martin. *Candida: The Natural Way* (Boston: Element Books. 1998), 10-11. This information is adapted from a *Candida* Questionnaire developed by William Crook, M.D., and included in his book *The Yeast Connection Handbook* (Jackson, TN: Professional Books, 1996), 15-19.

15 D. M. Blair, C. S. Hangee-Bauer, and C. Calabrese. "Intestinal Candidiasis, *Lactobacillus acidophilus* Supplementation and Crook's Questionnaire." *Journal of Naturopathic Medicine* 2 (1991), 33-37.

16 Tim Birdsall. "Gastrointestinal Candidiasis: Fact or Fiction?" *Alternative Medicine Review* 2:5 (1997), 346-348.

17 U.S. General Accounting Office. "FDA Strategy Needed to Address Animal Drug Residues in Milk." (Washington, DC: General Accounting Office, 1992). S. Begley. "The End of Antibiotics." *Newsweek* (March 28, 1994), 48. Lee Hitchcock, D.C. *Long Life Now* (Berkeley, CA: Celestial Arts, 1996), 67.

18 M. Rosenbaum, M.D., and M. Susser, M.D. *Solving the Puzzle of Chronic Fatigue Syndrome* (Tacoma, WA: Life Sciences Press, 1992), 131.

19 Joseph Pizzorno, N.D. and Michael T. Murray, N.D., eds. *A Textbook of Natural Medicine* (Seattle, WA: John Bastyr College Publications, 1988-89).

20 Michael T. Murray, N.D. "Probiotics: *Acidophilus, Bifidobacter,* and FOS." *American Journal of Natural Medicine* 3:4 (1996), 11-14. Elizabeth Lipski, M.S., C.C.N. *Digestive Wellness* (New Canaan, CT: Keats, 1996). John A. Catanzaro, N.D., and Lisa Green, B.Sc., "Microbial Ecology and Dysbiosis in Human Medicine." *Alternative Medicine Review* 2:3 (1997), 202-209. John A. Catanzaro, N.D., and Lisa Green, B.Sc., "Microbial Ecology and Probiotics in Human Health (Part II)." *Alternative Medicine Review* 2:4 (1997), 296-305. P.S. Moshchich et al. "Prevention of Dysbacteriosis in the Early Neonatal Period Using a Pure Culture of Acidophilic Bacteria." *Pediatriia* (1989), 25-30. S.J. Bhatia et al. "*Lactobacillus acidophilus* Inhibits Growth of Campylobacter pylori in vitro." *Journal of Clinical Microbiology* 27:10 (1989), 2328-2330.

21 W.J. Crinnion. "Clinical Trial Results on Neesby's Capricin." (Unpublished manuscript). Available from: Probiologic, Inc., 1803 132nd Avenue NE, Bellevue, WA 98005.

22 Paul Bergner, *The Healing Power of Garlic* (Rocklin, CA: Prima Publishing, 1996), 98-100.

23 Heinrich P. Koch, Ph.D, M.Pharm., and Larry D. Lawson, Ph.D. *Garlic: The Science and Therapeutic Application of Allium sativum L. and Related Species* (Baltimore, MD: Williams & Wilkins, 1996), 168-172.

24 Cass Ingram, D.O. *The Cure Is in the Cupboard: How to Use Oregano for Better Health* (Buffalo Grove, IL: Knowledge House, 1997), 14-16, 34, 50.

25 C.F. Carson and T.V. Riley. "Antimicrobial Activity of the Major Components of the Essential Oil of Melaleuca alternifolia." *Journal of Applied Bacteriology* 78:3 (1995), 264-269.

26 For additional information on tea tree oil, see: Eugene R. Zampieron, N.D., A.H.G., and Ellen Kamhi, Ph.D., R.N. *The Natural Medicine Chest* (New York: M. Evans, 1999).

Chapter 7

Eliminating Parasites

1 D. W. Bendig, M.D. "Diagnosis of Giardiasis in Infants and Children by Endoscopic Brush Cytology." *Journal of Pediatric Gastroenterology and Nutrition* 8:2 (1989), 204-206.

2 T.S. Bocanegra et al. "Musculoskeletal Syndromes in Parasitic Diseases." *Rheumatic Disease Clinics of North America* 19:2 (May 1993), 505-513.

3 R.Q. Sherry et al. "Reiter's Syndrome Associated with Cryptosporidial Gastroenteritis." *Journal of Rheumatology* 22:10 (October 1995), 1962-1963.

4 M. Letts et al. "Synovitis Secondary to Giardiasis in Children." *American Journal of Orthopedics* 27:6 (June 1998), 451-454.

5 Than-Saw et al. "Isolation of Entamoeba Histolytica from Arthritic Knee Joint." *Tropical and Geographical Medicine* 44:4 (October 1992), 355-358.

6 S.K. Lee et al. "Nine Cases of Strongyloidiasis in Korea." *Korean Journal of Parasitology* 32:1 (March 1994), 49-52.

7 P.E. McGill. "Rheumatic Syndromes Associated with Parasites," *Baillieres Clinical Rheumatology* 9:1 (February 1995), 201-13.

8 A. Di Pietro et al. "Parasitic Arthritis: A Case Report." *Pediatria Medica e Chirurgica* 18:2 (March/April 1996), 211-212.

9 R.P. Messner. "Arthritis Due to Tuberculosis, Fungal Infections, and Parasites." *Current Opinions in Rheumatology* 3:4 (August 1991), 617-20.

10 Patrick R. Murray, ed. *Manual of Clinical Microbiology* (Washington, DC: ASM Press, 1999).

11 Dan Bensky et al. *Chinese Herbal Medicine: Materia Medica* (Seattle, WA: Eastland Press, 1986), 630.

12 D. Mirelman et al. "Inhibition of Growth of Entamoeba Histolitica by Allicin, the Active Principle of Garlic Extract (Allium sativum)." *Journal of Infectious Disease* 156:1 (1987), 243-244.

13 S. Gupte. "Use of Berberine in the Treatment of Giardiasis." *American Journal of Diseases of Children* 129 (1975), 866.

14 Joseph Pizzorno, N.D. *Total Wellness* (Rocklin, CA: Prima Publishing, 1996), 79.

15 Martha Windholz, ed. *Merck Index: An Encyclopedia of Chemicals and Drugs* 9th ed. (Rahway, NJ: Merck, 1976), 1214.

16 "Antibiotic Alternative Proven Effective." *The GSE Report* 1:1, 1.

17 Earl Mindell, R.Ph., Ph.D. *Earl Mindell's Supplement Bible* (New York: Simon and Schuster, 1998), 63.

18 The Burton Goldberg Group. *Alternative Medicine: The Definitive Guide* (Tiburon, CA: Future Medicine Publishing, 1995), 782-787.

Chapter 8
Alleviating Leaky Gut Syndrome

1 H. Mielants et al. "Intestinal Mucus Permeability in Inflammatory Rheumatic Diseases II: Role of Disease." *Journal of Rheumatology* 81:3 (1991), 394-400.

2 Ibid.

3 R. Jenkins et al. "Increased Intestinal Permeability in Patients with Rheumatoid Arthritis: A Side Effect of Oral Non-Steroidal Anti-Inflammatory Drug Therapy?" *British Journal of Rheumatology* 26 (1987), 103-107. See also: J. F. Fries et al. "Toward an Epidemiology of Gastropathy Associated with Non-Steroidal Anti-Inflammatory Drug Use." *Gastroenterology* 96 (1989), 647-655.

4 I. Bjarnason et al. "The Leaky Gut of Alcoholism: Possible Route of Entry for Toxic Compounds." *The Lancet* 28:1 (January 1984), 179-182.

5 Jeffrey Bland, Ph.D. *Advancement in Clinical Nutrition* (Gig Harbor, WA: Healthcom, 1993-1994), 4-25.

6 H. Mielants. "Reflections on the Link Between Intestinal Inflammatory Joint Disease." *Journal of Rheumatology* 8:5 (1990), 523-524.

7 L.G. Darlington, M.D., et. al. "Diets for Rheumatoid Arthritis." *The Lancet* 333 (1991), 1209. See also: H. Lithell et al. "A Fasting and Vegetarian Diet Treatment Trial on Chronic Inflammatory Disorders." *Acta Dermato-Venereologica* 63 (1983), 397-403. L. Skoldstam et al. "Impaired Con A Suppressive Cell Activity in Patients with Rheumatoid Arthritis Shows Normalization During Fasting." *Scandinavian Journal of Rheumatology* 12:4 (1983), 369-373. T. Sundqvist et al. "Influence of Fasting on Intestinal Permeability and Disease Activity in Patients With Rheumatoid Arthritis Showing Normalization During Fasting." *Scandinavian Journal of Rheumatology* 11 (1982), 33-38.

8 A.M. Uden et al. "Neutrophil Function and

Clinical Performances After Total Fasting in Patients with Rheumatoid Arthritis." *Annals of Rheumatic Disease* 42 (1983), 45-51. See also: J. Palmblad et al. "Acute Energy Deprivation in Man: Effect on Serum Immunoglobulins Antibody Response Complement Factors Three and Four, Acute Phased Reactants and Interferon Producing Capacity of Blood Lymphocytes." *Clinical Experimental Immunology* 30 (1977), 55.

9 David Hoffman. *The Herb User's Guide* (Wellingborough, Northamptonshire, England: Thorsens Publishing Group, 1987), 44.

10 David Hoffman. *The Herb User's Guide* (Northamptonshire, England: Thorsens Publishers, 1987), 55.

11 John Lust. *The Herb Book* (New York: Bantam Books, 1974), 270.

12 P. Braquet. *Ginkgolides: Chemistry, Biology, Pharmacology and Clinical Perspectives, Vol. I* (Barcelona, Spain: J. Prous Science Publishers, 1988). See also: P. Braquet, ed. *Ginkolides: Chemistry Biology, Pharmacology and Clinical Perspectives, Vol. II* (Barcelona, Spain: J. Prous Science Publishers, 1989). E. W. Fungfeld, ed. *Rokan: Ginkgo Biloba* (New York: Springer Verlag, 1988).

13 Walter H. Lewis and Memry Elvin Lewis. *Medical Botany: Plants Effecting Man's Health* (New York: John Wiley and Sons, 1077).

15 Kerry Bone. *Phytosynergistic Prescribing: A Professional Proscribers Reference Guide to Herbal Formulas* (Lake Oswego, OR: Communications Medicus), 17, Formula 5.

15 Simon Y. Mills, M.A. *The Dictionary of Modern Herbalism* (Rochester, VT: Healing Arts Press, 1988), 138.

16 David Hoffman. *The Herb User's Guide* (Northamptonshire, England: Thorsens Publishers, 1987), 55.

17 Simon Y. Mills, M.A. *The Dictionary of Modern Herbalism* (Rochester, VT: Healing Arts Press, 1988), 58-59.

18 Steven Foster. *Chamomile* Botanical Series 307 (Austin, TX: American Botanical Council, 1991).

19 David Hoffman. *The New Holistic Herbal* (Rockport, MA: Element, 1991), 204.

20 V.P. Choundhry, M. Sabir, and V.N. Bhide. "Berberine in Giardiasis." *Indian Pediatrics* 9:3 (March 1972), 143-146.

21 Y. Kumazawa et al. "Activation of Peritoneal Macrophages by Berberine-Alkaloids in Terms of Induction of Cytostatic Activity." *International Journal of Immunopharma-cology* 6 (1984), 587-592.

22 R.R. van der Hulst et al. "Glutamine and the Preservation of Gut Integrity." *The Lancet* 334 (1993), 1363-1365.

23 H. Chun, M. Sasaki, Y. Fugiyama, and T. Bamba. "Effect of Anteral Glutamine on Intestinal Permeability and Bacterial Translocation after Abdominal Radiation Injury in Rats." *Journal of Gastroenterology* 32:2 (1997), 189-195.

24 R. Denno, J.D. Rounds, R. Faris, L.B. Holeiko, and D.W. Wilmore. "Glutamine-Enriched Total Parenteral Nutrition Enhances Plasma Glutathione in the Resting State." *Journal of Surgical Research* 61:1 (1996), 35-38.

25 C.J. Johnston, C.G. Meyer, and J.C. Srilakshmi. "Vitamin C Elevates Red Blood Cell Glutathione in Healthy Adults." *American Journal of Clinical Nutrition* 58 (1993), 103-105.

26 A. Witschi et al. "The Systemic Availability or Oral Glutathione." *European Journal of Clinical Pharmacology* 43 (1992), 667-669.

27 A.F. Burton and F.H. Anderson. "Decreased Incorporation of 14C-Glucosamine Relative to 3H-N-Acetylglucosamine in the Intestinal Mucosa of Patients with Inflammatory Bowel Disease." *American Journal of Gastroenterology* 78 (1983), 19-22.

28 G. Tate et al. "Suppression of Acute and Chronic Inflammation by Dietary Gamma Linoleic Acid." *Journal of Rheumatology* 16:6 (1989), 729-734.

29 S. Pullman-Moore et al. "Alteration of the Cellular Fatty Acid Profile and the Production of Eicosanoids in Human Monocytes by Gamma Linoleic Acid (GLA)." *Arthritis and Rheumatism* 33:10 (1990), 1526-1533.

30 N. Ishibashi et al. "*Bifidobacteria*: Research and Development in Japan." *Food Technology* 47:6 (1993), 126-134. See also: D.C. Hoover. "*Bifidobacteria*: Activity and Potential Benefit." *Food Technology* 47:6 (1993), 120-124.

Chapter 9

Allergies and Arthritis

1 M.A. Van de Laar et al. "Food Intolerance in Rheumatoid Arthritis II: Clinical and Histological Aspects." *Annals of Rheumatic Disease* 51:3 (1992), 303-306.

2 A.M. Denman et al. "Joint Complaints and Food Allergic Disorders." *Annals of Allergy* 51:2 Part 2 (1983), 260-263.

3 Marshall Mandell, M.D., and Anthony Conte, M.D. "Role of Allergy in Arthritis, Rheumatism, and Polysymptomatic Cerebral Visceral or Somatic Disorders: A Double-Blind Study." *Journal of the International Academy of Preventive Medicine* (July 1982). In: Marshall Mandell, *M.D. Dr. Mandell's Lifetime Arthritis Relief System* (New York: Coward-McCann, 1983), 84-86.

4 R.S. Panush et al. "Food-Induced (Allergic) Arthritis: Inflammatory Arthritis Exacerbated by Milk." *Arthritis and Rheumatism* 29:2 (February 1986), 220-226.

5 U. Bengtsson et al. "Survey of Gastrointestinal Reactions to Foods in Adults in Relation to Atopy Presence of Mucus in the Stools, Swelling of Joints, and Arthralgia in Patients with Gastrointestinal Reactions to Foods." *Clinical and Experimental Allergy* 26:12 (December 1996), 1387-1394.

6 D. Beri et al. "Effect of Dietary Restrictions on Disease Activity in Rheumatoid Arthritis." *Annals of Rheumatic Disease* 47:1 (January 1988), 69-72.

7 R.S. Pinals. "Arthritis Associated with Gluten-Sensitive Enteropathy." *Journal of Rheumatology* 13:1 (February 1986), 201-204.

8 James Braly, M.D. "Detecting Hidden Food Allergies." *Alternative Medicine* 24 (June/July 1998), 32.

9 *The Lancet* (June 14, 1997).

10 E. Lubrano et al. "The Arthritis of Celiac Disease: Prevalence and Pattern in 200 Adult Patients." *British Journal of Rheumatology* 35:12 (December 1996), 1314-1318.

11 Norman F. Childers, Ph.D. *A Diet to Stop Arthritis* (Somerville, NJ: Somerset Press, 1991).

12 Arthur Winter, M.D., F.I.C.S., and Ruth Winter, M.S. *Smart Food* (New York: St. Martin's Griffin, 1999), 77.

13 Michael Hodgson, M.D., M.P.H. "The Medical Evaluation" and "The Sick Building Syn-drome" in *Effects of the Indoor Environment on Health*. Cited in: *Occupational Medicine: State of the Art Reviews* 10:1 (January-March 1995), 167-194.

Chapter 10

Desensitize the Autoimmune Reaction

1 Joseph Pizzorno, N.D. *Total Wellness* (Rocklin, CA: Prima Publishing, 1996), 167-168.

2 Ibid.

3 D.T. Yu. "Pathogenesis of Reactive Arthritis." Internal Medicine 38:2 (February 1999), 97-101.

4 Richard Ravel, M.D. *Clinical Laboraroty Medicine* 6th ed. (St. Louis, MO: Mosby-Year Book, 1989), 377.

5 *Physicians' Desk Reference* (Montvale, NJ: Medical Economics, 1998), 1281-1282, 738-740.

6 D.E. Trentham et al. "Effects of Oral Administration of Type II Collagen on Rheumatoid Arthritis." *Science* 261:5129 (1993), 1727-1730. M. Baringa. *Science* 261 (1993), 1669-1670.

7 "Arthred." Available from: Allergy Research Group, P.O. Box 489, San Leandro, CA 94577; tel: 800-654-4432 or 510-639-4572; fax: 510-635-6730.

8 Stanley W. Jacobs, M.D., Ronald M. Lawrence, M.D., Ph.D., and Martin Zucker. *The Miracle of MSM* (New York: G.P. Putnam's Sons, 1999), 203-204.

9 Anthony DeFabio, M.A. and Gus J. Prosch, Jr., M.D. *Arthritis* (Franklin, TN: The Arthritis Trust of America, 1997), 298.

10 Martha M. Christy. *Your Own Perfect Medicine* (Scottsdale, AZ: Future Medicine, 1994), 28.

11 Ibid., 131.

12 C.W.M. Wilson, M.D. and A. Lewis, M.D. "Autoimmune Bucal Urine Therapy (AIBUT) Against Human Allergic Disease: A Physiologic Self-Defense Mechanism." *Law Hospital in Scotland* (1983).

13 Y. Deyong. "Clinical Observation of 144 Cases of Rheumatoid Arthritis Treated With Glycoside of Radix *Tripterygium wilfordii*." *Journal of Traditional Chinese*

Medicine 3 (1983), 125-129.

14 S.Z. Qian et al. "Effects of Tripterygium on Male Fertility." *Advances in Contraception* 4:4 (December 1988), 307-310.

15 D.S. Xu et al. *Chung Kuo Chung Hsi I Chieh Ho Tsa Chih* 16:1 (January 1996), 14-23.

16 Kerry Bone. *Clinical Applications of Ayurvedic and Chinese Herbs: Monographs for the Western Herbal Practitioner* (Warwick, Queensland, Australia: Phytotherapy Press, 1996), 118-119.

17 C.K. Atal et al. "Immunomodulating Agents of Plant Origin I: Preliminary Screening." *Journal of Ethnopharmacology* 18:2 (1986), 133-141.

18 T.M. Haqqi et al. "Prevention of Collagen-Induced Arthritis in Mice by a Polyphenolic Fraction From Green Tea." *Proceedings of the National Academy of Sciences* 96:8 (April 13, 1999), 4524-4529.

19 Paul Schulick. *Ginger: Common Spice & Wonder Drug* (Brattleboro, VT: Herbal Free Press, 1994), 21.

20 Ibid., 65.

21 Michael Murray. *The Healing Power of Herbs* 2nd ed. (Rocklin, CA: Prima Publishing, 1995), 140.

22 D. Chandra et al. "Anti-Inflammatory and Anti-Arthritic Activity of Volatile Oil of *Curcuma longa* (Haldi)." *Indian Journal of Medical Research* 60 (1972), 138-142.

23 Daniel J. McCarty et al. "Treatment of Pain Due to Fibromyalgia With Topical Capsaicin: A Pilot. *Seminars in Arthritis and Rheumatism* 23:6 Suppl. 3, 41-47.

Chapter II

Mind/Body Approaches to Arthritis

1 M. Scofield. *Work Site Health Promotion* (Philadelphia: Hanley & Belfus, 1990), 459.

2 Timothy D. Schellhardt. "Company Memo to Stressed-Out Employees: 'Deal With It'." *The Wall Street Journal* (October 2, 1996).

3 J.L. Marx. "The Immune System 'Belongs to the Body'." *Science* 277 (1985), 1190-1192.

4 Hans Selye, M.D. *Stress Without Distress* (New York: New American Library, 1975). J.D. Beasley and J. Swift. *Kellogg Report: The Impact of Nutrition, Environment, and Lifestyle on the Health of Americans* (Annandale-on-Hudson, NY: Institute of Health Policy and Practice, The Bard College Center, 1989).

5 M. Marcenaro et al. "Rheumatoid Arthritis, Personality, Stress Response Style, and Coping With Illness: A Preliminary Survey." *Annals of the New York Academy of Sciences* 876 (June 22, 1999), 419-425.

6 Arthur Guyton, MD. *Textbook of Medical Physiology* 7th Ed. (Philadelphia, PA, W. B. Saunders, 1986), 910.

7 Redford B. William, M.D. "Hostility and the Heart." In: Daniel Goleman, Ph.D., and Joel Gurin, eds. *Mind/Body Medicine* (Yonkers, NY: Consumer Reports Books, 1993), 66-67.

8 C. David Jenkins. "The Mind and the Body." *World Health* 47:2 (March/April 1994), 6-7.

9 Louise L. Hay. *You Can Heal Your Life* (Santa Monica, CA: Hay House, 1984), 132.

10 Emrika Padus and the Editors of *Prevention Magazine. Using Emotions to Heal: The Happy Mind, Healthy Body Connection to Self Healing* (Emmaus, PA: Rodale Press, 1986), 7-8.

11 Dennis Jaffe, Ph.D. *Healing From Within* (New York: Simon & Schuster, 1980), 70, 105.

12 Louise L. Hay. *You Can Heal Your Life* (Santa Monica, CA: Hay House, 1984).

13 Brian Tracy. *The Psychology of Achievement* (Niles, IL: Nightingale-Conant Corporation, 1987), 4.

14 R. A. Chalmers et al., eds. *Scientific Research on Maharishi's Transcendental Meditation and TM-Sidih Program: Collected Papers, Vol. 2-4* (Vlodrop, Netherlands: Maharishi Vedic University Press, 1989).

15 R.K. Wallace et al. "Physiological Effects of Transcendental Meditation." *Science* 167 (1970), 1751-1754. M.C. Dillbeck et al. "Physiological Differences between TM and Rest." *American Physiologist* 42 (1987), 879-881.

16 R. W. Cranson et al. "Transcendental Meditation and Improved Performance on Intelligence-Related Measures: A Longitu-dinal Study." *Personality and Individual Differences* 12 (1991), 1105-1116.

17 D.H. Shapiro and R.N. Walsh. *Meditation: Classic and Contemporary Perspectives* (New York: Aldine, 1984).

18 Jon Kabat-Zinn, Ph.D. *Full Catastrophe Living: Using the Wisdom of Your Body and Mind to Face Stress, Pain and Illness* (New York: Delacorte Press, 1990).

19 Shad Helmsetter, Ph.D. *What to Say When You Talk To Yourself* (Scottsdale, AZ: Grindle Press/Audio, 1986).

20 R. Dilts and T. Hallbom. *Beliefs: Pathways to Health and Well-Being* (Portland, OR: Metamorphous Press, 1990), 1-2.

21 J.C. Parker et al. "Effects of Stress Management on Clinical Outcomes in Rheumatoid Arthritis." *Arthritis and Rheumatism* 38:12 (1995), 1807-1818.

22 The Burton Goldberg Group. *Alternative Medicine: The Definitive Guide* (Tiburon, CA: Future Medicine Publishing, 1993), 77.

23 Leon Chaitow, N.D., D.O. *Amino Acids in Therapy: A Guide to the Therapeutic Application of Protein Constituents* (Wellingborough, Northhamptonshire, UK: Thorsens, 1985), 50-61.

24 N. Miller. "Learning of Visceral and Glandular Responses." *Science* 163:866 (January 1969), 434-445, 627.

25 The Burton Goldberg Group. *Alternative Medicine: The Definitive Guide* (Tiburon, CA: Future Medicine Publishing, 1993), 245.

26 William Lowe Mundy, M.D. *Curing Allergy With Visual Imagery* (Shawnee Mission, KS: Munday & Associates, 1993), 45.

27 The Burton Goldberg Group. *Alternative Medicine: The Definitive Guide* (Tiburon, CA: Future Medicine Publishing, 1993), 244.

28 J.W. Turner, Ph.D., and T.H. Fine, Ph.D. "Flotation/REST Used in the Treatment of Arthritis Pain." A paper presented at the Fourth Annual International Conference on REST, Washington, D.C. (1990). Roderick A. Borrie, Ph.D., et al. *Flotation/ REST for the Management of Rheumatoid Arthritis.* Proceedings of the Ninth Annual Conference on Interdisciplinary Health Care (Stony Brook, NY: SAHP/SUNY, 1988), 277-282. T.H. Fine and J.W. Turner, Jr. "Flotation REST and Chronic Pain." Presented at the International Congress of Psychology, Acapulco, Mexico (1984).

29 Peter Suedfeld, Ph.D., et al. "Water Immersion and Flotation: From Stress Experiment to Stress Treatment." *Journal of Environmental Psychology* 3 (1983), 147-155.

30 T.H. Fine, Ph.D., and J. W. Turner, Jr., Ph.D. "The Effect of Flotation/REST on EMG Biofeedback and Plasma Cortisol." In: T.S. Fine and J.W. Turner, Jr., eds. *Proceedings of the First International Conference on REST and Self Regulation* (Toledo, OH: IRIS, 1985), 148-155.

31 Based on clinical observations of Eugene R. Zampieron, N.D., A.H.G., Naturopathic Medical Center, Middlebury, CT (1993-1998).

32 Based on clinical observations of Eugene R. Zampieron, N.D., A.H.G., Naturopathic Medical Center, Middlebury, CT (1994 -1995).

33 Larry Dossey, M.D. *Healing Words: The Power of Prayer and the Practice of Medicine* (San Francisco: HarperCollins, 1993), 268.

34 Marilyn Elias. "Attending Church Found Factor in Longer Life." *USA Today* (August 8, 1999), 1A.

35 The John Templeton Foundation, P.O. Box 8322, Radnor, PA 19087; tel: 610-687-8942; e-mail: info@templeton.org; website: www.templeton.org.

36 R.B. Tisserand. *The Art of Aromatherapy* (Rochester, VT: Healing Arts Press, 1977).

37 G.H. Dodd. "Receptor Events in Perfumery." In: S. van Toller and G. H. Dodd, eds. *Perfumery: The Psychology and Biology of Fragrance* (London: Chapman and Hall, 1988).

38 J. Steele. "Brain Research and Essential Oils." *Aromatherapy Quarterly* 3 (Spring 1984), 5.

39 "Aromatherapy on the Wards: Lavendar Beats Benzodiazepines." *International Journal of Aromatherapy* 1:2 (1988), 1.

40 R.B. Tisserand. *The Art of Aromatherapy* (Rochester, VT: Healing Arts Press, 1977).

Chapter 12
The Arthritis Diet

1 Joseph Pizzorno, N.D. *Total Wellness* (Rocklin, CA: Prima Publishing, 1996), 264.

2 I. Hafstrom et al. "Effects of Fasting on Disease Activity, Neuotrophil Function, Fatty Acid Composition, and Leukotriene Biosynthesis in Patients With Rheumatoid Arthritis." *Arthritis and Rheumatology* 31:5 (May 1988), 585-92.

3 J. Kjeldsen-Kragh et al. "Changes in Laboratory Variables in Rheumatoid Arthritis Patients During a Trial of Fasting and One-Year Vegetarian Diet." *Scandinavian Journal of Rheumatology* 24:2 (1995), 85-93.

4 Sheldon Margen, M.D., and the Editors of the University of California at Berkeley *Wellness Letter. The Wellness Encyclopedia of Food and Nutrition* (New York: Rebus, 1992), 498. Udo Erasmus. *Fats That Heal, Fats That Kill* (Burnaby, British Columbia, Canada: Alive Books, 1993), 237.

5 L.G. Cleland et al. "Clinical and Biochemical Effects of Dietary Fish Oil Supplements in Rheumatoid Arthritis." *Journal of Rheumatology* 15:10 (October 1988), 1471-1475.

6 J.M. Kremer et al. "Dietary Fish Oil and Olive Oil Supplementation in Patients with Rheumatoid Arthritis. Clinical and Immunologic Effects." *Arthritis and Rheumatology* 33:6 (June 1990), 810-820.

7 Udo Erasmus. *Fats That Heal, Fats That Kill* (Burnaby, BC, Canada: Alive Books, 1993), 264.

8 Personal communication with Vincent Buyck, Sr., Ph.D., National College of Complementary Medicine and Sciences, Washington, D.C.

9 J.A. Dudek and E.R. Elkins, Jr. "Effects of Cooking on the Fatty Acid Profiles of Selected Seafoods." In A.P. Simopopulos, R.R. Kifer, R.E. Martin, eds. *Health Effects of Polyusaturated Fatty Acids in Seafoods* (New York: Academic Press, 1986), 431-450.

10 Ralph Golan, M.D. *Optimal Wellness* (New York: Ballantine Books, 1995), 50.

11 W.A. Newman Dorland, M.D. *American Illustrated Medical Dictionary* (Philadelphia: W.B. Saunders, 1946), 1122.

12 Udo Erasmus. *Fats That Heal, Fats That Kill* (Burnaby, BC, Canada: Alive Books, 1993), 112.

13 M. Azzini et al. "Fatty Acids and Antioxidant Micronutrients in Psoriatic Arthritis." *Journal of Rheumatology* 22:1 (January 1995), 103-108.

14 Julian Whitaker, M.D. *Health and Healing* 7:11 (November 1997), 1-3.

15 Eugene Zampieron, N.D., A.H.G., and Ellen Kamhi, Ph.D., R.N. *The Natural Medicine Chest* (New York: M. Evans, 1999), 179-182.

Chapter 13
Supplements for Arthritis

1 R.D. Semba. "Vitamin A, Immunity, and Infection." *Clinical Infectious Diseases* 19 (1994), 489-499.

2 A. Bendich. "Beta-Carotene and the Immune Response." *Proceedings of the Nutrition Society* 50 (1991), 263-274.

3 K.J. Rothman et al. "Teratogenecity of High Vitamin A Intake." *New England Journal of Medicine* 333 (1995), 1369-1373.

4 W.J. Blot et al. "Nutrition Intervention Trials in Linxian, China: Supplementation with Specific Vitamin/Mineral Combinations, Cancer Incidence, and Disease-Specific Mortality in the General Population." *Journal of the National Cancer Institute* 85 (1993), 1483-1491.

5 W. Kaufman. *The Common Form of Joint Dysfunction: Its Incidence and Treatment* (Brattleboro, VT: E.L. Hildreth, 1949).

6 J.R. DiPalma and W.S. Thayer. "Use of Niacin as a Drug." *Annual Review of Nutrition* 11 (1991), 169-187.

7 P.J. Bingley et al. "Nicotinamide and Insulin Secretion in Normal Subjects." *Diabetiologia* 36 (1993), 675-677.

8 E.C. Barton-Wright and W.A. Elliott. "The Pantothenic Acid Metabolism of Rheumatoid Arthritis." *The Lancet* ii (1963), 862-863.

9 General Practitioner Research Group. "Calcium Pantothenate in Arthritic Conditions." *Practitioner* 224 (1980), 208-211.

10 P.J. Collip et al. "Pyridoxine Treatment of

Childhood Asthma." *Annals of Allergy* 35 (1975), 93-97. K. Folkers et al. "Biochemical Evidence For a Deficiency of Vitamin B6 in Subjects Reacting to Monosodium Glutamate by the Chinese Restaurant Syndrome." *Biochemical and Biophysical Research Communications* 100 (1981), 972-977. R.D. Reynolds and C.L. Natta. "Depressed Plasma Pyridoxal-5-Phosphate Concentrations in Adult Asthmatics." *American Journal of Clinical Nutrition* 41 (1985), 684-688.

11 M.K. Bum et al. "Association of Vitamin B6 Status with Parameters of Immune Function in Early HIV-1 Infection." *Journal of AIDS* 4 (1991), 122-132.

12 G.F. Crowell and E.S. Roach. "Pyridoxine-Dependent Seizures." *American Family Physician* 27 (1983), 183-187.

13 M. Lipton, R. Mailman, and C. Numeroff. "Vitamins, Megavitamin Therapy, and the Nervous System." In: R. Wurtman and J. Wurtman, eds. *Nutrition and the Brain, Vol. 3* (New York: Raven Press, 1979), 183-264.

14 J. Martineau et al. "Vitamin B6, Magnesium, and Combined B6-Magnesium: Therapeutic Effects in Childhood Autism." *Biological Psychiatry* 20 (1985), 467-468.

15 M. Cohen and A. Bendich. "Safety of Pyridoxine: A Review of Human and Animal Studies." *Toxicology Letters* 34 (1986), 129-139.

16 G. Krystal, G.M. Morris, and L. Sokoloff. "Stimulation of DNA Synthesis by Ascorbate in Cultures of Articular Chondrocytes." *Arthritis and Rheumatism* 25 (1982), 318-325.

17 A. Mullen and C.W.M. Wilson. "The Metabolism of Ascorbic Acid in Rheumatoid Arthritis." *Proceedings of the Nutrition Society* 35 (1976), 8A-9A.

18 C.S. Johnston and B. Luo. "Comparison of the Absorption and Excretion of Three Commercially Available Sources of Vitamin C." *Journal of the American Dietetic Association* 94 (1994), 779-781.

19 H. Reichel, H.P. Koeffler, and A.W. Norman. "The Role of Vitamin-D Endocrine System in Health and Disease." *New England Journal of Medicine* 320 (1989), 980-981.

20 F.M. Gloth and H.D. Tobin. "Vitamin D Deficiency in Older People." *Journal of*

the American Geriatric Society 43 (1995), 822-828. F. Lore et al. "Vitamin D Metabolites in Postmenopausal Osteoporosis." *Hormone and Metabolic Research* 16 (1984), 58.

21 Meryl S. LeBoff et al. "Occult Vitamin D Deficiency in Postmenopausal U.S. Women with Acute Hip Fracture." *Journal of the American Medical Association* 281 (April 28, 1999), 1505-1511.

22 I. Machtey and L.Ouaknine. "Tocopherol in Osteoarthritis: A Controlled Pilot Study." *Journal of the American Geriatric Society* 26 (1978), 328-330.

23 R.L. Travers, G.C. Rennie, and R.E. Newnham. "Boron and Arthritis: The Results of a Double-Blind Pilot Study." *Journal of Nutrition in Medicine* 1 (1990), 127-132.

24 S.L. Meacham et al. "Effect of Boron Supplementation on Blood and Urinary Calcium, Magnesium, and Phosphorus, Urinary Boron in Athletic and Sedentary Women." *American Journal of Clinical Nutrition* 61 (1995), 341-345.

25 F.H. Nielsen. "Studies on the Relationship Between Boron and Magnesium Which Possibly Affects the Formation and Maintenance of Bones." *Magnesium and Trace Elements* 9 (1990), 61-69.

26 E,B, Finley and F.L. Cerklewski. "Influence of Ascorbic Acid Supplementation on Copper Status in Young Adult Men." *American Journal of Clinical Nutrition* 47 (1988), 96-101.

27 A.R. Gaby. *Preventing and Reversing Osteoporosis* (Rocklin, CA: Prima Publishing, 1994).

28 J. Thom et al. "The Influence of Refined Carbohydrate on Urinary Calcium Excretion." *British Journal of Urology* 50 (1978), 459-464.

29 R. Recker. "Calcium Absorption and Achlorhydria." *New England Journal of Medicine* 313 (1985), 70-73.

30 R.P. Heaney and C.M. Weaver. "Calcium Absorption From Kale." *American Journal of Clinical Nutrition* 51 (1990), 656-657.

31 B.P. Bourgoin et al. "Lead Content in 70 Brands of Dietary Calcium Supplements." *American Journal of Public Health* 83 (1993), 1155-1160.

32 J.A. Harvey et al. "Superior Calcium Absorption From Calcium Citrate Than Calcium Carbonate Using External

Forearm Counting." *Journal of the American College of Nutrition* 9 (1990), 583-587.

33 C. Zhou et al. "Clinical Observation of Treatment of Hypertension with Calcium." *American Journal of Hypertension* 7 (1994), 363-367.

34 Lavon Dunne. *The Nutrition Almanac* (New York: McGraw Hill, 1990).

35 Gail Darlington and Linda Gamlin. *Diet and Arthritis* (London, England: Vermilion, 1996).

36 W.R. Ghent et al. "Iodine Replacement in Fibrocystic Disease of the Breast." *Canadian Journal of Surgery* 36 (1993), 453-460.

37 J.M. Hitch. "Acneform Eruptions Induced by Drugs and Chemicals." *Journal of the American Medical Association* 200 (1967), 879-880.

38 W. Bezwoda et al. "The Importance of Gastric Hydrochloric Acid in the Absorption of Non-Heme Iron." *Laboratory and Clinical Medicine* 92 (1978), 108-116.

39 V. Gordeuk et al. "Iron Overload: Causes and Consequences." *Annual Review of Nutrition* 7 (1987), 485-508. P. Biemond et al. "Intra-articular Ferritin-Bound Iron in Rheumatoid Arthritis." *Arthritis and Rheumatism* 29 (1986), 1187-1193. J.T. Salonen et al. "High Stored Iron Levels are Associated With Excess Risk of Myocardial Infarction in Eastern Finnish Men." *Circulation* 80 (1992), 803-811.

40 C.L. Keen and S. Zidenberg-Cherr. "Manganese." In: M.L. Brown, ed. *Present Knowledge in Nutrition* 6th ed (Washington, DC: International Life Sciences Institute, 1990), 279-286.

41 B.M. Altura. "Basic Biochemistry and Physiology of Magnesium: A Brief Review." *Magnesium and Trace Elements* 10 (1991), 167-171.

42 T. Bohmer et al. "Bioavailability of Oral Magnesium Supplementation in Female Students Evaluated From Elimination of Magnesium in 24-Hour Urine." *Magnesium and Trace Elements* 9 (1990), 272-278. L. Gullestad et al. "Oral Versus Intravenous Magnesium Supplementation in Patients With Magnesium Deficiency." *Magnesium and Trace Element* 10 (1991), 11-16.

43 J.S. Lindberg et al. "Magnesium

Bioavailability From Magnesium Citrate and Magnesium Oxide." *Journal of the American College of Nutrition* 9 (1990), 48-55.

44 D.F.L. Money. "Vitamin E and Selenium Deficiencies and Their Possible Aetological Role in Sudden Infant Death Syndrome." *New Zealand Medical Journal* 71 (1970), 32-34.

45 O. Andersen and J.B. Nielsen. "Effects of Simultaneous Low-Level Dietary Supplementation with Inorganic and Organic Selenium on Whole-Body, Blood, and Organ Levels of Toxic Metals in Mice." *Environmental Health Perspectives* 102:Suppl. 3 (1994), 321-324.

46 M. Mutanen. "Bioavailability of Selenium." *Annals of Clinical Research* 18 (1086), 48-54.

47 Centers for Disease Control. "Selenium Intoxication." *Morbidity and Mortality Weekly Report* 33 (1984), 157.

48 A. Prasad. "Clinical, Biochemical and Nutritional Spectrum of Zinc Deficiency in Human Subjects: An Update." *Nutrition Reviews* 41 (1983), 197-208. T.E. Tuormaa. "Adverse Effect of Zinc Deficiency: A Review From the Literature." *Journal of Orthomolecular Medicine* 10 (1995), 149-162.

49 P.C. Mattingly and A.G. Mowat. "Zinc Sulphate in Rheumatoid Arthritis." *Annals of the Rheumatic Diseases* 41 (1982), 456-457.

50 Jason Theodosakis, M.D., M.S., M.P.H, Brenda Adderly, M.H.A., and Barry Fox, Ph.D. *The Arthritis Cure* (New York: St. Martin's Griffin, 1997), 35-36.

51 A.L. Var. "Double-Blind Clinical Evaluation of the Relative Efficacy of Ibuprofen and Glucosamine Sulfate in the Management of Osteoarthritis of the Knee in Out-Patients." *Current Medical Research and Opinion* 8 (1982), 145-149.

52 I. Setnikar et al. "Pharmacokinetics of Glucosamine in Man." *Arzneimittel-Forschung* 43 (1993), 1109-1113.

53 Luke Bucci, Ph.D. *Pain Free: The Definitive Guide to Healing Arthritis, Low-Back Pain, and Sports Injuries Through Nutrition and Supplements* (Fort Worth, TX: The Summit Group, 1995), 74.

54 M. Morrison. "Therapeutic Applications of Chondroitin-4-Sulfate: Appraisal of

Biologic Properties." *Folia Angiol* 25 (1977), 225–232.

55 John Anderson. "Quick-Acting Natural Arthritis Relief." *Alternative Medicine Digest* 20 (October/November 1997), 90.

56 D. Rothman et al. "Botanical Lipids: Effects in Inflammation, Immune Response, and Rheumatoid Arthritis." *Seminars in Arthritis and Rheumatism* (October 1995).

57 John Anderson. "S-Adenosyl-L-Methionine—Nutrient Duo Relieves Depression and Pain." *Alternative Medicine* 27 (December 1998/January 1999), 72.

58 H. Muller-Fassbender. "Double-Blind Clinical Trial of S-Adenosylmethionine Versus Ibuprofen in the Treatment of Osteoarthritis." *American Journal of Medicine* 83:Suppl. 5A (1987), 81-83.

59 S. Glorioso et al. "Double-Blind Multicentre Study of the Activity of S-Adenosylmethion-ine in Hip and Knee Osteoarthritis." *International Journal of Clinical Pharmacology Research* 5 (1985), 39-49.

60 Julian Whitaker. *Health and Healing* (December 1995), 4-5.

61 Earl Mindell. *The MSM Miracle* (New Canaan, CT: Keats, 1997), 12.

62 John Anderson. "New Zealand's Green-Lipped Mussel for Arthritis Relief." *Alternative Medicine Digest* 21 (December 1997/January 1998), 74-77.

63 "Consumer Bulletin: Sea Cucumbers." *Whole Foods* (October 1994).

64 R.A. Hazelton. "A Cure in Rheumatoid Arthritis: A Six-Month Placebo-Controlled Study." University of Queensland, Australia, August 1992.

65 M. Walker. "Biochemical Components of Sea Cucumber for Human Benefit." *Explore!* 3 (1992), 12–17. M. Walker. "Chinese Seafood Eases Arthritis." *Natural Health* (March/April 1993).

66 Kerry Bone. "Developments on Phytotherapy: *Boswellia serrata*." *The Modern Phytotherapist* 3:1 (Summer 1996). G.B. Singh et al. *Agents and Actions* 18 (1996), 407. M.L. Sharma et al. "Effect of Salai Guggal ex-*Boswellia serrata* on Cellular and Humoral Immune Responses and Leucocyte Migration." *Agents and Actions* 24:1-2 (1988), 161-164. M.L. Sharma et al. *International*

Journal of Immunopharmacology 11 (1989), 647.

67 G. Kesava Reddy and S.C. Dhar. "Effect of a New Non-Steroidal Anti-inflammatory Agent on Lysosomal Stability in Adjuvant-Induced Arthritis." *Italian Journal of Biochemistry* 36:4 (1987), 205-217.

68 Michael Tierra. *Planetary Herbology* (Santa Fe, NM: Lotus Press, 1988), 279.

69 S. Hiai et al. "Stimulation of the Pituitary-Adrenocortical Axis by Saikosaponina of *Bupleuri radix*." *Chemical and Pharmaceutical Bulletin* 29:2 (1981), 495-499.

70 Daniel J. McCarty et al. "Treatment of Pain Due to Fibromyalgia With Topical Capsaicin: A Pilot." *Seminars in Arthritis and Rheumatism* 23:6 Suppl. 3, 41-47.

71 Eugene Zampieron, N.D., A.H.G., and Ellen Kamhi, Ph.D., R.N. *The Natural Medicine Chest* (New York: M. Evans, 1999), 79-81.

72 E.S. Johnson et al. "Efficacy of Feverfew as Prophylactic Treatment of Migraine." *British Medical Journal* 291 (1985), 569-573.

73 Paul Schulick. *Ginger: Common Spice & Wonder Drug* (Brattleboro, VT: Herbal Free Press, 1994), 21.

74 Paul Schulick. *Ginger: Common Spice & Wonder Drug* (Brattleboro, VT: Herbal Free Press, 1994), 65.

75 Paul Schulick. *Ginger: Common Spice & Wonder Drug* (Brattleboro, VT: Herbal Free Press, 1994), 81.

76 K.C. Srivastava et al. "Ginger (Zingiber officinale) in Rheumatism and Musculoskeletal Disorders." *Medical Hypotheses* 39:4 (December 1992), 342-348.

77 David Hoffmann, M.N.I.M.H, A.H.G. *The Herb Users Guide* (Northamptonshire, England: Thorson's, 1986), 72.

78 Edward S. Ayensu, Ph.D., F.L.S. *Medicinal Plants of the West Indies* (Alogonac, MI: Reference Publications, 1981), 144.

79 D.D. Jamieson et al. "Comparison of the Central Nervous System Activity of the Aqueous and Lipid Extracts of Kava (*Piper methysticum*)." *Archives Internationales de Pharmacodynamie et de Therapie* 301 (1989), 66-80.

80 Steven Foster. *Herbs for Your Health* (Loveland, CO: Interview Press, 1996), 58-59.

81 H.M. Chang et al. *Pharmacology and*

Applications of Chinese Materia Medica, Vol. 1 (Singapore: World Scientific Publications, 1986).

82 Michael T. Murray. *The Healing Power of Herbs* (Rocklin, CA: Prima Publishing, 1995).

83 M.F. Chen et al. "Effect of Glycyrrhizin on the Pharmacokinetics of Prednisone Following Low Dosage of Prednisolone Hemisubstinate". *Endocrinologia Japonica* 37:3 (1990), 331-341.

84 Kerry Bone, M.N.I.M.H. *Phytosynergistic Prescribing for Professional Prescribers* (Lake Oswego, OR: Communications Medicus, 1994), 23.

85 Clinical observation of Eugene Zampieron, N.D., A.H.G. (1998). Dr. Zampieron is preparing fluid extracts of these plants and has begun a clinical trial.

86 S. Kuwano and K. Yamauchi. "Effect of Berberene on Tyrosine Decarboxylase Activity of Streptococcus faecalis." *Chemical and Pharmaceutical Bulletin* 8 (1960), 491-496.

87 Rao M.N. Sreejayan. "Nitric Oxide Scavenging by Curcuminoids." *Journal of Pharmacy and Pharmacology* 49 (1997), 105-107. F. Bonte et al. "Protective Effect of Curcuminoids on Epidermal Skin Cells Under Free Radical Stress." *Planta Medica* 63:3 (1997), 265-266.

88 D. Chandra et al. "Anti-Inflammatory and Anti-Arthritic Activity of Volatile Oil of Curcuma longa (Haldi)." *Indian Journal of Medical Research* 60 (1972), 138-142.

89 J. Shabert and N. Ehrlich. *The Ultimate Nutrients: Glutamine* (Garden City Park, NY: Avery Publishing Group, 1997).

90 Michael T. Murray. *The Healing Power of Herbs* (Rocklin, CA: Prima Publishing, 1995). S. Tanaka et al. "Effects of Toki (Angelica acutiloba) Extracts on Writhing and Capillary Permeability in Mice (Analgesic and Anti-Inflammatory Effects)." *Yakugaku Zasshi* 91 (1971), 1098-1104.

91 Dan Bensky et al. *Chinese Herbal Medicine Materia Medica* (Seattle, WA: Eastland Press, 1986), 408.

92 Daniel Reed. *A Handbook of Chinese Healing Herbs* (Boston: Shambhala, 1995).

93 Dan Bensky et al. *Chinese Herbal Medicine Materia Medica* (Seattle, WA: Eastland Press, 1986), 97. H.M. Chang et al. *Pharmacology and Applications of Chinese Materia Medica, Vol. 1* ([CITY]: World Scientific Publications, 1986), 470.

94 Kerry Bone. *Clinical Applications of Ayurvedic and Chinese Herbs: Monograms for the Western Herbal Practitioner* (Warwick, Queensland, Australia: Phytotherapy Press, 1996), 52.

95 R. Denno et al. "Glutamine-Enriched Total Parenteral Nutrition Enhances Plasma Glutathione in the Resting State." *Journal of Surgical Research* 61:1 (1996), 35-38.

96 R. Denno et al. "Decreased Concentration of Free Histidine in Serum in Rheumatoid Arthritis: An Isolated Amino Acid Abnormality Not Associated With Generalized Hypoaminoacidemia." *Journal of Rheumatology* 2:4 (1975), 384-392.

97 R. Denno et al. "Low Free Serum Histidine Concentration in Rheumatoid Arthritis: A Measure of Disease Activity." *Journal of Clinical Investigation* 55 (1975), 1164-1173.

98 R. Denno and M.G. Gerber. "Specificity of a Low Free Serum Histidine Concentration for Rheumatoid Arthritis." *Journal of Chronic Diseases* 30 (1977), 115-127.

99 R. Denno et al. "Treatment of Rheumatoid Arthritis With Histidine." *Arthritis and Rheumatism* 12 91969), 295.

100 A. Fox and B. Fox. *DPLA: To End Chronic Pain and Depression* (New York: Long Shadow Books, 1985).

101 R. Balagot et al. "Analgesia in Mice and Humans by D-Phenylalanine: Relation to Inhibition of Enkephalin Degradation and Enkephalin Levels." In: J.J. Bonica et al., eds. *Advances in Pain Research and Therapy* 5 (1983), 289-293. See also: K. Budd. "Use of D-Phenylalanine, an Enkephalinase Inhibitor, in the Treatment of Intractable Pain." *Advances in Pain Research and Therapy.*

102 L.W. Blau. "Cherry Diet Control for Gout and Arthritis." *Texas Report on Biology and Medicine* 8 (1950), 309-311.

103 Elson M. Haas, M.D. *Staying Healthy*

With Nutrition (Berkeley, CA: Celestial Arts, 1992), 272.

104 A. Bindoli, M. Valente, and L. Cavallini. "Inhibitory Action of Quercitin on Xanthine Oxidase and Xanthine Dehydrogenase Activity." *Pharmacological Research Communications* 17 (1985), 831-839.

105 J. Galvez. "Application of Natural Products in Experimental Models of Intestinal Inflammation in Rats." *Metabolism* 18:Suppl (1996), B7-B10.

106 J.P. Tarayre and H. Lauressergues. "Advantages of a Combination of proteolytic Enzymes, Flavonoids and Ascorbic Acid in Comparison With Non-Steroidal Anti-Inflammatory Agents." *Arzneimittel-Forschung* 27 (1977), 1144-1149.

107 B. Schwitters and J. Masquelier. *OPC in Practice: Bioflavonoids and Their Application* (Rome, Italy: Alfa Omega, 1993).

108 J. Masquelier, M.C. Dumon, and J. Dumas. "Stabilization of Collagen by Procyanidolic Oligomers." *Acta Ther* 7 (1981), 101-105.

109 E. Rubenstein et al. "Antibacterial Activity of the Pancreatic Fluid." *Gastroenterology* 88 (1985), 927-932.

110 I. Horger. "Enzyme Therapy in Multiple Rheumatic Diseases." *Therapiewoche* 33 (1983), 3948-3957. C. Steffen et al. "Enzyme Therapy in Comparison With Immune Complex Determinations in Chronic Polyarteritis." *Rheumatologie* 44 (1985), 51-56.

111 A. Cohen and J. Goldman. "Bromelain Therapy in Rheumatoid Arthritis." *Pennsyl-vania Medical Journal* 67 (1964), 27-30.

112 G. Uhli and J. Seifert. "The Effect of Proteolytic Enzymes (Traumanase) on Post-traumatic Edema." *Fortschritte der Medizin* 99 (1994), 554-556.

113 V. Balakrishnan, A, Hareendran, and C. Sukumaran Nair. "Double-Blind Cross-Over Trial of an Enzyme Preparation in Pancreatic Steatorrhea." *Journal of the Association of Physicians of India* 29 (1981), 207-209.

114 Gregory S. Kelly. "Bromelain: A Literature Review and Discussion of Its Therapeutic Applications." *Alternative Medicine Review* 1:4 (1996), 245.

115 V. Tretter V et al. "Fucose Alpha-1,3 Linked to the Core Region of Glycoprotein N-Glycans Creates an Important Epitope for IgE From Honeybee Venom Allergic Individuals." *International Archives of Allergy and Immunology* 102 (1993), 259-266. E. Batanero et al. "Cross-Reactivity Between the Major Allergen From olive pollen and Unrelated Glycoproteins: Evidence of an Epitope in the Glycan Moiety of the Allergen." *Journal of Allergy and Clinical Immunology* 97 (1996), 1264-1271.

116 A. Gutfreund, S. Taussig, and A. Morris. "Effect of Oral Bromelain on Blood Pressure and Heart Rate of Hypertensive Patients." *Harvard Medical Journal* 37 (1978), 143-146.

117 Diane Robertson. *Jamaican Herbs* (Montego Bay, Jamaica: DeSola Pinto, 1982).

118 T.J. De Witte et al. "Hypochlorhydria and Hypergastrinemia in Rheumatoid Arthritis." *Annals of Rheumatic Diseases* 38 (1979), 14-17. K. Henriksson et al. "Gastrin, Gastric Acid Secretion, and Gastric Microflora in Patients with Rheumatoid Arthritis." *Annals of Rheumatic Diseases* 45 (1986), 475-483.

119 T.J. De Witte et al. "Hypochlorhydria and Hypergastrinemia in Rheumatoid Arthritis." *Annals of Rheumatic Diseases* 38 (1979), 14-17. K. Henriksson et al. "Gastrin, Gastric Acid Secretion, and Gastric Microflora in Patients with Rheumatoid Arthritis." *Annals of Rheumatic Diseases* 45 (1986), 475-483.

Chapter 14

Exercises and Physical Therapies

1 Adaptation of a program designed by Visual Health Information, P.O. Box 44646, Tacoma, WA 98444; tel: 253-536-4922.

2 Sophia Delza. *Tai Chi-Chuan: Body and Mind in Harmony* (Albany, NY: SUNY Press, 1985), 1,3,6.

3 Burton Goldberg Group. *Alternative Medicine: The Definitive Guide* (Tiburon, CA: Future Medicine Publishing, 1993), 423-426.

4 Eugene Zampieron, N.D., A.H.G. Interview with Ameni Harris on WPKN, 89.5 FM's *The Natural House Call* (May 1998).

5 A.Thrash and C. Thrash. *Home Remedies:*

Hydrotherapy, Massage, Charcoal and Other Simple Treatments (Seale, AL: Thrash Publications, 1981), 102.

6 *Gurney's Inn, Resort and Spa Guidebook* (Montauk, NY: Holdens Publication, 1997).

7 Ibid.

8 Brian W. Fahey, Ph.D. *The Power of Balance: A Rolfing View of Health* (Portland, OR: Metamorphous Press, 1989), 39.

9 Michael Murray, N.D., Joseph Pizzorno, N.D., and Rick Kitaeff, N.D. *A Textbook of Natural Medicine: Non-Pharmacological Control of Pain IV* (Seattle, WA: Bastyr Publications, 1986), 2.

10 Ron Lawrence, M.D., Ph.D., and Paul J. Rosch, M.D., F.A.C.P. *Magnet Therapy: The Pain Cure Alternative* (Rocklin, CA: Prima Publishing, 1998), 117.

11 Cervical Spine Mobility Stretching Charts. Available from: Visual Health Information, P.O. Box 44646, Tacoma, WA 98444; tel: 253-536-4922; fax: 253-536-4944

12 Julie Friedberger. *Office Yoga* (Glasgow, Scotland: Thorsons, 1991), 23.

13 D.L. Berkson. "Osteoarthritis, Chiropractic and Nutrition." *Medical Hypothesis* 36:4 (1991), 356-367.

Index

BOOKS *your health* depends on

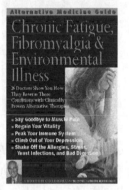
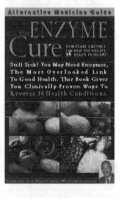
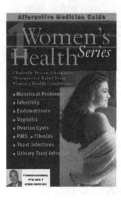
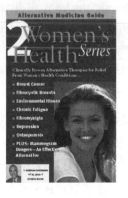
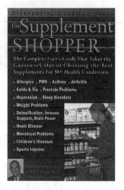

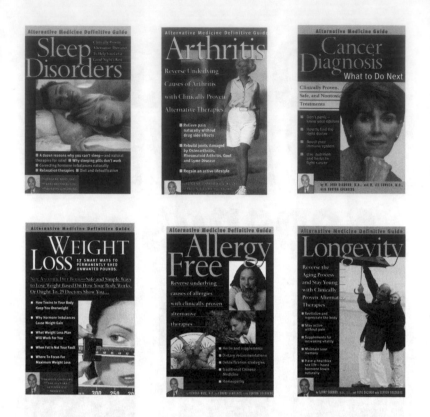

These titles are part of our *Alternative Medicine Guide* paperback series—healing-edge advice that may mean the difference between sickness and robust health. We distill the advice of hundreds of leading alternative physicians from all disciplines and put it into a consumer-helpful format—medical knowledge without the jargon. Essential reading before—or instead of—your next doctor's visit. Because you need to know your medical alternatives.

To order, call 800-841-BOOK or visit www.alternativemedicine.com. You can also find our books at your local health food store or bookstore.

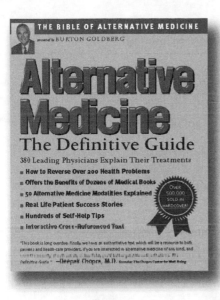